RNA TUMOR VIRUSES, ONCOGENES, HUMAN CANCER AND AIDS:

On the Frontiers of Understanding

DEVELOPMENTS IN ONCOLOGY

F.J. Cleton and J.W.I.M. Simons, eds.: Genetic Origins of Tumour Cells. 90-247-2272-1.
J. Aisner and P. Chang, eds.: Cancer Treatment Research. 90-247-2358-2.
B.W. Ongerboer de Visser, D.A. Bosch and W.M.H. van Woerkom-Eykenboom, eds.: Neuro-oncology: Clinical and Experimental Aspects. 90-247-2421-X.
K. Hellmann, P. Hilgard and S. Eccles, eds.: Metastasis: Clinical and Experimental Aspects. 90-247-2424-4.
H.F. Seigler, ed.: Clinical Management of Melanoma. 90-247-2584-4.
P. Correa and W. Haenszel, eds.: Epidemiology of Cancer of the Digestive Tract. 90-247-2601-8.
L.A. Liotta and I.R. Hart, eds.: Tumour Invasion and Metastasis. 90-247-2611-5.
J. Banoczy, ed.: Oral Leukoplakia. 90-247-2655-7.
C. Tijssen, M. Halprin and L. Endtz, eds.: Familial Brain Tumours. 90-247-2691-3.
F.M. Muggia, C.W. Young and S.K. Carter, eds.: Anthracycline Antibiotics in Cancer. 90-247-2711-1.
B.W. Hancock, ed.: Assessment of Tumour Response. 90-247-2712-X.
D.E. Peterson, ed.: Oral Complications of Cancer Chemotherapy. 0-89838-563-6.
R. Mastrangelo, D.G. Poplack and R. Riccardi, eds.: Central Nervous System Leukemia. Prevention and Treatment. 0-89838-570-9.
A. Polliack, ed.: Human Leukemias. Cytochemical and Ultrastructural Techniques in Diagnosis and Research. 0-89838-585-7.
W. Davis, C. Maltoni and S. Tanneberger, eds.: The Control of Tumor Growth and its Biological Bases. 0-89838-603-9.
A.P.M. Heintz, C. Th. Griffiths and J.B. Trimbos, eds.: Surgery in Gynecological Oncology. 0-89838-604-7.
M.P. Hacker, E.B. Double and I. Krakoff, eds.: Platinum Coordination Complexes in Cancer Chemotherapy. 0-89838-619-5.
M.J. van Zwieten, The Rat as Animal Model in Breast Cancer Research: A Histopathological Study of Radiation- and Hormone-Induced Rat Mammary Tumors. 0-89838-624-1.
B. Löwenberg and A. Hogenbeck, eds.: Minimal Residual Disease in Acute Leukemia. 0-89838-630-6.
I. van der Waal and G.B. Snow, eds.: Oral Oncology. 0-89838-631-4.
B.W. Hancock and A.M. Ward, eds.: Immunological Aspects of Cancer. 0-89838-664-0.
K.V. Honn and B.F. Sloane. Hemostatic Mechanisms and Metastasis. 0-89838-667-5.
K.R. Harrap, W. Davis and A.N. Calvert, eds.: Cancer Chemotherapy and Selective Drug Development: 0-89838-673-X.
V.D. Velde, J.H. Cornelis and P.H. Sugarbaker, eds.: Liver Metastasis. 0-89838-648-5.
D.J. Ruiter, K. Welvaart and S. Ferrone, eds.: Cutaneous Melanoma and Precursor Lesions. 0-89838-689-6.
S.B. Howell, ed.: Intra-Arterial and Intracavitary Cancer Chemotherapy. 0-89838-691-8.
D.L. Kisner and J.F. Smyth, eds.: Interferon Alpha-2: Pre-Clinical and Clinical Evaluation. 0-89838-701-9.

RNA TUMOR VIRUSES, ONCOGENES, HUMAN CANCER AND AIDS:
On the Frontiers of Understanding

Proceedings of the International Conference on RNA Tumor Viruses in Human Cancer, Denver, Colorado, June 10-14, 1984

edited by

Philip Furmanski
Jean Carol Hager
Marvin A. Rich

AMC Cancer Research Center
Denver, Colorado

Martinus Nijhoff Publishing
a member of the Kluwer Academic Publishers Group
Boston/Dordrecht/Lancaster

Distributors for North America:
Kluwer Academic Publishers
190 Old Derby Street
Hingham, MA 02043

Distributors for all other countries:
Kluwer Academic Publishers Group
Distribution Centre
P.O. Box 322
3300 AH Dordrecht
THE NETHERLANDS

Library of Congress Cataloging in Publication Data

International Conference on RNA Tumor Viruses in Human Cancer (1984: Denver, Colo.)
RNA tumor viruses, oncogenes, human cancer and AIDS.

(Developments in oncology)
Includes bibliographies and index.
1. Viral carcinogenesis—Congresses. 2. Viruses, RNA—Congresses. 3. Oncogenes—Congresses. 4. Acquired immune deficiency syndrome—Etiology—Congresses. 5. Cancer—Genetics aspects—Congresses. I. Furmanski, Philip, 1946- . II. Hager, Jean Carol, 1943- . III. Rich, Marvin A. IV. Title. V. Title: R.N.A. tumor viruses, oncogenes, human cancer and AIDS. VI. Series. [DNLM: 1. Acquired Immunodeficiency Syndrome—etiology—congresses. 2. Neoplasms—etiology—congresses. 3. Oncogenes—congresses. 4. Retroviridae—congresses.
W1 DE998N / QW 166 I606r 1984]
RC268.57.I573 1984 616.99'4071 84-25515
ISBN-13:978-1-4612-9620-1 e-ISBN-13:978-1-4613-2583-3
DOI: 10.1007/978-1-4613-2583-3

Softcover reprint of the hardcover 1st edition 1985

DEDICATION

As in all scientific advances, the achievements that move us toward a true understanding of the nature and cause of cancer through studies of the RNA tumor viruses were made by standing on "the shoulders of giants". This volume is dedicated to three individuals who, by their own germinal discoveries in the laboratory and their unstinting efforts in the promotion, support and coordination of research, were driving forces behind much of the progress in this area.

Twenty-five years ago, they isolated the agents that comprise the FMR group of murine leukemia viruses. Their discoveries stimulated an effort involving hundreds of laboratories throughout the world, resulting in thousands of scientific publications, each adding incrementally to our knowledge of cancer development.

The importance of their findings is evidenced also by contributions of the FMR viruses to such diverse areas as differentiation, immunology, genetics, biochemistry and molecular biology.

But these eminent scientists served the cancer research effort in a larger capacity -- the initiation, promotion and direction of the world-wide scientific battle against cancer.

It is for their discoveries, their insights, their energies and their accomplishments that this volume is dedicated to:

PIONEERS IN TUMOR VIROLOGY

Dr. Charlotte Friend
Discoverer - The Friend Murine Leukemia Virus
Professor and Director
Center for Experimental Cell Biology
Mount Sinai School of Medicine

Dr. John B. Moloney
Discoverer - The Moloney Murine Leukemia Virus
Former Associate Director for Viral Oncology,
Chairman, Virus Cancer Program,
Former Assistant Director
National Cancer Institute

Dr. Frank J. Rauscher, Jr.
Discoverer - The Rauscher Murine Leukemia Virus
Former Director
National Cancer Institute,
Senior Vice President for Research
American Cancer Society

CONTENTS

CONTRIBUTORS

Stuart A. Aaronson, Laboratory of Cellular and Molecular Biology, National Cancer Institute, Bethesda, Maryland, 20205

Igbal Ali, Laboratory of Tumor Immunology and Biology, National Cancer Institute, Bethesda, Maryland, 20205

Suresh Arya, Laboratory of Tumor Cell Biology, Division of Cancer Treatment, National Cancer Institute, Bethesda, Maryland, 20205

Richard Ascione, Laboratory of Molecular Oncology, National Cancer Institute, Frederick Cancer Research Facility, Frederick, Maryland, 21701

Therese Astier-Gin, INSERM U. 117, 229 crs de l'Argonne, 33076 Bordeaux, France

Christopher S. Barker, Department of Microbiology, University of Alabama, Laboratory for Special Cancer Research, Birmingham, Alabama, 35294

Francoise Barre-Sinoussi, Laboratory of Virology, Institut Pasteur, Paris, France

John W. Berg, Department of Epidemiology, AMC Cancer Research Center, Denver, Colorado, 80214; and Departments of Pathology, Biometrics and Preventive Medicine, University of Colorado School of Medicine, Denver, Colorado, 80262

James Bradac, Laboratory for Special Cancer Research, Department of Microbiology, University of Alabama, Birmingham, Alabama, 35294

Claudine Bruck, Department of Molecular Biology, University of Brussels, Genese, Belgium

Francoise Brun-Vezinet, Hopital Claude Bernard, Paris, France

Arsene Burny, Faculty of Agronomy, Gembloux, and Department of Molecular Biology, University of Brussels, Genese, Belgium

Cirilo D. Cabradilla, Division of Viral Diseases, Center for Infectious Diseases, Centers for Disease Control, Atlanta, Georgia, 30333

Robert Callahan, Laboratory of Tumor Immunology and Biology, National Cancer Institute, Bethesda, Maryland, 20205

Arnaldo Caruso, Laboratory of Tumor Immunology and Biology, National Cancer Institute, Bethesda, Maryland, 20205

Subatndra Chatterjee, Laboratory for Special Cancer Research, Department of Microbiology, University of Alabama, Birmingham, Alabama, 35294

Jean-Claude Chermann, Department of Virology, Institut Pasteur, Paris, France

Ing-Ming Chiu, Laboratory of Tumor Immunology and Biology, National Cancer Institute, Bethesda, Maryland, 20205

Brent Cochran, Harvard Medical School, Boston, Massachusetts, 02115

Maurice Cohen, National Cancer Institute, Frederick Cancer Research Facility, Frederick, Maryland, 21701

David L. Cohn, Denver Disease Control Service, Denver Department of Health and Hospitals, Denver, Colorado, 80204-4507

Jonathan A. Cooper, The Salk Institute, San Diego, California, 92138

Dominique Couez, Department of Molecular Biology, University of Brussels, Genese, Belgium

Carlo M. Croce, The Wistar Institute of Anatomy and Biology, Philadelphia, Pennyslvania, 19104

Tom Curran, Molecular Biology and Virology Laboratory, The Salk Institute, San Diego, California, 92138

Kathleen C. Davis, Conrad D. Stephenson Laboratory for Research in Immunology, Department of Medicine, National Jewish Hospital and Research Center, Denver, Colorado, 80206

Annelies de Klein, Department of Cell Biology and Genetics, Erasmus University, 3000 DR Rotterdam, The Netherlands

Guy de The, Centre National de la Recherche Scientifique, Universite Claude Bernard, Laboratoire D'Epidemiologie et Immunovirologie des Tumeurs, Faculty of Medicine Alexis Carrel, Rue G. Paradin, 69372 Lyon, Cedex 2, France

Jacqueline Deschamps, ULB, Department Chimie Biologique, 1640 Rhode-Ste-Genese, Belgique; and Laboratory of Molecular Biology, University of Brussels, Genese, Belgium

Ron Desrosiers, Laboratory for Special Cancer Research, Department of Microbiology, University of Alabama, Birmingham, Alabama, 35294

Bruce S. Dobozin, Conrad D. Stephenson Laboratory for Research in Immunology, Department of Medicine, National Jewish Hospital and Research Center, Denver, Colorado, 80206

Kevin Doherty, Laboratory of Molecular Immunobiology, Dana-Farber Cancer Institute, Boston, Massachusetts, 02115

Peter H. Duesberg, Department of Molecular Biology and Virus Laboratory, University of California, Berkeley, California, 94720

Max Essex, Department of Microbiology, Harvard School of Public Health, Boston, Massachusetts, 02115

Paul M. Feorino, Division of Viral Diseases, Center for Infectious Diseases, Centers for Disease Control, Atlanta, Georgia, 30333

Peter J. Fischinger, National Cancer Institute, Bethesda, Maryland, 20205

Christos Flordellis, Laboratory of Molecular Oncology, National Cancer Institute, Frederick Cancer Research Facility, Frederick, Maryland, 21701

Donald P. Francis, Division of Viral Diseases, Center for Infectious Diseases, Centers for Disease Control, Atlanta, Georgia, 30333

Robert C. Gallo, Laboratory of Tumor Cell Biology, Division of Cancer Treatment, National Cancer Institute, Bethesda, Maryland, 20205

Murray B. Gardner, Department of Pathology, University of California, Davis, California, 95817

Jacques Ghysdael, Laboratory of Molecular Biology, University of Brussels, Genese, Belgium

Raymond Gilden, National Cancer Institute, PRI-Frederick Cancer Research Facility, Frederick, Maryland, 21701

Jean-Claude Gluckman, U.E.R. Pitie-Salpetriere, Paris, France

Kathy Gould, The Salk Institute, San Diego, California, 92138

Diane Gregoire, Laboratory of Molecular Biology, University of Brussels, Genese, Belgium

John Groffen, Oncogene Science Inc., Mineola, New York, 11501

Gerard Grosveld, Department of Cell Biology and Genetics, Erasmus University, 3000 DR Rotterdam, The Netherlands

Bernard J. Guillemain, INSERM U. 117, 229 crs de l'Argonne, 33076 Bordeaux, France

Beatrice Hahn, Laboratory of Tumor Cell Biology, Division of Cancer Treatment, National Cancer Institute, Bethesda, Maryland, 20205

Patricia Horan Hand, Laboratory of Tumor Immunology and Biology, National Cancer Institute, Bethesda, Maryland, 20205

William D. Hardy, Jr., Laboratory of Veterinary Oncology, Memorial Sloan Kettering Cancer Center, New York, New York, 10021

Nora Heisterkamp, Oncogene Science Inc., Mineola, New York, 11501

Edward A. Hoover, Department of Pathology, College of Veterinary Medicine and Biomedical Science, Colorado State University, Fort Collins, Colorado, 80523

Toby Horn, Laboratory of Tumor Immunology and Biology, National Cancer Institute, Bethesda, Maryland, 20205

Charles R. Horsburgh, Jr., Conrad D. Stephenson Laboratory for Research in Immunology, Department of Medicine, National Jewish Hospital and Research Center, Denver, Colorado, 80206

Eric Hunter, Laboratory for Special Cancer Research, Department of Microbiology, University of Alabama, Birmingham, Alabama, 35294

Tony Hunter, The Salk Institute, San Diego, California, 92138

Franklyn N. Judson, Denver Disease Control Service, Denver Department of Health and Hospitals, Denver, Colorado, 80204-4507

V. S. Kalyanaraman, Division of Viral Diseases, Center for Infectious Diseases, Centers for Disease Control, Atlanta, Georgia, 30333

Nancy C. Kan, Laboratory of Molecular Oncology, National Cancer Institute, Frederick Cancer Research Facility, Frederick, Maryland, 21701

Kathleen Kelly, Immunology Branch, National Cancer Institute, Bethesda, Maryland, 20205

Richard Kettmann, ULB, Department Chimie Biologique, 1640 Rhode-Ste-Genese, Belgium; Faculty of Agronomy, Gembloux; and Department of Molecular Biology, University of Brussels, Genese, Belgium

Charles H. Kirkpatrick, Conrad D. Stephenson Laboratory for Research in Immunology, Department of Medicine, National Jewish Hospital and Research Center, Denver, Colorado, 80206

David Klatzmann, U.E.R. Pitie-Salpetriere, Paris, France

Michiko Koga, Roswell Park Memorial Institute, Buffalo, New York, 14263

Mary-Ann Lane, Laboratory of Molecular Immunobiology, Dana-Farber Cancer Institute, and Harvard Medical School, Boston, Massachusetts, 02115

James A. Lautenberger, Laboratory of Molecular Oncology, National Cancer Institute, Frederick Cancer Research Facility, Frederick, Maryland, 21701

Philip Leder, Department of Genetics, Harvard Medical School, Boston, Massachusetts, 02115

Douglas R. Lowy, Laboratory of Cellular Oncology, National Cancer Institute, Bethesda, Maryland, 20205

Marc Mammerickx, National Institute for Veterinary Research, Uccle, Belgium

Robert Z. Mamoun, INSERM U. 117, 229 crs de l'Argonne, 33076 Bordeaux, France

Malcolm A. Martin, Laboratory of Molecular Microbiology, National Institute of Allergy and Infectious Diseases, National Institutes of Health, Bethesda, Maryland, 20205

A. Dusty Miller, Molecular Biology and Virology Laboratory, The Salk Institute, San Diego, California, 92138

Luc Montagnier, Department of Virology, Institut Pasteur, Paris, France

Raffaella Muraro, Laboratory of Tumor Immunology and Biology, National Cancer Institute, Bethesda, Maryland, 20205

Peter C. Nowell, Department of Pathology and Laboratory Medicine, University of Pennsylvania School of Medicine, Philadelphia, Pennsylvania, 19104

Michael Nunn, The Salk Institute, San Diego, California, 92138

Catherine D. O'Connell, National Cancer Institute, Frederick Cancer Research Facility, Frederick, Maryland, 21701

Takis S. Papas, Laboratory of Molecular Oncology, National Cancer Institute, Frederick Cancer Research Facility, Frederick, Maryland, 21701

Kent Penley, Denver Disease Control Service, Denver Department of Health and Hospitals, Denver, Colorado, 80204-4507

Mikulas Popovic, Laboratory of Tumor Cell Biology, Division of Cancer Treatment, National Cancer Institute, Bethesda, Maryland, 20205

Daniel Portetelle, Faculty of Agronomy, Gembloux; and Department of Molecular Biology, University of Brussels, Genese, Belgium

Miltos C. Psallidopoulos, Laboratory of Molecular Oncology, National Cancer Institute, Frederick Cancer Research Facility, Frederick, Maryland, 21701

Arnold B. Rabson, Laboratory of Molecular Microbiology, National Institute of Allergy and Infectious Diseases, National Institutes of Health, Bethesda, Maryland, 20205

Nicole Rebeyrotte, INSERM U. 117, 229 crs de l'Argonne, 33076 Bordeaux, France

Marvin S. Reitz, Jr., Laboratory of Tumor Cell Biology, Division of Cancer Treatment, National Cancer Institute, Bethesda, Maryland, 20205

Roy Repaske, Laboratory of Molecular Microbiology, National Institute of Allergy and Infectious Diseases, National Institutes of Health, Bethesda, Maryland, 20205

Nancy Rice, National Cancer Institute, LBI-Frederick Cancer Research Facility, Frederick, Maryland, 21701

Patricia E. Rickmann, Conrad D. Stephenson Laboratory for Research in Immunology, Department of Medicine, National Jewish Hospital and Research Center, Denver, Colorado, 80206

Joan Robbins, Laboratory of Tumor Immunology and Biology, National Cancer Institute, Bethesda, Maryland, 20205

Keith C. Robbins, Laboratory of Cellular and Molecular Biology, National Cancer Institute, Bethesda, Maryland, 20205

Charles E. Rogler, Liver Research Center and Departments of Medicine and Cell Biology, Albert Einstein College of Medicine, Bronx, New York, 10461

Christine Rouzioux, Hopital Claude Bernard, Paris, France

Ugo G. Rovigatti, Laboratory of Molecular Oncology, National Cancer Institute, Frederick Cancer Research Facility, Frederick, Maryland, 21701

S. Zaki Salahuddin, Laboratory of Tumor Cell Biology, Division of Cancer Treatment, National Cancer Institute, Bethesda, Maryland, 20205

Kenneth P. Samuel, Laboratory of Molecular Oncology, National Cancer Institute, Frederick Cancer Research Facility, Frederick, Maryland, 21701

M. G. Sarngadharan, Laboratory of Tumor Cell Biology, Division of Cancer Treatment, National Cancer Institute, Bethesda, Maryland, 20205

Jeffrey Schlom, Laboratory of Tumor Immunology and Biology, National Cancer Institute, Bethesda, Maryland, 20205

Jorge Schupbach, Laboratory of Tumor Cell Biology, Division of Cancer Treatment, National Cancer Institute, Bethesda, Maryland, 20205

Peter H. Seeburg, Genentech, Inc., South San Francisco, California, 90007

Toshio Seyama, Research Institute for Nuclear Medicine and Biology, Hiroshima University, Hiroshima 734, Japan

David A. Shafritz, Liver Research Center and Departments of Medicine and Cell Biology, Albert Einstein College of Medicine, Bronx, New York, 10461

George Shaw, Laboratory of Tumor Cell Biology, Division of Cancer Treatment, National Cancer Institute, Bethesda, Maryland, 20205

Morris Sherman, Liver Research Center and Departments of Medicine and Cell Biology, Albert Einstein College of Medicine, Bronx, New York, 10461

B. I. Sahai Srivastava, Roswell Park Memorial Institute, Buffalo, New York, 14263

Paul E. Steele, Laboratory of Molecular Microbiology, National Institute of Allergy and Infectious Diseases, National Institutes of Health Bethesda, Maryland, 20205

Henry A. F. Stephens, Laboratory of Molecular Immunobiology, Dana-Farber Cancer Institute and Harvard Medical School, Boston, Massachusetts, 02115

Robert Stephens, National Cancer Institute, LBI-Frederick Cancer Research Facility, Frederick, Maryland, 21701

John R. Stephenson, Oncogene Science Inc., Mineola, New York, 11501

Charles Stiles, Harvard Medical School, Boston, Massachusetts, 02115

Ann Thor, Laboratory of Tumor Immunology and Biology, National Cancer Institute, Bethesda, Maryland, 20205

Matthew B. Tobin, Laboratory of Molecular Immunobiology, Dana-Farber Cancer Institute, Boston, Massachusetts, 02115

Charles Van Beveren, Molecular Biology and Virology Laboratory, The Salk Institute, San Diego, California, 92138

Inder M. Verma, Molecular Biology and Virology Laboratory, The Salk Institute, San Diego, California, 92138

Dennis K. Watson, Laboratory of Molecular Oncology, National Cancer Institute, Frederick Cancer Research Facility, Frederick, Maryland, 21701

Maureen Weeks, National Cancer Institute, Bethesda, Maryland, 20205

John W. Wills, Department of Microbiology, University of Alabama, Laboratory for Special Cancer Research, Birmingham, Alabama, 35294

Berthe M. Willumsen, University of Copenhagen, Microbiology Institute, Copenhagen, Denmark

Flossie Wong-Staal, Laboratory of Tumor Cell Biology, Division of Cancer Treatment, National Cancer Institute, Bethesda, Maryland, 20205

David Wunderlich, National Cancer Institute, Bethesda, Maryland, 20205

Kazuyoshi Yanagihara, Research Institute for Nuclear Medicine and Biology, Hiroshima University, Hiroshima 734, Japan

Kenjiro Yokoro, Research Institute for Nuclear Medicine and Biology, Hiroshima University, Hiroshima 734, Japan

PREFACE

We stand today on the threshold of a new understanding of cancer. Primarily through the powerful tools of molecular biology, unified hypotheses explaining the origins of the disease are emerging and rapidly being validated. This volume, which presents the latest findings from laboratories throughout the world on the role of RNA tumor viruses in cancer, is a celebration of these achievements and a prediction of further progress leading ultimately to the control of the disease.

It is important in this context to recall the natural history or life cycle of RNA cancer virology. From the earliest days of the science, when viruses were first recognized as distinct biologic agents of etiologic significance, their role in cancer was proposed and hotly debated. The critical early discoveries, even those made as recently as 25 years ago, were met with rejection; not skepticism or cautious restraint, but outright rejection. During the 60's, there was a gradual acceptance of the association between viruses and cancer, the result of landmark studies in experimental systems, and this led to a frenzy of activity in the field. There followed another period of doubt and uncertainty, due to the difficulty in attempting to apply directly, and in retrospect inappropriately, the tenets of infectious disease to human cancers, only to have the field resurrected, revitalized and redirected by the explosion of progress in molecular biology and genetics.

Until this renaissance in RNA tumor virology, a unified explanation for the origin of cancer was beyond our reach. But now we are approaching a true molecular understanding of malignant transformation. Very much of this quantum leap forward has been made possible by the contributors to this volume.

Yet major questions remain to be answered. We must turn these same tools of molecular biology and tumor virology, so valuable in dissecting and analyzing the causes of cancer, to the task of understanding other equally critical aspects of the cancer problem: progression, heterogeneity and the metastatic process. These are absolutely crucial to our solving the clinical difficulties of cancer: detection, diagnosis and effective treatment. Thus, our intent is that this volume, in addition to presenting the state-of-the-art in RNA tumor virology, will serve as a stimulus to those in the field and others interested in the pathophysiology of cancer for the attack and resolution of these problems. It is through these efforts that we will achieve our final goal -- the complete control of cancer.

We gratefully acknowledge assistance in the preparation of this volume by Susan Guyer, Cathrine Allen and Carol Rains, and the generous support of the AMC Cancer Research Center and the National Institutes of Health through grant CA-38586 from the National Cancer Institute.

Philip Furmanski
Jean Carol Hager
Marvin A. Rich

RNA TUMOR VIRUSES, ONCOGENES,
HUMAN CANCER AND AIDS:
On the Frontiers of
Understanding

1

Myc, a Genetic Element that is Shared by a Cellular Gene (proto-*myc*) and by viruses with one (MC29) or two (MH2) *onc* genes

T. S. Papas[1], N. C. Kan[1], D. K. Watson[1], J. A. Lautenberger[1], C. Flordellis[1], K. P. Samuel[1], U. G. Rovigatti[1], M. C. Psallidopoulos[1], R. Ascione[1], and P. H. Duesberg[2]; [1]National Cancer Institute-FCRF, National Institutes of Health, Frederick, MD 21701 and [2]Department of Molecular Biology, University of California, Berkeley, California 94740

INTRODUCTION

The transforming (*onc*) genes of several avian carcinoma viruses including MC29, MH2, CMII, and OK10 and of a normal cellular gene (proto-*myc*) share a common structural domain termed *myc*. Proto-*myc* consists of three exons, a largely non-coding 5' exon joined with two coding exons of 1.6 kb. The *myc*-related gene of MC29 is a hybrid consisting of 1.5 kb derived from the 5' half of the *gag* gene of nondefective retroviruses and 1.6 kb derived from the two 3' exons of the proto-*myc* gene. The *myc* gene of MH2 consists of a 5' *gag*-derived exon of 6 codons and a 3' exon corresponding to the two 3' exons of the proto-*myc* gene. In addition, MH2 contains a second gene termed Δ*gag*-*mht* with transforming potential. The two genes of MH2 are throught to cooperate in neoplastic transformation (1, 2).

Here we have analyzed and compared the *myc*-related genes of MC29 and MH2 viruses and of the normal cell to understand why the viral genes have obligatory transforming function when expressed in avian cells, whereas proto-*myc* is regularly expressed in normal cells without apparent transforming function (3, 4).

In complementary studies we have analyzed the relationship between the *myb* sequences present in avian myeloblastosis virus (AMV), avian erythroblastosis virus (E26), and a cellular gene termed proto-*myb*. The *myb*-containing viruses have a narrower oncogenic spectrum than the viruses that contain *myc*. The *myb*-containing viruses cause only leukemia *in vivo* and transform hematopoietic cells *in vitro*. They do not cause solid tumors and do not transform fibroblasts in culture (Table 1).

TABLE I

ONCOGENIC PROPERTIES OF AVIAN ACUTE LEUKEMIA VIRUSES

Virus Strain	Neoplastic growth induced in vivo			Cell Types Transformed in vitro	Viral onc sequences
	Sarcoma	Carcinoma	Acute Leukemia		
	(Fibrosarcoma=F) (Hepatocytoma=H)	(Renal Adenocarcinoma=RC) (Carcinoma=C)	(Myelocytomatosis=M) (Erythroblastosis=E) (Myeloblastosis=My)	(Fibroblastic=f) (Epitheloid=ep) (Myeloid=m) (Erythroid=e)	
MC29-subgroup					
MC29	F, H	C, RC	M, E	f, ep, m, e	myc
MH2	F, H	C, RC	M, E	f, ep, m, e	myc, mht
OK10	F, H	C, RC	M, E	f, ep, m, e	myc
CMII	F, H	C, RC	M, E	f, ep, m, e	myc
AMV-subgroup					
AMV	-	-	My	m	myb
E26	-	-	My, E	m, e	myb, ets
AEV-subgroup					
AEV	F	C	M, E	f, e	erb A, erb B

RESULTS AND DISCUSSION

Sequence analysis of MC29 and chicken and human proto-myc oncogenes. We have cloned (5) and sequenced the MC29 v-myc gene as well as the chicken cellular myc and the human cellular myc homologs (6, 7, 8,). We have aligned these sequences on the basis of their nucleotide homology, and based on the sequence homology (9) we have constructed a model that is depicted in Fig. 1.

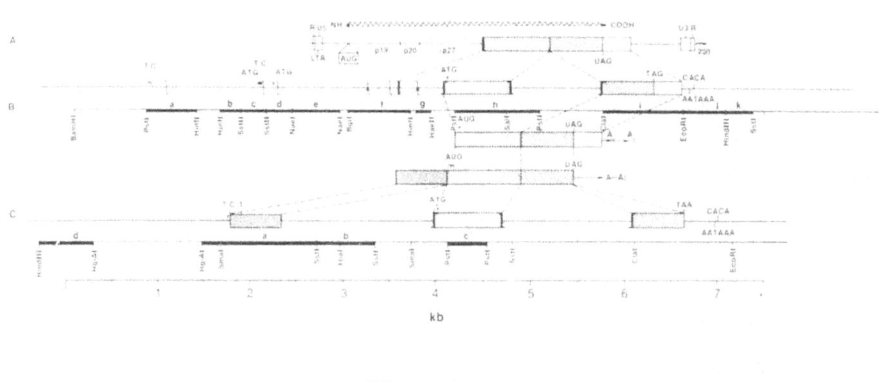

Figure 1

The highlights of this work are the following:

1. MC29 is a defective virus, because it lacks the entire polymerase (pol) gene, part of the gag gene, and 71 amino acids from the NH_2-terminus of the envelope (env) gene. Instead of these retroviral genetic elements MC29 contains the cell-derived myc sequence.

2. An open reading frame is observed extending from the first ATG initiation codon located at the 5' end of the gag gene into the myc sequence. This open reading frame is designated as the hatched area in Fig. 1.

3. Nucleotide sequence comparison of MC29 and cellular myc genes reveals a stretch of 12 nucleotides shared by the virus and the chicken cell, but not shared by the human proto-myc gene. A perfect consensus donor-acceptor splice signal is located at the 3' border of the 12 nucleotide-region. This splice signal has probably functioned in linking up the 12-nucleotide sequence with the 5' end of the second exon of chicken proto-myc when MC29 virus was generated. Thus the 5' end of this 12-mer defines the 5' recombination point between the helper virus and chicken proto-myc gene.

4. Both chicken and human proto-myc genes contain at least two coding exons interrupted by an intron of about 1 Kb. These exons are defined by consensus donor-acceptor splice signals and by the absence of introns in the v-myc sequence.

5. The two exons in the chicken and human proto-myc genes share a common reading frame which is terminated by a conserved translation termination signal: TAG in v-myc and chicken proto-myc, and TAA in human proto-myc.

6. Using the following approaches we have been able to demonstrate that mRNA from normal cells may be generated from proto-myc sequences:

a) By direct examination of the nucleotide sequence of cloned myc genes consensus trancriptional signals were detected.

b) By utilization of ^{32}P-DNA probes derived from specific fragments of cloned myc DNA, and by hybridization studies using mRNA extracted from appropriate cells a major proto-myc mRNA species of 2.5 kb and minor species up to 4 kb were detected.

c) By comparison of myc-related sequences isolated from genomic DNA libraries and from cDNA libraries proto-myc mRNAs were identified (10).

7. The chicken and human proto-myc genes are distinctive cellular eukaryotic genes, possessing all the characteristic signals of a eukaryotic

gene. Both genes are trancriptionally active. Furthermore, comparison of human and mouse proto-*myc* sequences reveals a highly conserved region in the largely non-coding 5' exon (11).

In general, data derived from these approaches lead one to the conclusion that the human proto-*myc* locus is possibly less complex than that of the chicken. When compared to each other the chicken and human proto-*myc* genes comprise constant and variable domains. The constant region consists of the major coding exons, while the variable regions consist of the introns and the exon sequences upstream from the two major coding exons. The integrity of these two coding exons may be important for the viability of the cell and also for certain kinds of tumors, because in neoplastic avian systems such as chicken bursal lymphomas, where promoter insertion has been observed, promoters do not disrupt the coding regions conserved between chicken and man (12). Similarly in Burkitt lymphomas where chromosomal breakage occurs within the *myc* gene, the constant region always remains undisturbed (13).

Comparison of the gene products predicted from the nucleotide sequences of the human and chicken proto-*myc* and the MC29 v-*myc* genes is shown schematically in Fig. 1. The *myc* domain of the virus differs by seven amino acids from that encoded by the chicken cell. There is a much greater amino acid variation between human proto-*myc* and chicken proto-*myc* genes. This variation occurs primarily in the coding region flanking the splice junctions and is consistent with a higher rate of evolutionary change occurring in the exon regions nearest the diverging introns. Consistent with this contention, one observes that the introns of chicken and human proto-*myc* genes have completely diverged from each other. The viral gene differs from the cellular gene primarily in the 5' end region. Here in addition to the *myc*-related sequence, the viral genome contains about 1.5 Kb of specific sequences from the viral *gag* gene. Sequence analysis of the chicken proto-*myc* locus reveals an open reading frame which is shared with the MC29 *myc* gene. An mRNA may be generated from the cellular gene which in turn can be putatively translated into a protein product.

To assist with the identification of the normal cellular protein, we raised an antiserum against a synthetic peptide deduced from the 5' end of the *myc* sequence, and an antiserum against a *myc*-containing protein encoded by an expression vector in *E. coli* (14). These antisera have been shown to be immunoreactive with viral and cellular myc proteins. Recently it has been reported that the MC29 transforming protein is localized in the nucleus of the transformed cell (15). We have therefore determined the authenticity of our antisera as to whether they are able to functionally localize the MC29 transforming antigen. We have shown that our antisera can indeed localize a myc-related protein in the nucleus of MC29-transformed cells(14). Furthermore, we have labeled MC29-transformed Q8 quail cells and chicken embryo fibroblasts (CEF) with ^{35}S-methionine, and have immunoprecipitated cell lysates using antisera directed against both the synthetic and bacterial products. Both types of antisera precipitate the viral p110 gag-myc protein in MC29-transformed cells, and a cellular protein migrating at 55K daltons (p55) in the normal chicken cell. The latter protein cannot be detected using preimmune antisera. To verify that these two proteins, p110 gag-myc and p55, share similar peptides, the immunoprecipitated proteins were purified and digested with trypsin. Their tryptic peptides were mixed together and identified on two-dimentional fingerprints. In these instances we observe no differences between their tryptic peptide components (data not shown). We therefore conclude that the p55 protein is a normal cellular homolog of the MC29 transforming protein. Utilizing two different approaches, micro-amino acid sequencing and nucleotide sequencing, we are attempting to confirm the origin of this normal cellular protein and to identify the presence of additional exon(s) located upstream from the first major coding exon.

Molecular Structure of MH2. We have molecularly cloned the MH2 provirus and determined its exact genetic structure by nucleotide sequence analysis shown in Fig. 2 (1,2).

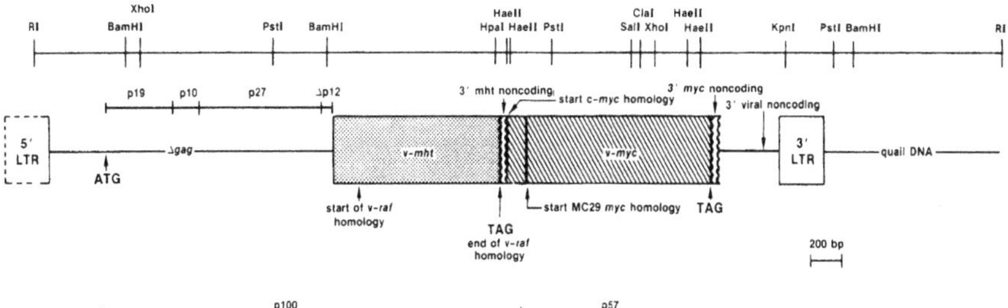

Figure 2

Unexpectedly this analysis revealed an MH2-specific sequence of 1.2 Kb, termed mht, which is totally unrelated to the myc sequence (7,8). The nucleotide sequence of MH2 viral genome indicates that the gag region and the mht gene form an open reading frame starting in the gag and terminating at a TAG stop codon near the 3' end of mht. This open reading frame contains 894 amino acids capable of accounting for a protein migrating at 100K dalton. This prediction is in accord with the size of the p100 gag-mht fusion protein observed in MH2-transformed cells (16).

MC29, MH2 and MSV 3611: Comparison of Molecular Structures. By nucleotide sequence comparison one observes that the myc sequence of MH2 has 182 nucleotides not found in the MC29 myc sequence, but present in the cellular proto-myc gene flanking the first major coding exon. This region consists of the 3' end of the intron preceeding the first of the two major exons and contains an RNA splice acceptor site in the chicken cell. Thus the myc sequence of the MH2 genome includes the cellular splice acceptor site which can be used to generate the 2.6 Kb subgenomic mRNA (17). This spliced subgenomic RNA species is subsequently translated into a 57K dalton protein, the myc-containing protein detected in MH2-transformed cells (17). In additon the myc sequence of MH2 differs from that of MC29 in 33 substitutions out of 419 amino acids, and a deletion of 4 amino acids in the MH2 myc sequence.

When the mht sequence of MH2 was compared with the onc-specific raf sequence of murine sarcoma virus (MSV) 3611, a striking homology was observed (Fig. 3) (18).

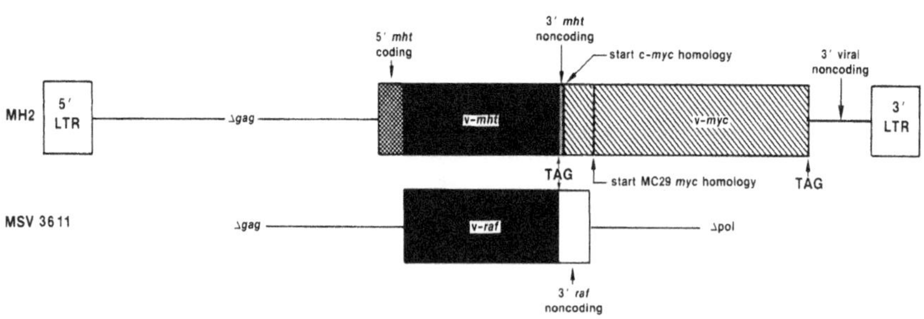

Figure 3

The sequence homology between the two onc-genes is 80 percent. Most of the observed nucleotide changes are third base substitutions. The raf sequence of MSV 3611 differs from the mht sequenc of MH2 by having 19 amino acid substitutions and one inserted proline. The bulk of these amino acid changes occurs at the 3' half of the respective onc genes. Significantly the homology between these two oncogenes at the deduced amino acid level is 94 percent. This region of homology is flanked on both sides by MH2- and MSV 3611-specific sequences, with essentially no homology between the two viruses. As shown in Fig. 3, at the 5' side, the homology begins 174 bp 3' to the gag-mht junction in MH2. Thus the first 58 amino acids of mht preceding the start of homology with raf are MH2-specific. At the 3' side, the two sequences share a common termination codon at position 1186 and diverge beyond this point. It is concluded from these studies that MH2 virus has two nonstructural genes with oncogenic potential. Further work is necessary to determine whether each of these genes is oncogenic by itself, or whether they cooperate with each other to affect transformation.

To further assess the biological activity and determine the possible cooperativity of the two onc-genes, we established a DNA transfection assay using chicken embryo fibroblasts (CEF) as recipient cells. Primary cultures of CEF have been cotransfected with molecularly cloned MH2 proviral and helper virus (RAV-1) DNA. Foci of the transformed cells were observed between ten and twenty days after transfection. The cells were further passaged several times in order to achieve massive transformation. In figure 4, DNA from the transformed cultures (lanes 2 and 4) and from cultures transformed with no DNA (lane 1) and with helper viral DNA (lane 3) were purified and cleaved with Eco R1, blotted onto a nitrocellulose filter, and probed with v-myc or v-mht DNA (Fig. 4, panels A and B, respectively).

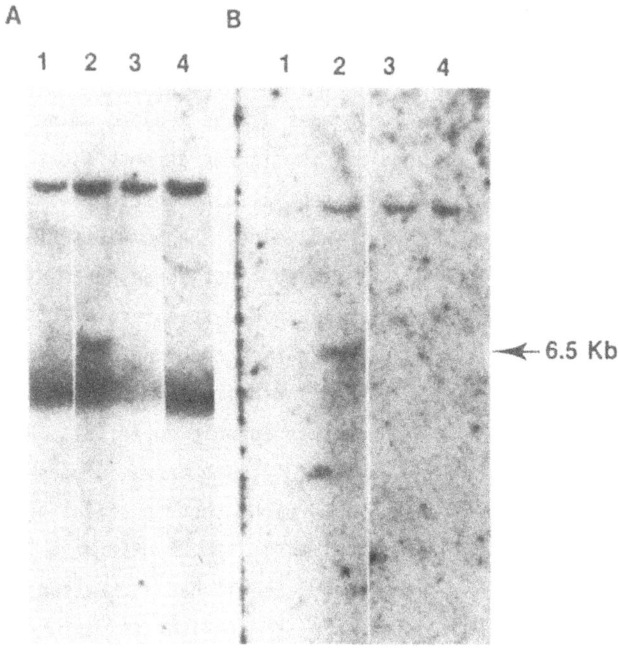

Figure 4

Results indicate that cells transformed by MH2 DNA, in addition to containing the cellular proto-<u>myc</u> and proto-<u>mht</u> genes, contain a ~ 6.5 Kb band representative of the entire MH2 sequence. Furthermore, the transforming virus released subsequent to cotransfection has been identified by T1 oligonucleotide fingerprinting as of MH2 viral RNA (Fig. 5).

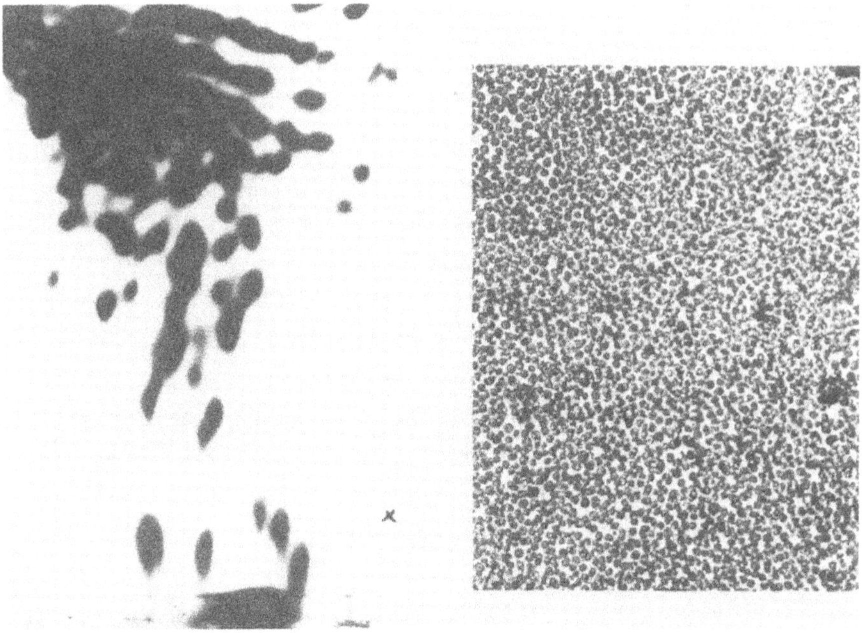

Figure 5

Now that we have an assay established, we can selectively delete regions in mht, myc and/or gag in order to assess their biological activities in the CEF transfection system.

The observation that the onc-specific sequences of MH2 and MSV 3611 are essentially colinear and 94 percent homologous at the amino acid level represents the closest homology found so far among onc-sequences of retroviruses from different taxonomic groups. The Δgag-mht and Δ gag-raf genes differ only in the 174 mht-specific nucleotides and in their gag regions (Fig. 3). The coincidence that a sequence conserved in two different animal species appears in taxonomically-unrelated retroviruses argues that only a limited number of cellular sequences can, upon transduction into a retroviral vector, function as an onc gene. Furthermore, conservation of these sequences in different animal species suggests that these sequences belong to functionally important cellular genes. There is however no evidence at this time that the cellular proto-mht/raf genes possess any oncogenic potential of their own.

The observation that mht is a segment of a normal celllular gene is demonstratable in two ways: (a) A 3.8 Kb cellular mht-related mRNA was detected by Northern-blot hybridization using RNA purified from normal chicken cells (7). The chicken proto-mht gene may therefore contain a coding region of about 3.8 Kb, whereas the tranduced segment of the 1.2 Kb mht sequence in MH2 probably only represents a subset of the proto-mht gene. (b) Clones derived from a normal chicken genomic DNA library contain the 174 bp v-mhtspecific nucleotides which are not present in the v-raf gene. The 174 bpsegment in v-mht is represented in the normal cellular gene by three exons (Flordellis et. al., in preparation). The first exon consists of 146 bp and only 32 bp at its 3' end were transduced into the MH2 genome. The 5' border of the 32 bp-segment thus represents the 5' recombination point between the helper virus and cellular-mht gene. Comparison of chicken proto-mht and the gag sequence flanking the v-mht in MH2 reveals no homology. It is therefore concluded that the recombination probably occurred at the DNA level by an illegitimate recombination process. DNA sequence analysis indicates that the 5' three exons in proto-mht are flanked by canonical consensus donor-acceptor splice signals. The sizes of the second and third exons are 28 bp and 128 bp respectively. The open reading frame of the three proto-mht exons is identical to that of the v-mht. Comparing the sequences of proto-mht to v-mht, we find no nucleotide changes in the first two exons. There are three point mutations in the third exon, only one of which encodes a different amino acid. The 174 bp of v-mht are dispersed within three defined domains throughout a 4 kb genomic region. This data is consistent with the conclusion that the mht sequence of MH2 is only a segment of the normal cellular proto-onc gene. In similar experiments involving MC29 and AMV viruses, we have also observed differences among the sizes of proto-onc genes, their corresponding proto-onc transcripts, and the _onc_-specific sequences transduced by retroviruses. These results support the overall scheme that retroviral _onc_-genes are subsets of proto-_onc_ genes (Table 2).

TABLE II

CELLULAR GENES TRANSDUCED BY AVIAN ACUTE LEUKEMIA VIRUSES

Cellular Gene	Transcript (kb)	Virus	Segment Transduced (kb)
myc	2.5	MC29	1.4
		MH2	1.5
mht	3.8	MH2	1.2
myb	4.0	AMV	1.2
		E26	0.8
ets	7.4	E26	1.5

Based upon the foregoing data we can then summarize our conclusions as follows:

1. Viral _onc_ genes appear to be subsets of proto-_onc_ genes.
2. Most viral _onc_ genes are genetic hybrids: sequences derived from a proto-_onc_ gene are usually linked to sequences derived from one or more retroviral essential genes.
3. The number of cellular proto-_onc_ genes is limited, because MH2 and MSV 3611 as well as other retroviruses from different taxonomic groups, have transduced the same _onc_ gene sequences from different animal species.
4. Specific deletions and linkage of the same proto-_onc_ sequences to retroviral vector elements affect the oncogenic potential of the resultant viruses. The differences in the transformational abilities of MH2 and MSV 3611 viruses serve as examples.

REFERENCES

1. Kan N, Flordellis C, Garon C, Duesberg P, Papas T: Avian carcionoma virus MH2 contains a specific sequence, mht, and shares the myc sequence with MC29, CM11 and OK10 viruses. Proc Natl Acad Sci(80): 6566-6570, 1983.
2. Kan N, Flordellis C, Mark G, Duesberg P, Papas T: Nucleotide sequence of avian carcinoma virus MH2: Two potential onc genes, one related to avian virus MC29 and the other related to murine sarcoma virus 3611. Proc Natl Acad Sci(81): 3000-3004, 1984.
3. Eva A, Robbins K, Anderson P, Srinivasan A, Ronick S, Reddy E, Ellmore N, Galen A, Lautenberger J, Papas T, Westin E, Wong-Staal F, Gallor R, Aaronson S: Cellular gene analogous to retorviral onc genes are transcribed in human tumor cells. Nature(295): 116-119, 1982.
4. Kelly K, Cochran V, Stiles C, Leder P: Cell-specific regulation of the c-myc gene by lymphocyte mitogens and platelet-derived growth factor. Cell(35): 603-610.
5. Lautenberger J, Schultz R, Garon C, Tsichlis P, Papas T: Molecular cloning of avian myelocytomatosis virus (MC29) transforming sequences. Proc Natl Acad Sci(78): 1518-1522, 1981.
6. Reddy E, Reynolds K, Watson D, Schulz R, Lautenberger J, Papas T: Nucleotide sequence analysis of the proviral genome of avian myelocytomatosis virus (MC29). Proc Natl Acad Sci(80): 2500-2504, 1983.
7. Watson D, Reddy E, Duesberg P, Papas T: Nucleotide sequence analysis of the chicken c-myc gene reveals homologous and unique coding regions by comparison wiith the transforming gene of avian myelocytomatosis virus MC29, gag-myc. Proc Natl Acad Sci(80): 2146-2150, 1983.
8. Watson, D, Psallidopoulos M, Samuel D, Dalla Favera R, Papas T: Nucleotide sequence analysis of human c-myc locus, chicken homologue, and myelocytomatosis virus MC29 transforming gene reveals a highly conserved gen product. Proc Natl Acad Sci(80): 3642-3645, 1983.

9. Papas T, Kan N, Watson D, Flordellis C, Psallidopoulos M, Lautenberger J, Samuel K, Duesberg P: myc-related genes in viruses and cells. In: Levin A, Topp W, Vande Woude GF, Watson JD (eds) Cancer Cell.

10. Watt R, Stanton L, Marcu K, Gallo R, Croce C, Rovera G: Nucleotide sequence of cloned cDNA of human c-myc oncogene. Nature(303): 725-728, 1983.

11. Bernard O, Cory S, Gerondakis S, Webb E, Adams J: Sequence of the murine and human cellular myc oncogenes and two modes of myc transcription resulting from chromosome translocation in B lymphoid tumours. The EMBO Journal(2): 2375-2383, 1983.

12. Hayward W, Shih C, Goodenow M, Wiman K, Hayday A, Saito H, Tonegawa S: Mechanisms of c-myc activation in avian and human B-cell lymphomas. In: Ahmad F, Black S, Schultz J, Scott W, Whelan W (eds) Advances in Gene Technology: Human Genetic Disorders. ICSU Press, Miami, Florida 1984, pp 12-15.

13. Gelmann E, Psallidopoulos M, Papas T, Dalla Favera R: Identification of reciprocal translocation sites within the c-myc oncogene and immunoglobulin μ locus in a Burkitt lymphoma. Nature(306): 799-803, 1983.

14. Lautenberger J, Court D, Papas T: High-level in Escherichia coli of the carboxy-terminal sequences of the avian myelocytomatosis virus (MC29) v-myc protein. Gene(23):75-84.

15. Hann S, Abrams H, Rohrschneider L, Eisenman R: Proteins encoded by v-myc and c-myc oncogenes: Identification and localization in acute leukemia virus transformants and Bursal lymphoma cell lines. Cell(34): 789-798, 1983.

16. Hu S, Moscovici C, Vogt P: The defectiveness of Mill Hill 2, a carcinoma-inducing avian oncovirus. Virology(89): 162-178, 1978.

17. Pachl C, Beigalke B, Linial M: RNA and protein encoded by MH2 virus: Evidence for subgenomic expression of v-myc. J of Virology(45): 133-139, 1983.

18. Kan N, Flordellis C, Mark G, Duesberg P, Papas T: A common onc gene sequence transduced by avian carcinoma virus MH2 and by murine sarcoma virus 3611. Science(223): 813-816, 1984.

2

VIRAL AND CELLULAR *FOS* GENE

I. M. VERMA, T. CURRAN, A. D. MILLER, AND C. VAN BEVEREN

The Salk Institute, San Diego, California

A remarkable discovery of the past few years is the fact that many acutely oncogenic retroviruses contain sequences as an integral part of their genome which have homologs in normal cells (1). Acquisition of normal cellular sequences by retroviruses, usually at the expense of genes required for replication, enables them to induce neoplasias in vivo and transformation of a wide variety of cells in vitro (2). Such acquired cellular sequences have been termed as cellular protooncogenes or c-*onc* while their viral homologs are referred to as viral oncogenes or v-*onc*. To date nearly 20 unique v-*onc* genes have been identified which have cellular counterparts (3). Some c-*onc* genes have been identified by DNA transfection studies (4). The c-*onc* gene sequences are remarkably well conserved during evolution (5).

If all normal cells contain c-*onc* genes, why are most cells not tumor cells? Two general themes are commonly advanced to counter this conundrum. 1) *Quantitative modulation*: When the threshold levels of c-*onc* gene product in a normal cell undergoes quantitative changes (for instance, elevated levels), it has the potential to affect the cellular metabolic processes in a manner that leads to cellular transformation. Examples of this mechanism will include transformation by LTR-activated c-*mos* gene (6) and enhanced c-*myc* expression in ALV-induced chicken bursal tumors (7); 2) *Qualitative alterations*: The product of c-*onc* gene undergoes mutation with respect to normal c-*onc* gene product. For instance, a single bp changes in c-*ras* gene product makes it a transforming gene (8,9). We would like to propose that while qualitative and quantitative modes discussed alone may explain certain types of neoplasia, the majority of neoplastic growth can perhaps be best explained by a third model, which we refer to as an inappropriate expression model. Below we would furnish the example of the *fos* gene, which we have used as a model system.

FBJ murine osteosarcoma virus (FBJ-MuSV) was isolated from a spontaneous tumor and causes exclusively bone tumors (10). The candidate oncogene of FBJ-MuSV is termed *fos* which encodes a protein of 381 amino acids (11,12). The cellular counterpart of v-*fos* gene has been molecularly cloned from both mouse and human cells (13). The c-*fos* gene product encodes a protein of 380 amino acids (12). When compared to v-*fos* gene product, the first 332 amino acids are nearly identical but the remainder of 48 amino acids at the C-terminus are totally different (12). Despite these structural differences, both v-*fos* and c-*fos* proteins can transform fibroblasts and have a nuclear localization (14, 15). Below we will describe the molecular structure of the v-*fos* and c-*fos* genes, their transforming capabilities, the nature of their encoded proteins and expression in normal cells.

RESULTS

Molecular architecture of the fos gene. Figure 1 shows a diagrammatic sketch of v-*fos* and c-*fos* genes based on their complete nucleotide sequence. The salient features can be summarized as follows. 1)FBJ-MuSV proviral DNA contains 4,026 nucleotides which include two long terminal repeats (LTRs) of 617 nucleotides each, 1,639 nucleotides of acquired cellular sequences (v-*fos*) and a portion of the *env* gene (see Fig. 1). 2) Both the initiation and termination codons of the v-*fos* protein lie in the acquired sequences which encode a proteion of 381 amino acids, having a molecular weight of 41,601. 3) In cells transformed by FBJ-MuSV, a phosphoprotein of an apparent MW of 55 kDa (p55) on SDS-PAGE has been identified as the transforming protein (16). The discrepancy in size is likely due to the unusual amino acid composition of the *fos* protein (10% proline), since the v-*fos* protein expressed in bacteria has a similar estimated molecular weight (17). 4) The sequences in c-*fos* which are homologous to v-*fos* are interrupted by four regions of non- homology, three of which represent bonafide introns. 5) The 104 nucleotide long fourth region, which is present in both mouse and human c-*fos* genes, represents sequences which have been deleted during the biogenesis of the v-*fos* gene. The additional 104 nucleotides in the c-*fos* gene transcripts do not increase the predicted size of the c-*fos* protein because of a switch to a different reading frame. 6) The c-*fos* protein is 380 amino acids which is remarkably similar to the size of the

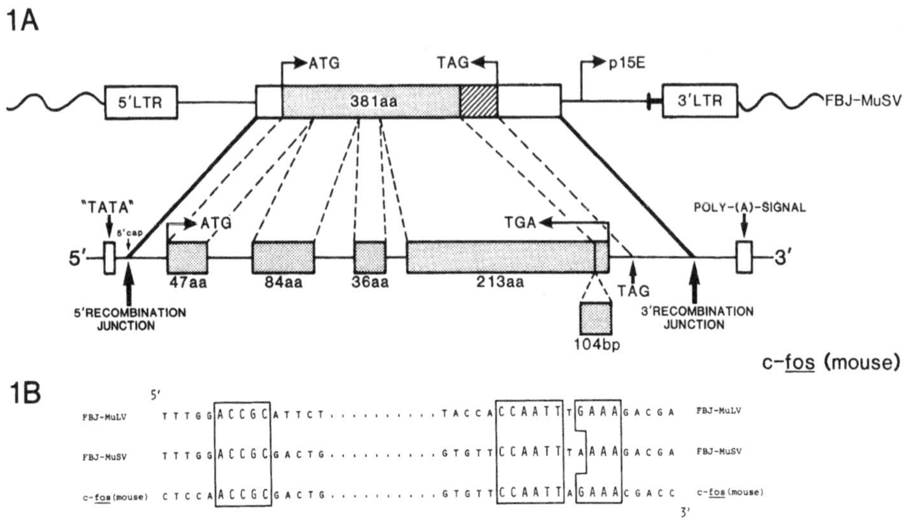

FIGURE 1. A) Molecular architecture of FBJ-MuSV proviral DNA and mouse c-*fos* gene. The organization of FBJ-MuSV is shown in the upper lane. The large open box indicates the acquired cellular sequences; the initiation and termination codons of v-*fos* proteins (solid bars) are indicated. The stippled region (░) indicates the C-terminal 49 amino acids of v-*fos* protein encoded in a different reading frame due to deletion of 104 bp of c-*fos* sequences. The 5' and 3' recombination junctions are indicated by a solid line. The position of p15E protein is indicated. The solid boxes in the c-*fos* gene are the exons and the number of amino acids encoded by each exon is given. The 104 bp sequence that has been deleted in the v-*fos* sequences is indicated with a triangle. Unlike the v-*fos* protein, the c-*fos* protein terminates at a TGA codon. The position of the TAG codon which acts as chain terminator of v-*fos* protein is shown by a thin arrow (↑). The position of the "TATA" box, 5'-cap, putative polyadenylation signal and recombination junctions (⬆) are indicated. B) Nucleotide sequences at the 5' and 3' junctions of FBJ-MuLV, FBJ-MuSV and mouse c-*fos* gene. Boxed areas indicate sequence homology.

v-fos protein (381 amino acids). 7) In the first 332 amino acids, the v-*fos* and mouse c-*fos* proteins differ only at 5 amino acids, while the remaining 48 amino acids of c-*fos* are encoded in a different reading frame in v-*fos*. Thus, the v-*fos* and c-*fos* proteins, though largely similar, have different C-termini (Fig. 1A). 8) The mouse and human c-*fos* genes share greater than 90% sequence homology, differing in only 24 residues out of a total of 380 amino acids (Fig. 2) (18).

FBJ-MuSV arose by recombination between the parental FBJ-MuLV and c-*fos* sequences. Nucleotide sequence analysis of the 5'- and 3'-junctions of v-*fos* substitution reveals that the putative parents of

```
                     10        20        30        40        50        60
                           *              :               *    *  *     :
v-fos        MMFSGFNADYEASSFRCSSASPAGDSLSYYHSPADSFSSMGSPVNTQDFCADLSVSSANF
c-fos(human) MMFSGFNADYEASSSRCSSASPAGDSLSYYHSPADSFSSMGSPVNAQDFCTDLAVSSANF
c-fos(mouse) MMFSGFNADYEASSSRCSSASPAGDSLSYYHSPADSFSSMGSPVNTQDFCADLSVSSANF
                                                          *    *  *

                     70        80        90       100       110       120
                   *            *         :     * * **     *  **   **   :
             IPTVTATSTSPDLQWLVQPTLVSSVAPSQTRAPHPYGLPTQSAGAYARAEMVKTVSGGRA
             IPTVTAISTSPDLQWLVQPALVSSVAPSQTRAPHPFGVPAPSAGAYSRAGVVKTMTGGRA
             IPTVTAISTSPDLQWLVQPTLVSSVAPSQTRAPHPYGLPTQSAGAYARAGMVKTVSGGRA
                                *               * * **     *   *   **

                    130       140       150       160       170       180
                                          :                         *     :
             QSIGRRGKVEQLSPEEEEKRRIRRERNKMAAAKCRNRRRELTDTLQAETDQLEDKKSALQ
             QSIGRRGKVEQLSPEEEEKRRIRRERNKMAAAKCRNRRRELTDTLQAETDQLEDEKSALQ
             QSIGRRGKVEQLSPEEEEKRRIRRERNKMAAAKCRNRRRELTDTLQAETDQLEDEKSALQ

                    190       200       210       220       230       240
                                          :                    **         :
             TEIANLLKEKEKLEFILAAHRPACKIPDDLGFPEEMSVASLDLTGGLPEASTPESEEAFT
             TEIANLLKEKEKLEFILAAHRPACKIPDDLGFPEEMSVASLDLTGGLPEVATPESEEAFT
             TEIANLLKEKEKLEFILAAHRPACKIPDDLGFPEEMSVASLDLTGGLPEASTPESEEAFT
                                                               **

                    250       260       270       280       290       300
                         *       **   *   :               *    **       :
             LPLLNDPEPKPSLEPVKSISNVELKAEPFDDFLFPASSRPSGSETSRSVPNVDLSGSFYA
             LPLLNDPEPKPSVEPVKSISSMELKTEPFDDFLFPASSRPSGSETARSVPDMDLSGSFYA
             LPLLNDPEPKPSLEPVKSISNVELKAEPFDDFLFPASSRPSGSETSRSVPDVDLSGSFYA
                         *       **   *                   *     *

                    310       320       330       340       350       360
                     *       *            :  ****************************
             ADWEPLHSNSLGMGPMVTELEPLCTPVVTCTPLLRLPELTHAAGPVSSQRRQGSRHPDVP
             ADWEPLHSGSLGMGPMATELEPLCTPVVTCTPSCTAYTSSFVFTYPEADSFPSCAAAHRK
             ADWEPLHSNSLGMGPMVTELEPLCTPVVTCTPGCTTYTSSFVFTYPEADSFPSCAAAHRK
                     *       *               *  *

                    370       380
             *************** ******
             LPELVHYREEKHVFPQRFPST
             GSSSNEPSSDSLSSPTLLAL
             GSSSNEPSSDSLSSPTLLAL
```

FIGURE 2. Comparison of c-*fos*(human), c-*fos*(mouse) and v-*fos* gene products. Amino acids are indicated by the single-letter code; those that differ between the c-*fos*(human) and v-*fos* genes are shown above the sequences, while those that differ between the c-*fos*(human) and c-*fos*(mouse) genes are shown below. The carboxyl-terminal 48 amino acids of the c-*fos*(human) and c-*fos*(mouse) gene products are totally different from those of the v-*fos* protein.

FBJ-MuSV share a 5' nucleotide sequence at the 5'-end and 10 out of 11 nucleotides at the 3'-end (Fig. 1B). Sequences involved in recombination at the 5'-end lie in the untranslated region of FBJ-MuLV and immediately downstream from the predicted 5'-end of c-*fos* mRNA. Recombination at the 3'-end involved the p15E region of the FBJ-MuLV *env* gene and the 3'-untranslated region of the c-*fos* gene. The 104 bp sequence in c-*fos*

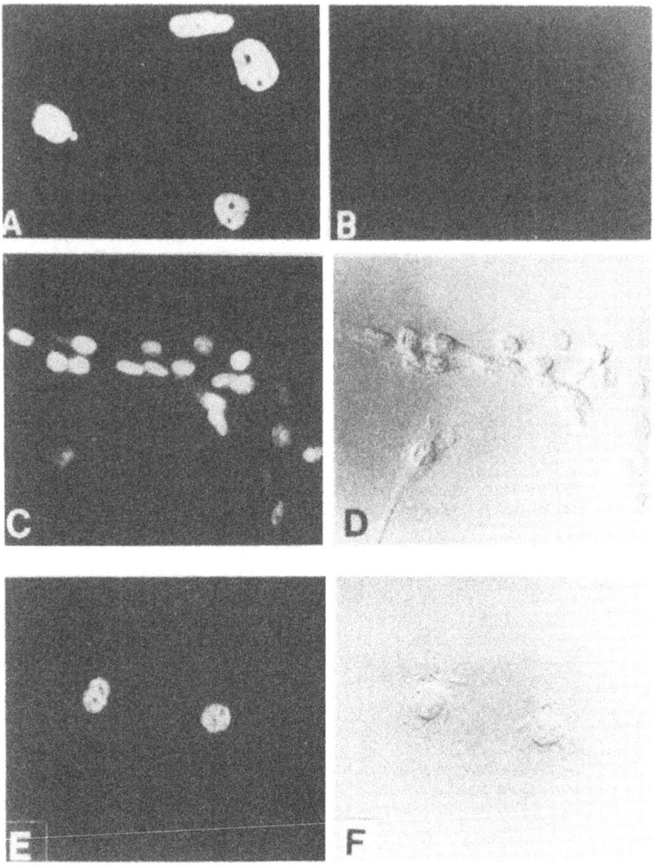

FIGURE 3. Indirect immunofluorescence labeling of *fos* proteins. Cells are grown on coverslips and processed for indirect immunofluorescence as described (15). The second antibody in each case was rhodamine-conjugated rabbit anti-rat IgG. A) CHO dhfr - cells transfected with pSV dhfr-*fos* and selected for resistance in 4 x 10^{-6} M methotrexate, stained with TBRS; B) same cells stained with normal rat serum; C) 208F rat cells transformed by the VMV construct (contains 83% of v-*fos* protein and the C-terminus of c-*fos* protein) stained with TBRS; D) the same field as in C but viewed under Nomarski optics; E) amnion cells stained with TBRS; and F) same field as in E viewed under Nomanski optics.

gene that has been deleted from the v-*fos* sequence is bounded by a 5 nucleotide inverted repeat which could be looped out in the formation of FBJ-MuSV.

v-fos and c-fos are nuclear proteins: Both the v-*fos* and c-*fos* proteins have been localized in the nucleus, both by immunofluorescence staining and immunoprecipitation with tumor bearing antisera (TBRS)(15).

Figure 3 shows the results of immunofluorescence labeling of CHO cells containing amplified v-*fos* gene product. Similar results were obtained when RS2 cells (rat nonproducer cells transformed by FBJ-MuSV) were stained with TBRS. The c-*fos* protein was localized in the nuclei of normal mouse amnion cells and in the nuclei of cells transformed by recombinant plasmid which expresses the c-*fos* gene product. However, $p55^{c\text{-}fos}$ undergoes more extensive post-translational modification in the nucleus than does $p55^{v\text{-}fos}$. Both the v-*fos* and c-*fos* proteins form a complex with p39 cellular protein. Immunofluorescence data indicate that the level of $p55^{c\text{-}fos}$ in normal mouse amnion cells is similar to that found in fibroblasts transformed by the v-*fos* or c-*fos* protein (15). Recently we have analyzed FBR-MuSV which also contains the *fos* oncogene (19,20). Nucleotide sequence analysis revealed that the FBR-MuSV genome encodes a *gag-fos* fusion protein as compared to the FBJ-MuSV encoded $p55^{v\text{-}fos}$ protein. Figure 4 shows the comparison of the *fos* proteins encoded by c-*fos* genes, FBJ-MuSV and FBR-MuSV. The FBR-MuSV *gag-fos* fusion protein retains only 236 amino acids of *fos*-derived sequences as compared to 381 amino acids of FBJ $p55^{v\text{-}fos}$ and 380 amino acids of c-*fos*. The FBR-*fos* lacks sequences encoding the first 24 and the last 98 amino acids of the c-*fos* gene product (20). Furthermore, the substituted region has undergone two in-frame deletions of 39 and 27 nucleotides (13 and 9 amino acids, respectively). The FBR-MuSV encoded $p75^{gag\text{-}fos}$ fusion protein is also localized in the nucleus and complexes with p39 cellular protein.

Transformation by v-fos and c-fos: The FBJ-MuSV proviral DNA induces *foci* in rat 208F cells (11). In comparison to many other oncogenes, FBJ-MuSV does not readily form *foci* in NIH/3T3 cells. The c-*fos* gene (mouse or human), on the other hand, is unable to induce foci in fibroblasts, even after linking of LTR sequences. Figure 5 shows the results obtained by a series of recombinants designed to delineate the region of the *fos* gene required to transform fibroblasts in vitro. Results can be summarized as follows: 1) Both v-*fos* and c-*fos* proteins are capable of inducing morphological transformation of fibroblasts. Thus the altered C-termini doesn't influence the ability to transform cells. This is not surprising since FBR-MuSV encoded $p75^{gag\text{-}fos}$ protein lacks 98 amino acids at the C-terminus. 2) To activate c-*fos* gene, two manipulations are required: a) addition of LTR sequences, presumably to

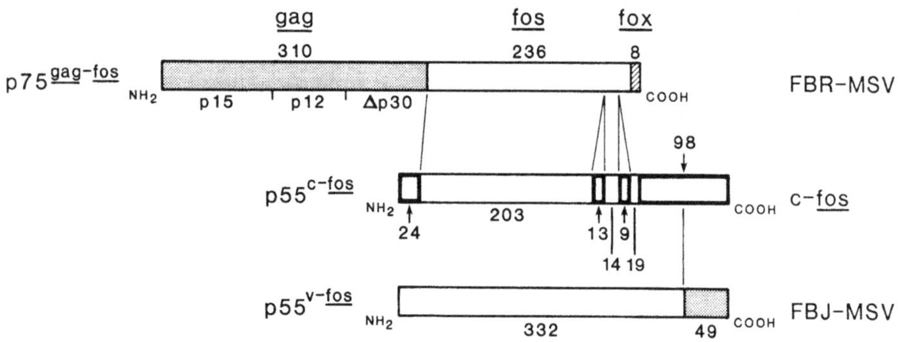

FIGURE 4. Comparison of *fos* proteins. A schematic comparison of p75*gag-fos*, p55c-*fos* and p55v-*fos* proteins is shown. In p75, the *gag*-encoded portion is indicated with a stippled box, and that encoded by v-*fos* is shown by the hatched box (for details see ref. 20). The region of p55c-*fos* indicated by thickened boxes and vertical arrows are those portions deleted in p75*gag-fos*. The hatched region in p55v-*fos* is the C-terminal portion which differs from that of p55c-*fos*. The numbers refer to the number of amino acids encoded by each region.

provide transcriptional enhancer elements, and b) disruption of 3' interacting sequences. This interaction most likely involves the 104 bp c-*fos* specific sequences. The mechanisms by which the 3'-interactions manifest their influence is not understood, but it appears to act at the level of translation since little or no *fos* protein is observed (14). In cells co-transfected with a selectable marker and a recombinant construct unable to induce transformation, the c-*fos* transcripts can be observed. Thus a novel mechanism, perhaps acting by influencing translation is the most likely explanation of the inability of c-*fos* genes to transform.

Expression of c-fos gene: The c-*fos* gene is expressed at the highest levels in extraembryonal tissue and more specifically in amnion cells (Fig. 6). Figure 6 shows the expression of c-*fos* in a variety of extraembryonal tissues. As shown in Figure 3, the c-*fos* protein can be

TRANSFORMING POTENTIAL OF c-fos GENE

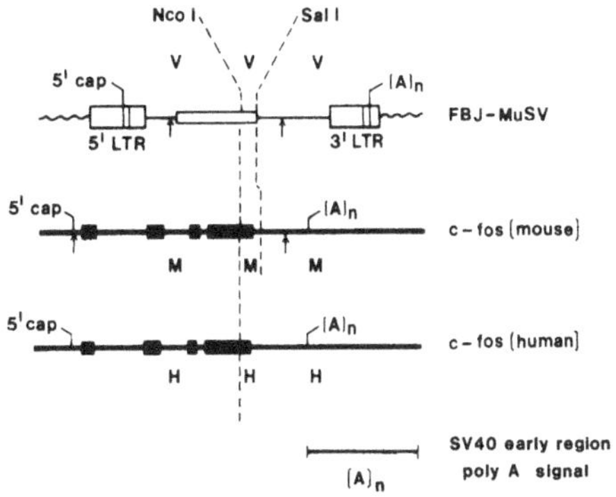

Clone	Transformation
V V V	+
M M M	−
M M V	+
M V V	+
V M V	+
M V M	−
V V M	+
V M M	−

Clone	Transformation
H H H	−
H V V	+
V H H	−
M M $(A)_n$	−
V M $(A)_n$	+

FIGURE 5. Transforming ability of v- and c-fos recombinants. The top line depicts the FBJ-MuSV provirus. The v-fos coding region is shown by an open box in the middle of the provirus. Rat DNA sequences surrounding the provirus are shown by wavy lines. The middle and lower lines depict the mouse and human c-fos genes respectively, with the c-fos coding regions shown by closed boxes. The coding regions of each of the c-fos genes are separated by 3 introns. The restriction endonucleases NcoI and SalI divide the v-fos and mouse c-fos genes into three regions, and the human c-fos gene into two regions, as shown. RNA 5' cap and polyadenylation signals are shown. The regions of these plasmids are described in "Experimental Procedures" of ref. 14. The arrows in the FBJ-MuSV provirus and in the c-fos gene indicate the positions of recombination between the mouse gene and the helper retrovirus which generated FBJ-MuSV. V = viral sequences; M = c-fos (mouse); H = c-fos (human) sequences, and $(A)_n$ is sequences containing putative polyadenylation sequences. Clones were tested for their transforming ability by transfection onto rat 208F cells as described (14). (+) indicates transformation efficiency of about 200 foci/μg DNA; (-) indicates transforming efficiency of <10 foci/μg of DNA.

identified in day 17 mouse amnion. Recently expression of c-fos gene has been observed in some bone marrow cells. It appears that c-fos may be expressed at high levels during induction of monocytes to macrophages. Growth factors, like PDGF, also induce expression of the fos gene.

DISCUSSION

FBJ-MuSV induces osteosarcomas in mice and transforms fibroblasts in vitro (10,11). The highest expression of c-fos gene is observed in normal amnion cells and perhaps some hematopoietic cells. We would like to propose that c-fos protein does not transform amnion cells because this cell type is either resistant to transformation by fos protein or it lacks targets with which fos protein interacts to induce transformation. The fibroblasts, on the other hand, are susceptible to transformation by

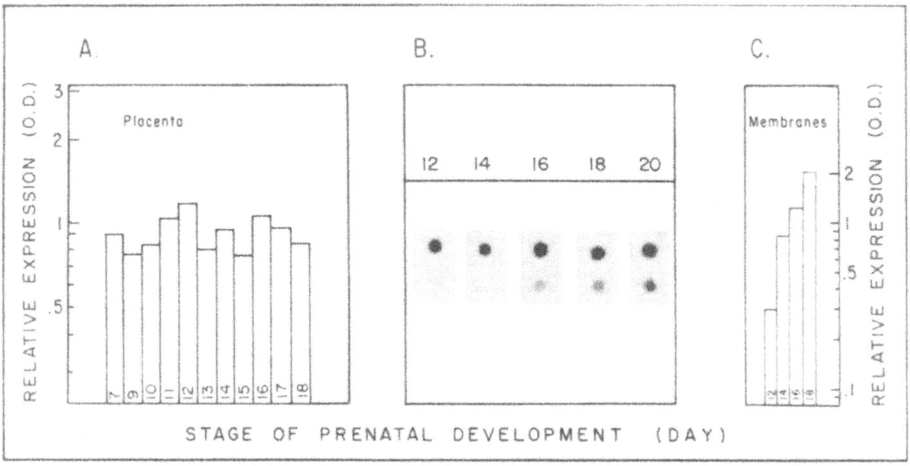

FIGURE 6. c-*fos* transcripts during mouse prenatal development. A) Placenta, day 7-18; B) outer (upper lane) and inner (lower lane) placenta; and C) extraembryonal membranes (including amnion and visceral yolk sac).

fos protein. No c-*fos* gene transcripts have been observed in fibroblasts. Thus fibroblasts constitute an inappropriate cell type for expression of the *fos* gene and consequently its gene product can cause transformation either directly or by interacting with other substrates present in the fibroblasts. Since the amount of c-*fos* protein in amnion cells appears to be equal to or higher than that in cells transformed by v-*fos* or c-*fos* gene constructs (Fig. 3), it is unlikely that quantitative changes influence the transforming ability of the c-*fos* gene. Since the v-*fos* and c-*fos* proteins have different C-termini, they are qualitatively different proteins, yet they both can induce transformation. Thus, transformation by *fos* genes is a consequence of expression in an inappropriate cell type rather than quantitative modulation or qualitative differences.

Induction of neoplasias by inappropriate expression may be a more frequent phenomenon than has previously been recognized. The *sis* oncogene product has been shown to be essentially identical to platelet-derived growth factor (PDGF) (21,22). Simian sarcoma virus (SSV) causes gliomas and fibrosarcomas, while the normal site of expression of PDGF is in megakaryocytes (23). This is perhaps an example of inappropriate expression of the *sis* gene in fibroblastic or glial cells. Another example of inappropriate expression is provided by the recent findings that the *erbB* oncogene is part of EGF receptor gene (24). Avian erythroblastosis virus (AEV), containing the *erbB* gene, causes erythroid leukemias, yet hematopoietic cells are normally devoid of EGF receptors. Thus, expression of *erbB* gene in myeloid cells, an inappropriate tissue for expression of EGF receptors, can lead to neoplastic transformation.

It seems that knowledge of the expression of cellular protooncogenes, in particular the identification of the cell type expressing a particular cell type, is crucial to understanding the mechanism of neoplastic transformation by oncogenes. Additionally, knowledge of the substrates with which oncogenic proteins interact is equally central to unlocking the mechanism involved in cancer.

ACKNOWLEDGMENTS

We thank C. Goller for help in the preparation of the manuscript. This work was supported by grants from the American Cancer Society and the National Institutes of Health. T. Curran is supported by a Damon Runyon-Walter Winchell Cancer Fund Fellowship (DRG 551). A. D. Miller is supported by a fellowship from the Leukemia Society of America.

REFERENCES

1. Bishop JM. Cellular oncogenes and retroviruses. Ann. Rev. Biochem. (52):301-354, 1983.
2. Bishop JM, Varmus HE. Functions and origins of retroviral transforming transforming genes. **In** Weiss R. (ed) Molecular Biology of Tumor Viruses (2nd ed). Cold Spring Harbor Laboratory, Cold Spring Harbor, New York, 1982, 999-1108.
3. Müller R, Verma IM. Expression of cellular oncogenes. Curr. Topics Microbiol. Immunol. (112):73-115, 1984.
4. Cooper GM. Cellular transforming genes. Science (218): 801-806, 1982.
5. Shilo BZ, Weinberg RA. DNA sequences homologous to vertebrate oncogenes are conserved in **Drosophila melanogaster**. Proc. Natl. Acad. Sci. USA (78):6789-6792, 1981.
6. Oskarsson M, McClements W, Blair DG, Maizel JV, Vande Woude GF. Properties of a normal mouse cell DNA sequence (sarc) homologous to the src sequence of Moloney sarcoma virus. Science (207):1222-1234, 1980.
7. Hayward WS, Neel BG, Astrin SM. Activation of a cellular onc gene by promoter insertion in ALV-induced lymphoid leukosis. Nature (290):475-480, 1981.
8. Tabin CJ, Bradley SM, Bargmann I, Weinberg RA, Papageorge, AG, Scolnick EM, Dhar R, Lowy DR, Chang EH. Mechanism of activation of a human oncogene. Nature (300):143-149, 1982.

9. Reddy EP, Reynolds RK, Santos E, Barbacid M. A point mutation is responsible for the acquisition of transforming properties by the T24 human bladder carcinoma oncogene. Nature (300):149-152, 1982.
10. Finkel MP, Biskis BO, Jinkins PB. Virus induction of osteosarcomas in mice. Science (151):698-701, 1966.
11. Curran T, Peters G, Van Beveren C, Teich NM, Verma IM. The FBJ murine osteosarcoma virus: identification and molecular cloning of biologically active proviral DNA. J. Virol. (44):674-682, 1982.
12. Van Beveren C, van Straaten F, Curran T, Müller R, Verma IM Nucleotide sequence analysis of FBJ-MuSV provirus and c-fos(mouse) gene reveals that viral and cellular fos gene products have different carboxy termini. Cell (32):1241-1255, 1983.
13. Curran T, MacConnell WP, van Straaten F, Verma IM. Structure of the FBJ murine osteosarcoma virus genome: Molecular cloning of its associated helper virus and the cellular homolog of the v-fos gene from mouse and human cells. Mol. Cell. Biol. (3):259-268, 1983.
14. Miller AD, Curran T, Verma IM. C-fos protein can induce cellular transformation: a novel mechanism of activation of a cellular oncogene. Cell (36):51-60, 1984.
15. Curran T, Miller AD, Zokas LM, Verma IM. Viral and cellular fos gene products are located in the nucleus. Cell (36):259-268, 1984.
16. Curran T, Teich NM. Candidate product of the FBJ murine osteosarcoma virus oncogene: characterization of a 55,000 dalton phosphoprotein. J. Virol. (42):114-122, 1982.
17. MacConnell WP, Verma IM. Expression of FBJ-MSV oncogene (fos) product in bacteria. Virology (131):367-374, 1984.
18. Van Straaten F, Müller R, Curran T, Van Beveren C, Verma IM. Nucleotide sequence of a human c-onc gene: deduced amino acid sequence of human c-fos protein. Proc. Natl. Acad. Sci. USA (80):3183-3187, 1983.
19. Curran T, Verma IM. FBR murine osteosarcoma virus. I. Molecular analysis and characterization of a 75,000 Da gag-fos fusion product. Virology (135):218-228, 1984.
20. Van Beveren C, Enami S, Curran T, Verma IM. FBR murine osteosarcoma virus. II. Nucleotide sequence of the provirus reveals that the genome contains sequences acquired from two cellular genes. Virology (135):229-243, 1984.
21. Waterfield MD, Scrace GT, Whittle N, Stroobant P, Johnsson A, Wasteson A, Westermark B, Heldin C-H, Huang JS, Dual TF. Platelet-derived growth factor is structurally related to the putative transforming protein $p28^{sis}$ of simian sarcoma virus. Nature (304):35-39, 1983.
22. Doolittle RF, Hunkapiller MW, Hood LE, Devare SG, Robbins KC, Aaronson SA, Antoniades HN. Simian sarcoma virus onc gene, v-sis, is derived from gene (or genes) encoding a platelet-derived growth factor. Science (221):275-277, 1983.
23. Devare SG, Reddy EP, Law JD, Robbins KC, Aaronson SA. Nucleotide sequence of simian sarcoma virus genome: demonstration that its acquired cellular sequences encode the transforming gene product of $p28^{sis}$. Proc. Natl. Acad. Sci. USA (80):731-735, 1983.
24. Downward J, Yarden Y, Mayes E, Scrace G, Totty N, Stockwell P, Ullrich A, Schlessinger J, Waterfield MD. Close similarity of epidermal growth factor and v-erb-B oncogene protein sequences, Nature (307)521-527, 1984.

3

P21 *ras* TRANSFORMING PROTEIN: SIGNIFICANCE OF THE CARBOXY TERMINUS

Berthe M. WILLUMSEN[1,2] and Douglas R. LOWY[3]

[1]Fibiger Institute, Copenhagen, Denmark. [2]Present address: University of Copenhagen, Microbiology Institute, Copenhagen, Denmark. [3]Laboratory of Cellular Oncology, National Cancer Institute, Bethesda, Maryland

INTRODUCTION

The p21 *ras* genes form a multigene family that is conserved in evolution (reviewed in ref. 1). These genes were first detected and studied in two rodent-derived acute transforming retroviruses, Harvey (Ha) and Kirsten (Ki) murine sarcoma viruses (MuSV); both viruses are highly oncogenic in vivo and induce tumorigenic transformation of established cell lines in vitro. As is true for other acute transforming retroviruses, the transforming capacity of each virus resides in its viral oncogene (v-*onc*). The v-*onc* of Ha-MuSV and Ki-MuSV is a v-*ras* gene that was transduced from a cellular (c) *ras* gene. The 21 kd *ras* encoded proteins of both viruses share antigenic determinants. However, under stringent hybridization conditions, the *ras* sequences of Ha-MuSV and Ki-MuSV base pair with different restriction endonuclease fragments of genomic DNA from a given animal species, indicating that different c-*ras* genes gave rise to Ha-MuSV and Ki-MuSV v-*ras* genes. Molecular cloning and DNA sequencing of v-*ras* and c-*ras* genes have directly confirmed this conclusion (2-9). The mammalian genome contains at least three biologically active *ras* genes: c-ras^H (similar to Ha-MuSV *ras*), c-*ras*^{K} (similar to Ki-MuSV *ras*), and c-*ras*^{N} (first detected in a human *n*euroblastoma cell line). Versions of these three genes are apparently present in all vertebrate species. ras genes have also been detected in invertebrate eukaryotes, including yeast, which contain two genes that are closely related to the mammalian ras genes (10,11).

Altered forms of all three mammalian c-ras genes have been detected in human and animal tumors by virtue of the capacity of these activated ras genes to induce tumorigenic transformation of NIH 3T3 mouse cells (reviewed in ref. 12); the normal versions (proto-oncogenes) of these genes do not induce such transformation, unless their transcriptional activity is markedly enhanced (1,13). The observation that cellular transforming genes (tumor oncogenes) found in a wide variety of tumors are activated c-ras genes has added to interest in the biology of this gene family.

All mammalian ras genes encode closely related proteins that are approximately 21 kd (p21). DNA sequence analysis indicates that the ras genes have maintained a remarkable degree of evolutionary conservation in their amino acid sequence (3-9). Each mammalian ras gene encodes a 188 or 189 amino acid product; the rodent and human ras^H genes encode identical 189 amino acid p21 protein. The two yeast genes are larger (309 and 322 amino acids), but their larger size is localized principally to sequences in one region near the C-terminus (10, 11). The N-terminal 165 amino acids of the three human ras genes share about 90% homology with each other; the yeast and mammalian ras genes share more than 80% homology over this region. By contrast, there is only about 20% homology among the 24 amino acids located at the C-terminus of the mammalian genes. Similar heterogeneity has been noted in this region among the yeast genes; the much longer length of this region in the yeast proteins accounts for most of the difference in the size between the mammalian and yeast proteins (14). Compared with their normal versions, the activated c-ras genes contain single point mutations either in glycine-12 or glutamine-61, each leading to an amino acid substitution (12). Each v-ras gene contains at least two point mutations: for example, the v-ras^{H} gene of Ha-MuSV is mutated at amino acids 12 and 59.

The normal function of ras genes and the reason for their multiplicity remains unknown. Yeast cells from which either of the two ras genes have been disrupted remain viable; however, haploid spores with disruptions of both genes fail to grow (15). The only known biochemical activity common to all p21 proteins is their capacity to non-covalently bind guanine nucleotides (16,17). An additonal property of the p21 proteins encoded by Ha-MuSV and Ki-MuSV is that they can be autophosphorylated in vitro by guanine nucleotides at threonine-59 (18). A significant proportion of the viral p21 protein is also phosphorylated in vivo on the same threonine residue, leading to a p21 doublet in immunoprecipitates of the viral p21. The c-ras genes are not phosphorylated significantly, since they encode the normal alanine at amino acid 59.

The primary translation product of each ras gene undergoes at least three post-translational modifications, which may be interrelated. The protein is initially made on cytosol-associated associated free ribosomes (19). This precursor (pro p21) is processed to a form which has a slightly faster mobility in SDS-polyacrylamide gels. This processing event is associated with the tight binding of lipid to the protein (20) and its migration to the inner face of the plasma membrane (21). The amino acid(s) to which the lipid is bound has not been determined, nor is it known what post-translational changes in the protein account for its altered migration rate in gels; lipid binding and/or peptide cleavage might each play a role. Formic acid and V8 protease digestion studies have suggested that the change in migration rate is not due to alterations at the N-terminus of the protein (19).

The possible relevance of these various biochemical features of p21 to its biological activity has not yet been established, although such data would clearly help to elucidate functional aspects of the protein. With this goal in mind, we and our colleagues have begun to study defined mutants of the Ha-MuSV v-*ras*^{H} gene (22,23). The initial mutants we have studied contain various lesions in sequences encoding amino acids located at or near the C-terminus of the protein. Our results indicate cysteine-186 (located four amino acids from the C-terminus) is absolutely required for the gene to transform NIH 3T3 cells. The transforming activity of the mutants correlates with the capacity of their p21 proteins to undergo processing, bind lipid, and migrate to the membrane.

MATERIALS AND METHODS

Cells and DNA mediated gene transfer. The NIH 3T3 cells, tk$^-$ NIH 3T3 cells, and DNA transfection procedure have been previously described (22). The tk$^-$ cells were maintained on 100 ug/ml BrdUrd until used. Plasmid DNA in tk$^-$ cells were selected in HAT medium.

DNA clones. DNA mutants were constructed as previously described (22,23). Briefly, the starting clone (pBW276) is a DNA that contains the Ha-MuSV transforming region (the viral regulatory element [the long terminal repeat] and v-*ras*), the Herpes simplex virus thymidine kinase (tk) gene as a selectable marker for NIH 3T3 tk$^-$ cells, the TN5 neo^R gene for prokaryotic selection, and a prokaryotic origin of replication (from pBR322). Three classes of p21 mutants were constructed: premature chain termination mutants by introduction of an in frame TGA stop codon via insertion of a BclI linker (CTGATCAG) upstream from the authentic p21 stop codon; in frame deletion mutants (containing a restriction endonuclease linker inserted at the site of the deletion, leading to an insertion of three new amino acids in each mutant p21 at the site of the deletion); and two point mutants generated by site-directed mutagenesis, substituting Ser-186 and Thr-187 for Cys-186 and Val-187, respectively.

RESULTS

Premature termination mutants. We first studied the transforming activity of the p21 premature termination mutants (Table)(22). The mutants, which had lost only the 3-5 amino acids located at the C-terminus, encoded wild type amino acids except for the extreme C-terminus. Each mutant also encoded an additional one-three amino acids at its C-terminus because of the method used to introduce the premature stop codon. When tested in the NIH 3T3 transformation assay, none of the premature termination mutants tested could transform the cells. These negative data suggested that amino acids located at the C-terminus were required for transformation, although the introduction of the one or two new C-terminal amino acids might also have been responsible for the transformation-defective phenotype of the mutants. As a positive control, a mutant (pBW601) encoding the wild type p21, but from which the bases located immediately downstream from the nucleotide following the wild type p21 stop codon had been deleted, retained its transforming activity. These results indicated as expected that the sequences located immediately downstream from the p21 coding sequences were not required for transformation.

Deletion mutants. We also examined several in frame deletion mutants whose mutations involved amino acids upstream from the extreme C-terminus (Table). Each of these mutants encoded wild type amino acids upstream and downstream from the site of the deletion, as well as three new amino acids at the deletion as a result of the technique used to generate the mutants. When the capacity of these mutants to transform the NIH 3T3 cells was tested, the mutants fell into two phenotypes: those from which amino acids 166-179 were deleted were transformation-competent (they induced foci as efficiently as the wild type gene), while those which retained only amino acids 187-189 at the C-terminus were transformation-defective. Thus a stretch of amino acids

Table. Focus formation by p21 deletion mutants.

Clone No.	aa 160 Carboxy End of P21 aa 189	Focus Formation
Wild type controls:		
pBW 276	VREIRQHKLRKLNPPDESGPGCMSCKCVLSter	YES
pBW 601	------------------------------ter	YES
Premature termination mutants:		
pBW 769	--------------------------LISter	NO
pBW 277	---------------------------TPter	NO
pBW 603	-------------------------Pter	NO
Internal deletion mutants:		
pBW 672	------ PDQ ------------------ter	YES
pBW 739	------ PDQ ----------ter	YES
pBW 754	------ PDQ ---ter	NO
pBW 757	------------- PDQ ----------ter	YES
pBW 756	------------- PDQ ---ter	NO
pBW 755	--------------------- PDQ ---ter	NO

Table legend: Amino acids 160-189 for p21 are given for the starting clone (276); ter = termination codon. In the mutants, the symbol (-) means that this amino acid is the same as in the starting clone; a blank space means the amino acid is deleted; the letters indicate new amino acids introduced in construction of the mutant. Foci were counted at two weeks. All clones that gave rise to foci yielded $10^{2.8}$-$10^{3.4}$ foci per ug DNA (data from ref. 22).

located upstream from the extreme C-terminus was not required for transformation. In agreement with the data obtained from the premature termination mutants, the results also suggested that amino acids at the extreme C-terminus were required for transformation.

Mutant p21 proteins. We then characterized the p21 proteins encoded by the different classes of mutants.(22) The mutants contained a linked tk gene that could be used as a selectable phenotypic marker in tk^- cells independently of the transforming activity of the DNA; selection by this technique permitted analysis of tranformation-defective p21. When cells containing the DNAs were metabolically labeled with ^{35}S-methionine and extracts were immunoprecipitated with anti-p21 monoclonal antibody, (24)a p21 doublet whose migration rate differed from that of wild type p21 was detected for each mutant (data not shown). These preliminary results ruled out the possibility that the transformation-defective mutants either did not express p21 protein (through a possible cloning artefact) or encoded an unstable p21.

We also sought to determine if the p21 proteins by the mutants bound lipid similarly to the wild type protein. Although the p21 encoded by the transformation-competent mutants did label when cells with these mutants were grown in the presence of ^3H-palmitic acid, the p21 encoded by the premature termination or deletion mutants that were transformation-defective did not label with ^3H-palmitic acid (Fig.1). Since the lipid has previously been present on the forms of p21 located on the membrane, but not on the cytosol associated wild type pro p21, these results suggested that the p21 synthesized by the transformation-defective mutants might not be found on the plasma membrane.

This possilbility was tested by metabolically labeling cells with ^{35}S-methionine, fractionating the the cell homogenates into a supernatant-cytosol fraction and a membrane-

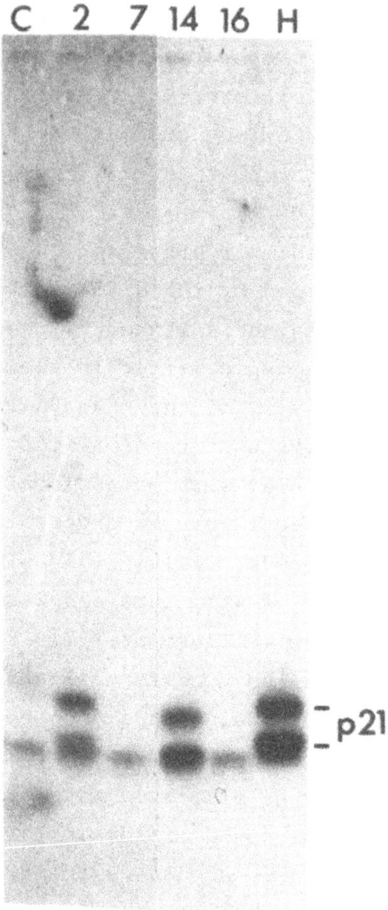

FIGURE 1. Lipid binding of mutant p21 proteins. Mass cultures of cells converted to tk^+ by the mutant DNAs were metabolically labeled overnight in growth medium containing ^3H-palmitic acid (20). Extracts of whole cells were prepared and precipitated with p21 monoclonal antibody Y13-259 (24). Immunoprecipitates were analyzed by electrophoresis in 15% SDS-polyacrylamide gels and bands were visualized by autoradiography for 7 days. Lane C = control cells; 2, 14, H = transformation-competent DNAs pBW601, pBW757, and Ha-MuSV wild type, respectively; 7, 16 = transformation-defective DNAs pBW603 and 755, respectively. The band that migrates just ahead of the non-phosphorylated form of viral p21 and is visualized in all lanes, including that containing the control cell precipitates, represents an endogenous form of p21 (data from ref. 22).

pellet fraction, and subjecting each fraction to p21 immunoprecipitation (Fig. 2). As expected, more than 90% of the mature wild type p21 forms were were found in the pellet fraction. Similar results were also obtained with transformation-competent mutants. However, p21 encoded by the premature termination and deletion mutants that were transformation-defective were found exclusively in the cytosol fraction.

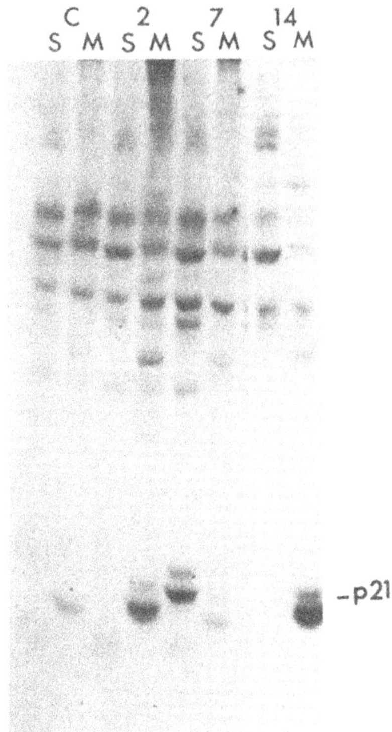

FIGURE 2. Fractionation of mutant p21 proteins. DNAs were metabolically labeled with methionine. Hypotonic swelling of the cells was followed by homogenization and low speed centrifugation to remove nuclei. The supernatant was fractionated by centrifugation at 100,000 x g min into a pellet particulate fraction containing the plasma membranes and a supernatant cytosol fraction as described (29). Fractions were precipitated with monoclonal p21 antibody YA6-172 (24) and analyzed as in Fig. 1. The lanes labeled S and M contain precipitates from the supernatant and membrane fractions, respectively. The number above each pair of lanes refers to the same DNA clone as in Fig. 1 (data from ref. 22).

Therefore the transformation-defective mutant p21 does not migrate to the plasma membrane.

Ser-186 point mutant. When the predicted C-terminal amino acids of the various ras genes are examined, a cysteine (amino acid 186 for ras^H) located four amino acids from the C-terminus is the only amino acid common to each gene (3-9). This cysteine is then followed in each gene by two hydrophobic amino acids (leucine, isoleucine, or valine). Given the demonstrated importance of the C-terminus for the transforming activity of the protein, its lipid binding, and membrane localization, conservation of this cysteine suggested that it might be required for mediating these functions. Clone pBW769, which may be viewed as a mutant from which Cys-186 has been deleted, also suggests that this cysteine might be essential. The presence of the two downstream hydrophobic amino acids suggested that this hydrophobic domain might also be required; results obtained with premature termination mutant pBW277 were consistant with this possibility.

The possible importance of Cys-186 and Val-187 was tested by generating two point mutants: one encoded Ser-186, the other Thr-187 (23). These amino acid substitutions were chosen because they introduce relatively minor changes in the side chain of the substituted amino acid. The Thr-187 mutant was transformation-competent, while the Ser-186 mutant was transformation-defective. When the p21 proteins encoded by these two mutants were analyzed (Fig. 3), they were phenotypically similar to the previously studied C-terminus mutants. The Ser-186 mutant p21 failed to bind lipid and wes found exclusively in the cytosol, while the Thr-187 protein bound lipid and was localized to the membrane (23). These results indicate an important role for Cys-186. The biologically active Thr-187 mutant demonstrates that the requiremwent for a hydrophobic domain in amino acids 187 and 188 is not absolute.

DISCUSSION

These studies have identified a crucial role for the C-terminus of p21 (22,23). Three different classes of mutants

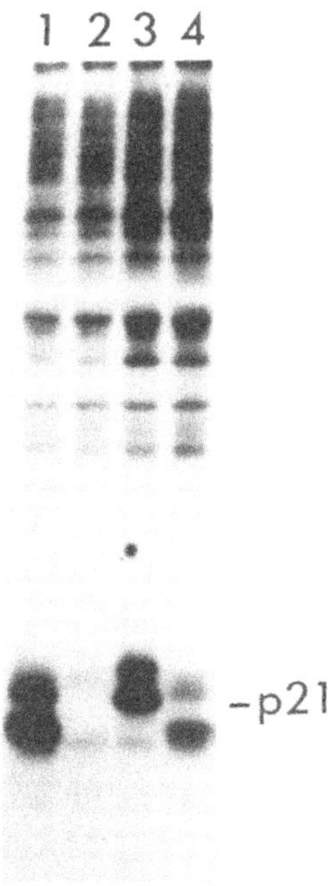

FIGURE 3. Immunoprecipitation of methionine labeled v-*ras*^{H} Ser-186 point mutant. Cultures were metabolically labeled for for 24 hours. Immunoprecipitation with p21 monoclonal antibody and gel electrophoresis were as for Fig. 2. Lanes 1 and 4 = wild type Ha-MuSV DNA; 2 = control cells; 3 = Ser-186 mutant (data from ref. 23).

with lesions exclusively in this region of the protein have been characterized: premature chain termination, in frame deletion, and point mutants. At least one member of each mutant class was unable to transform NIH 3T3 cells. The p21 encoded by each transformation-defective mutant displayed a similar phenotype: each failed to bind lipid and remained in the cytosol. This was true even for the transformation-defective Ser-186 mutant, which encodes a primary translation product that differs from the Cys-186 wild type gene only by specifying an oxygen atom in serine instead of the sulfur atom of cysteine. We have also found that the p21 encoded by these transformation-defective mutants does not undergo the post-translational processing that increases the electrophoretic migration rate of the mature p21 (23). Note here, for example, that the p21 encoded by the transformation-defective Ser-186 mutant migrated significantly more slowly than the wild type protein (Fig. 3), although both genes encode a 189 amino acid translation product. These results link the processing step to the lipid binding and membrane localization of the protein.

The data obtained with the deletion mutants also indicate that deletion of some amino acids located upstream from the extreme C-terminus do not affect the transforming activity of the viral DNA. The observation that p21 encoded by these sequences undergo post-translational processing, bind lipid, and localize to the membrane further strengthens the conclusion that these functions are important to the transforming activity of the virus. We infer that the the C-terminus enables p21 to carry out these functions. Since C-terminal mutants that cannot perform these functions also fail to transform NIH 3T3 cells, our results suggest that these post-translational alterations are required for the biological activity of the protein.

Although guanine nucleotide binding has not been measured directly for the mutants, the p21 encoded by even the transformation-defective mutants is phosphorylated in vivo similarly to wild type p21. Since phosphorylation of p21 is mediated by guanosine nucleotides in vitro (25), we infer that the nucleotide binding domain(s) of the protein is not affected by the C-terminal mutations. This observation is consistent with the hypothesis that the nucleotide binding region of p21 is located toward the N-terminus, while the C-terminus functions principally to enable the pro p21 to migrate from the cytosol to its biologically active location in the membrane.

Our experiments have been confined to the v-*ras*^{H} encoded protein, but the data are also relevant to c-*ras* genes. It has been experimentally determined that the normal and activated forms of the c-*ras* proteins undergo post-translational processing and membrane localization similar to that observed for the viral protein (17,26). Furthermore, the C-terminal amino acids encoded by the human and rodent c-*ras*^{H} genes are identical to those of the viral gene. The finding that the protein encoded by the transformation-defective Ser-186 mutant is phenotypically similar to p21 encoded by the other transformation-defective mutants implies that this residue helps to mediate these post-translational functions. The conservation of this cysteine in each *ras* gene stronly suggests that this region subserves a similar function in these genes.

These results cannot by themselves explain how the conserved Cys-186 at the C-terminus helps to mediate these post-translational functions. Cysteine residues usually create a specific conformation via disulfide linkage to another cysteine residue. Although Cys-186 may function in this manner, no other cysteine residues are conserved in all *ras* genes (3-9). Alternatively, the lipid may be linked to the sulfur of Cys-186. This could occur via a direct esther linkage, as proposed by Bolanowski et al. from their palmitic acid labeling studies of sea urchin lipoproteins (27), or via a thio-ether linkage to diacylglycerol, as has been found previously for the membrane associated murein lipoprotein of *E. coli* (28).

REFERENCES

1. Ellis RW, Lowy DR, Scolnick EM: The viral and cellular *ras* gene family. *In* Klein G (ed) Oncogene Studies, Advances in Viral Oncology (Vol. 1), Raven Press, New York, 1982, pp 107-126.

2. Chang EH, Gonda MA, Ellis RW, Scolnick EM, Lowy DR: Human genome contains four genes homologous to transforming genes of Harvey and Kirsten murine sarcoma viruses. Proc Natl Acad Sci USA (79): 4848-4852, 1982.

3. Dhar R, Ellis RW, Shih TY, Oroszlan S, Shapiro B, Maizel J, Lowy D, Scolnick EM: Nucleotide sequence of the p21 transforming protein of Harvey murine sarcoma virus. Science (217): 934-937, 1982.

4. Tsuchida N, Ryder T, Ohtsubo E: Nucleotide sequence of the oncogene encoding the p21 transforming protein of Kirsten murine sarcoma virus. Science (217): 937-938, 1982.

5. Capon DJ, Chen EY, Levinson AD, Seeburg PH, Goeddel DV: Complete nucleotide sequences of the T24 human bladder carcinoma oncogene and its normal homologue. Nature (302): 33-37, 1983.

6. Reddy EP: Nucleotide sequence analysis of the T24 human bladder carcinoma oncogene. Science (220): 1061-1063, 1983.

7. McGrath JP, Capon DJ, Smith DH, Chen EY, Seeburg PH, Goeddel DV, Levinson AD: Structure and organization of the human Ki-*ras* proto-oncogene and a related processed pseudogene. Nature (304): 501-506, 1983.

8. Shimizu K, Birnbaum D, Ruley MA, Fasano O, Suard Y, Edlund L, Taparowsky E, Goldfarb M, Wigler M: Structure of the Ki-*ras* gene of the human lung carcinoma cell line Calu-1. Nature (304): 497-500, 1983.

9. Taparowsky E, Shimizu K, Goldfarb M, Wigler M: Structure and activation of the human N-*ras* gene. Cell (34): 581-586, 1983.

10. Dhar R, Nieto A, Koller R, DeFeo-Jones D, Scolnick EM: Nucleotide sequence of two *ras*^{H} related-genes isolated from the yeast *Saccharomyces cerevisiae*. Nucleic Acids Res (12): 3611-3618, 1984.

11. Powers S, Kateoka T, Fasaro O, Goldfarb M, Strathern J, Broach J, Wigler M: Genes in S. cerevisiae encoding proteins with domains homologous to the mammalian *ras* proteins. Cell (36): 607-612, 1984.

12. Land H, Parada LF, Weinberg RA: Cellular oncogenes and multistep carcinogenesis. Science (222): 771-778, 1983.

13. Chang EH, Furth ME, Scolnick EM, Lowy DR: Tumorigenic transformation of mammalian cells induced by a normal human gene homologous to the oncogene of Harvey murine sarcoma virus. Nature (297): 479-483, 1982.

14. Papageorge AG, Defeo-Jones D, Robinson P, Temeles G, Scolnick EM: *Saccharomyces cerevisiae* synthesizes proteins related to the p21 gene product of *ras* genes found in mannals. Mol Cell Biol (4): 23-29, 1984.

15. Tatchell K, Chaleff DT, DeFeo-Jones D, Scolnick EM: Requirement of either of a pair of *ras*-related genes of *Saccharomyces cerevisiae* for spore viability. Nature (309): 523-527, 1984.

16. Scolnick EM, Papageorge AG, Shih TY: Guanine nucleotide-binding activity as an assay for src protein of rat-derived murine sarcoma viruses. Proc Natl Acad Sci USA (76): 5355-5359, 1979.

17. Papageorge A, Lowy DR, Scolnick EM: Comparative biochemical properties of p21 ras molecules coded for by viral and cellular ras genes. J Virol (44): 509-519, 1982.

18. Shih TY, Stokes PE, Smythers GW, Dhar R, Oroszlan S: Characterization of the phosphorylation sites and the surrounding amino acid sequences of the p21 transforming proteins coded for by the Harvey and Kirsten strains of murine sarcoma viruses. J Biol Chem (257): 11767-11773, 1982.

19. Shih TY, Weeks MO, Gruss P, Dhar R, Oroszlan S, Scolnick EM: Identification of a precursor in the biosynthesis of the p21 transforming protein of Harvey murine sarcoma virus. J Virol (42): 253-261, 1982.

20. Sefton BM, Trowbridge IS, Cooper JA, Scolnick EM: The transforming proteins of Rous sarcoma virus, Harvey sarcoma virus and Abelson virus contain tightly bound lipid. Cell (31): 465-474, 1982.

21. Willingham MC, Pastan I, Shih TY, Scolnick EM: Localization of the src gene product of the Harvey strain of MSV to plasma membrane of transformed cells by eletron microscopic immunocytochemistry. Cell (19): 1005-1014, 1980.

22. Willumsen BM, Christensen A, Hubbert NL, Papageorge AG, Lowy DR: The p21 ras C-terminus is required for transformation and membrane association. Nature (1984) in press.

23. Willumsen BM, Norris A, Papageorge AG, Hubbert NL, Lowy DR: Harvey murine sarcoma virus p21 ras protein: biological and biochemical significance of the cysteine nearest the carboxy terminus. Manuscript submitted.

24. Furth ME, Davis LJ, Fleurdelys B, Scolnick EM: Monoclonal antibodies to the p21 products of the transforming gene of Harvey murine sarcoma virus and of the cellular ras gene family. J Virol (43): 294-304, 1982.

25. Gibbs JB, Ellis RW, Scolnick EM: Autophosphorylation of a v-Ha-ras p21 is modulated by amino acid residue 12. Proc Natl Acad Sci USA (81): 2674-2678, 1984.

26. Finkel T, Channing JDer, Cooper GM: Activation of ras genes in human tumors does not affect localization, modification, or nucleotide binding properties of p21. Cell (37): 151-158, 1984.

27. Bolanowski MA, Earles BJ, Lennarz WJ: Fatty acylation of proteins during development of sea urchin embryos. J Biol Chem (259): 4934-4940, 1984.

28. Hantke K, Braun V: Covalent binding of lipid to protein: diglyceride and amide-linked fatty acid at the N-terminal end of the murein-lipoprotein of the *Escherichia coli* out membrane. Eur J Biochem (34): 284-296, 1973.

29. Courtneidge SA, Levinson AD, Bishop JM: The protein encoded by the transforming gene of avian sarcoma virus ($pp60^{src}$) and a homologous protein in normal cells ($pp60^{proto\text{-}src}$) are associated with the plasma membrane. Proc Natl Acad Sci USA (77): 3783-3787, 1980.

4

PROTEIN PHOSPHORYLATION AT TYROSINE IN NORMAL AND TRANSFORMED CELLS

JONATHAN A. COOPER, KATHY GOULD AND TONY HUNTER

The Salk Institute, San Diego, California

Retroviruses incorporating each of the oncogenes v-*src*, v-*fps* (a chicken gene whose mammalian homologue is v-*fes*), v-*abl*, v-*yes* or v-*fgr* (apparently the *yes* gene with added actin sequences) share the ability to increase the content of phosphotyrosine in the proteins of cells they transform (reviewed [1,2]). The transforming proteins encoded by these five genes are active tyrosine protein kinases *in vitro*, so it is assumed that much of the increase in tyrosine phosphorylation observed in the transformed cells is catalyzed directly by the retroviral transforming proteins, although it is possible that additional, cellular, tyrosine protein kinases are activated. However, tyrosine protein kinase activation is not a universal correlate of transformation. Cells transformed by chemicals, some tumor oncogenes, DNA tumor viruses, and many retroviruses have "normal" low levels of phosphotyrosine in their proteins (3). Even some retroviruses whose oncogenes have considerable sequence homology to the v-*src*-family of oncogenes do not increase cellular protein phosphotyrosine content detectably. Notable among these are the viruses that contain v-*mil* (a chicken gene whose mammalian homologue is v-*raf*), v-*ros*, v-*fms*, and v-*mos* (4-9). Paradoxically, the v-*ros* product is an active tyrosine protein kinase when isolated by immunoprecipitation yet cells transformed by UR2 virus, which encodes a *gag*-*ros* fusion protein, have only slightly enhanced levels of phosphotyrosine (9; Sefton BM, personal communication). One of the v-*src*-related oncogenes, v-*erb*^{B}, does induce a small (50%) increase in phosphate esterified to protein tyrosine hydroxyls (3), even though its protein product appears to be ineffective as a tyrosine protein kinase *in vitro*. Past failures to detect protein kinase activity in the v-*erb*^{B} protein may however be due to inadequacies of the *in vitro* assay, since it is now clear that the cellular homologue of this protein is an acknowledged tyrosine protein kinase.

Normal cells contain tyrosine protein kinases, as evinced by the detection of phosphotyrosine in normal cell proteins, and the high levels of phosphotyrosine obtained if cells are lysed and incubated with ATP (10). Included among these normal cell tyrosine protein kinases are the cellular homologues of the v-src family of oncogene products, including the c-src, c-yes, and c-fps/fes proteins, one or more of which is to be found in most adult and embryonal tissues (reviewed [1]). An important functional class of normal cell tyrosine protein kinases includes the cell-surface receptors for epidermal growth factor (EGF), platelet-derived growth factor (PDGF), insulin and the type 1 insulin-like growth factors (IGF-1)(reviewed [2]). The EGF receptor was first shown to be an EGF-stimulated protein kinase, and later found to be specific for tyrosine (11). Recently, the growth factor receptor category of tyrosine protein kinases converged with the retroviral transforming protein class with the discovery that the gene for the EGF receptor is the cellular homologue of the v-erb^B gene (12). The viral transforming protein lacks most of the extracellular domain of the EGF receptor, and thus is probably not responsive to EGF. We suspect that the viral protein may be a constitutive protein kinase, no longer dependent on EGF, which transforms by supplying a continuous mitogenic signal. In this regard, v-erb^B transformed cells show only subtle morphological changes but have some features of normal cells exposed to EGF, such as increased glucose utilization. The absence of a marked increment in phosphotyrosine in v-erb^B transformed cells may indicate that the transforming protein has retained much of the protein specificity of its cellular parent.

We have attempted to delve deeper into the processes of cell transformation and growth factor action by analyzing events occurring in transformed cells and in normal cells exposed to growth factors. Guided by the enzymatic activities of some transforming proteins and growth factor receptors, we have looked specifically for proteins whose phosphotyrosine content is increased by transformation by appropriate viruses, or by mitogens. It should be noted, however, that there is no direct evidence that any of the substrate proteins found by ourselves and others mediates any of the changes associated with the transformed state. Although it seems safe to assume that phosphorylation of a protein at tyrosine could regulate its function, it is possible that protein phosphorylation at tyrosine is merely a readily-assayed side reaction, and the primary function of the transforming protein and receptor kinases may be the phosphorylation of some non-proteinaceous substrate. Recently it has been reported that the v-*src* and v-*ros* kinases can phosphorylate polyhydric alcohols such as glycerol, diacylglycerol and phosphatidyl inositol (13,14). In transformed cells, the synthesis of mono- and diphosphoinositides is accelerated: however, it is difficult to assess whether this is a direct consequence of phosphatidyl inositol phosphorylation by the v-*src* kinase until phosphatidyl inositol metabolism is measured under a range of cell growth conditions.

The search for phosphotyrosine in cell proteins

Transformation of cells by v-*src* results in the phosphorylation of many cell proteins at tyrosine (15,16). We have used two approaches to search for particular proteins that may be modified in this way. A third avenue of great potential is to isolate these proteins by binding to phosphotyrosine-specific antibodies (17,18). Our experiments have involved the isolation of candidate phosphoproteins by immunoprecipitation, and the systematic survey of total cellular phosphoproteins by two-dimensional gel electrophoresis.

The first approach is limited by the number of cellular proteins for which antisera are available and the persistence of the investigator. The transforming proteins encoded by v-*src*, v-*fps*, v-*fes*, v-*abl*, v-*yes* and v-*fgr* all contain phosphotyrosine when immunoprecipitated from transformed cells. So in some cases do their cellular homologues isolated from normal cells. Another phosphotyrosine-containing protein was detected in this fashion: pp50 is a cell protein that is found in immunoprecipitates of the v-*src* and several other transforming proteins and is phosphorylated at serine and tyrosine (19). pp50 is complexed with the transforming protein and a heat shock protein, and may function in ferrying the transforming protein to the membrane (20,21). Sefton *et al* (22) surveyed six cyto-skeletal proteins by immunoprecipitation, and found that vinculin contained more phosphotyrosine when isolated from v-*src*-transformed cells than when isolated from normal cells. However, even in the transformed cells only one vinculin molecule in 50 contains phosphotyrosine. The significance of this may become clearer as *in vitro* assays of vinculin function are perfected, since it has been reported that it is possible to phosphorylate purified vinculin with a v-*src* protein fragment (23). To date, vinculin phosphorylation does not correlate perfectly with measurable aspects of cell morphology (24). Another protein studied by immunoprecipitation is the EGF receptor. It becomes more highly phosphorylated after EGF treatment of the cells, and some of this increased phosphorylation occurs at a single tyrosine residue (25), possibly amino acid number 845 in the complete sequence (26).

Our second approach using two-dimensional gel electrophoresis is limited by the separation power of the system. In particular, proteins that are too scarce, too acidic, too basic, too hydrophobic or too heterogeneous to focus as a discrete spot are liable to be overlooked (27). Since it would be impractical to analyze separately the phosphoamino acids of all resolvable phosphoproteins, we have chosen phosphoproteins for analysis if their phosphate content, judged from labeling of the cells to equilibrium with $^{32}P_i$, increases after transformation or exposure to growth factors. Clearly, proteins whose total phosphate content changes little may have been overlooked. Another problem is that when cells are labeled to equilibrium with $^{32}P_i$ most of the radioactivity is found in nucleic acid. Brief nuclease treatment of the sample can remove some of this, but exhaustive treatment is deemed unwise since protein phosphorylation or dephosphorylation can occur after cell lysis. Incubation of the gels in alkali before autoradiography has the dual benefits of reducing the background due to radioactive RNA and removing greater than 70% of phosphate linked to serine in cell proteins, without greatly affecting the phosphate linked to threonine or tyrosine (27). Many newly phosphorylated proteins are readily detectable in transformed cells by this technique, but it is likely that some phosphoproteins of interest are not detected, since some tyrosine phosphates are labile to alkali. For example, exposure of pp50 to alkali releases the phosphate as acid-soluble material.

Substrates for viral tyrosine protein kinases

The first phosphoprotein target for retroviral transforming proteins was detected in a two-dimensional gel survey of phosphoproteins by Radke and Martin (28). This phosphoprotein, known as pp36, contained more phosphate in v-*src*-transformed than normal cells. It was later found that the phosphate in pp36 was linked to tyrosine and serine (29,30). Among the phosphoproteins discovered since pp36 there appear to be no examples of protein species that are phosphorylated only at tyrosine. However, in most instances the individual phosphotyrosine-containing molecules do not contain phosphoserine, and vice versa. This may be deduced from two dimensional gel analysis, by comparing the isoelectric point of the denatured phosphoprotein and the isoelectric point of its apoprotein. Chemical modification of the apoprotein permits the number of charges introduced by phophorylation to be estimated. In most cases, the displacement in isoelectric point is equivalent to 1.5-2 charges, as expected for adding a single phosphate. The growth factor receptors and retroviral tyrosine protein kinases are exceptions to this generalization, since isolation of the phosphotyrosine-containing molecules with anti-phosphotyrosine sera yields proteins that contain both phosphoserine and phosphotyrosine (18). For both types of substrates there must be mechanisms for activating serine protein kinases that have the same targets as tyrosine protein kinases. In v-src-transformed cells, both specificities must be activated, or encoded, by v-src. It seems most likely that the tyrosine protein kinase that phosphorylates p36 is in fact the v-src protein, since the phosphorylation occurs at the authentic site with purified substrate and kinase in vitro (30), and this protein kinase and p36 are in proximity on cell membranes. The nature of the serine protein kinase is unknown, but it is unlikely to be the v-src protein since no tyrosine protein kinase has been found to phosphorylate serine. Serine protein kinases activated in transformed cells also phosphorylate other proteins that are not phosphorylated at tyrosine, including, for example, ribosomal protein S6 (31).

Our analysis of v-src-transformed cells, using alkaline hydrolysis to remove background radioactivity from two-dimensional gels, showed that several phosphoproteins in addition to pp36 contained phosphotyrosine. Two of these are now known to be glycolytic/gluconeogenic enzymes catalyzing consecutive steps near the end of glycolysis: phosphoglycerate mutase and enolase (32). Phosphorylation of a third enzyme, lactate dehydrogenase, also occurs in v-src-transformed cells, and to a greater extent in v-fes-transformed cells (32). Phosphorylation of all three enzymes can occur in vitro, with an immunoprecipitated transforming protein as a source of protein kinase activity (33). Unfortunately, it is not known whether

Table 1. Sequences surrounding tyrosines phosphorylated in transformed cells.[a]

Protein	Sequence
P120gag-abl	**Arg**.Leu.Met.Thr.Gly.**Asp**.Thr.**TYR**.Thr.Ala.**His**.Ala.Gly.Ala.Gly
pp60v-src	**Arg**.Leu.Ile.**Glu**.**Asp**.Asn.**Glu**.**TYR**.Thr.Ala.**Arg**.Gln.Gly.Ala.**Lys**
P90gag-yes	**Arg**.Leu.Ile.**Glu**.**Asp**.Asn.**Glu**.**TYR**.Thr.Ala.**Arg**.Gln.Gly.Ala.**Lys**
P140gag-fps	**Arg**.Gln.**Glu**.**Glu**.**Asp**.Gly.Val.**TYR**.Ala.Ser.Thr.Gly.Gly.Met.**Lys**
P85gag-fes	**Arg**.**Glu**.**Glu**.Ala.**Asp**.Gly.Val.**TYR**.Ala.Ala.Ser.Gly.Gly.Leu.**Arg**
P110gag-fes	**Arg**.**Glu**.Ala.Ala.**Asp**.Gly.Ile.**TYR**.Ala.Ala.Ser.Gly.Gly.Leu.**Arg**
Lactate dehydrogenase	**Lys**.Gln.Val.Val.**Asp**.Ser.Ala.**TYR**.**Glu**.Val.Ile.**Lys**.Leu.**Lys**.Gly
Enolase	Ser.Gly.Ala.Ser.Thr.Gly.Ile.**TYR**.**Glu**.Ala.Leu.**Glu**.Leu.**Arg**.

[a]The sequences of the seven amino acids preceding and the seven amino acids following tyrosines that are phosphorylated in appropriate transformed cells are shown. In all cases the target tyrosine is indicated **TYR**, acidic residues are in heavy type and underlined, and basic residues are in heavy type. Sequencing of the phosphorylation sites in lactate dehydrogenase and enolase is described in reference 33, which also lists references to the sequences of the retroviral transforming proteins.

tyrosine phosphorylation affects enzymatic activity of enolase, phosphoglycerate mutase or lactate dehydrogenase. It may seem trivial to assay separately the phosphorylated enzyme and nonphosphorylated enzyme, but the stoichiometry of phosphorylation *in vivo* is only 1-5%, and in our *in vitro* reactions the extent of phosphorylation is even lower. It may be possible to drive the *in vitro* system to completion by using larger amounts of a soluble tyrosine protein kinase and high concentrations of ATP. This will be a useful approach for the future.

Phosphorylation of enolase and lactate dehyrogenase occurs primarily at the same site in the transformed cell and *in vitro*, and these sites have been sequenced (33; Table 1). Acidic residues are commonly found adjacent to phosphorylation sites utilized by tyrosine protein kinases in intact cells. Acidic tyrosine-containing peptides are also substrates for tyrosine protein kinases *in vitro*. It is clear that primary structure is not the only determinant of phosphorylation specificity, however, since some proteins that are good substrates *in vitro* appear not to be phosphorylated *in vivo*. Most probably, interactions with other proteins and subcellular location are important. For example, the soluble enzymes enolase and

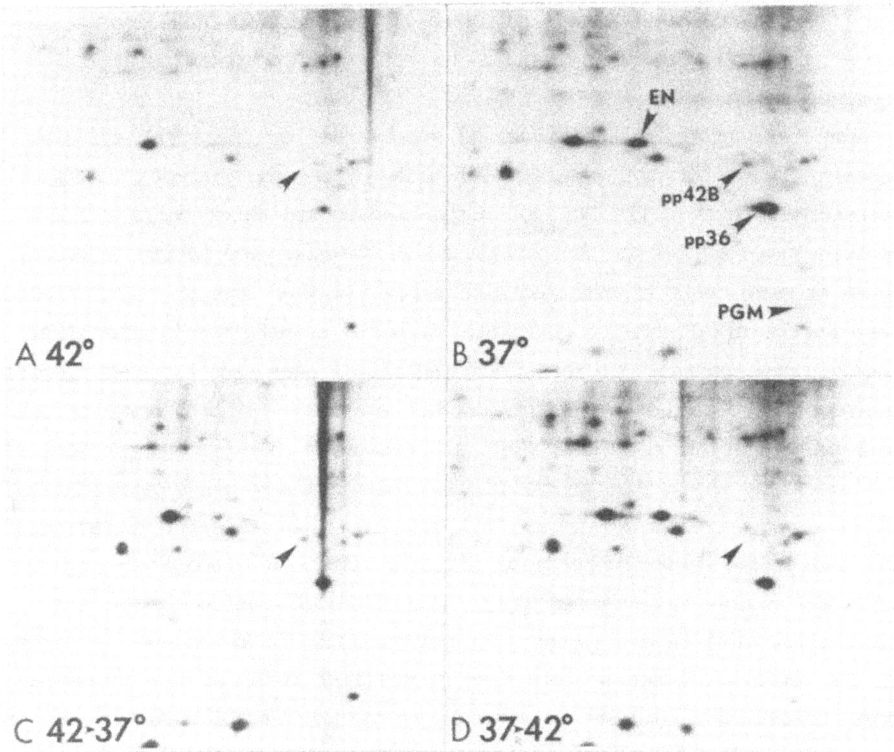

Figure 1. Phosphoproteins of chick embryo cells infected with temperature-sensitive virus.
Chick embryo cells were infected with Rous sarcoma virus mutant tsNY68 at 37°C. When the cultures appeared transformed, two were transferred to 42°C. All cultures were labeled for 12 hr with 1 mCi $^{32}P_i$ in 1 ml of phosphate-free Dulbecco medium supplemented with 4% total calf serum. 30 min before the end of the labeling period, one culture was transferred from 42°C to 37°C (C), and one from 37°C to 42°C (D). The other cultures were kept at 42°C (A) or 37°C (B). Samples were prepared and analyzyed essentially as described (27). Autoradiographs of alkali-treated two-dimensional gels are shown. The arrowheads in panel B point to phosphoproteins discussed in the text: EN, enolase; pp42B (also indicated on panels A, C and D); pp36; and PGM, phosphoglycerate mutase.

phosphoglycerate mutase are phosphorylated slowly in cells after activation of a thermolabile v-*src* protein by lowering the cell culture temperature, whereas the membrane-bound p36 is phosphorylated rapidly (28; Figure 1). When the protein kinase is inactivated by raising the temperature, p36 is dephosphorylated rapidly but enolase and phosphoglycerate mutase are dephosphorylated slowly (Figure 1). Thus turnover of phosphate on enolase and phosphoglycerate mutase, catalyzed by phosphatases and kinases, is slower than on p36. This applies to both the phosphotyrosine and phosphoserine.

Some cell proteins are preferred substrates for one viral tyrosine protein kinase but not another. Vinculin is phosphorylated in v-*src*-transformed chick cells but not v-*fps*-transformed chick cells (22). A protein known as p81 is phosphorylated at tyrosine and serine in human, mouse or mink cells transformed with v-*fes* (34,35). This protein contains very little alkali-stable phosphate in cells transformed by the other retroviruses studied. Our recent studies of p81 have made use of a specific antiserum developed by Anthony Bretscher against a chicken brush border cell protein of about 80 kDal (36). It transpires that the two proteins are the same, and the antiserum can be used both to study p81 localization and as an alternative to two-dimensional gel electrophoresis for isolation of p81 and pp81. Immunofluorescence staining shows p81 localized in the cortical region of cultured cells, concentrated noticeably in the microvilli. This is consistent with the purification by Anthony Bretscher of the cognate chicken protein from microvillar cores of the intestinal brush border (36). Studies by several groups have established that p36 is also found below the plasma membrane (37-40). p36 and p81 also share the property of becoming extensively phosphorylated at tyrosine when the unusual human tumor cell line, A431, which has several million EGF receptors per cell, is treated with EGF (25,41). Possibly the proximity of p36 and p81 to the EGF receptor ensures their phosphorylation. The subcellular location of the v-*fes* protein has not been studied in detail, but most of the v-*src*-family transforming proteins have at least a tenuous association with the membrane. p36 and p81 can be phosphorylated at tyrosine *in vitro*, when membranes from A431 cells are incubated with EGF and ATP.

Table 2. Agents that transiently stimulate phosphorylation of pp42B.[a]

Mitogenic agent	Cell types studied; Comments
Defined growth factors:	
EGF	A431, 3T3, NRK and chick fibroblasts; 3T3 cells lacking EGF receptors do not respond
PDGF	3T3, rat and chick fibroblasts
Fibroblast growth factor	3T3 cells
IGF-1	chick cells
Tumor promoters:	
Teleocidin	chick cells, 3T3 cells; non-mitogenic phorbol is inactive
TPA	
Diacylglycerol	
Proteases:	
Trypsin	chick cells; non-mitogenic chymotrypsin and proteolytically-inactive thrombin do not stimulate
Thrombin	

[a]References 42-46 and unpublished results.

Protein phosphorylations instigated by growth factors

p36 and p81 are not phosphorylated in all cell types in response to EGF. The only proteins that we have found phosphorylated after EGF treatment in all cell types studied are in the size range of 40-45 kDal (42,43). Michael Weber and colleagues have separated total cellular proteins into 60 size fractions by SDS polyacrylamide gel electrophoresis and analyzed their phosphoamino acids. They have reported that the major increase in phosphotyrosine following exposure to EGF occurs in proteins of 40-43 kDal (44). It is thus possible that the proteins we have identified on two-dimensional gels are the quantitatively major substrates for the EGF receptor in most cell types. These same 40-45 kDal proteins are also phosphorylated, on tyrosine and serine and in some cases threonine, when cells are exposed to other mitogens (Table 2). Active mitogens include factors whose receptors are known to possess tyrosine protein kinase activity - PDGF, EGF and IGF-1 - and factors whose receptors are most likely not tyrosine protein kinases - thrombin, trypsin and tumor promoters (43-46; unpublished data). The latter mitogens must stimulate phosphorylation at tyrosine by an indirect mechanism, perhaps by interaction with the PDGF, EGF, insulin or IGF-1 receptor, or with a cellular homologue of a viral oncogene tyrosine protein kinase. The fact that the mitogens tested can all stimulate phosphorylation of the 40-45 kDal proteins at tyrosine points to a possible involvement of these substrate proteins in the mitogenic response, or in some aspect of that response such as augmented metabolite uptake. It should be noted, however, that the dose of mitogen necessary for 50% maximal protein phosphorylation exceeds the dose required for mitogenic stimulation, often by an order of magnitude. Also, the stimulation of tyrosine phosphorylation is transient, and the phosphorylation of the 40-45 kDal proteins decays to control level by 2-4 hrs after mitogen addition. Perhaps a low threshold level of phosphorylation is adequate to set in motion other events that lead to mitogenesis.

We are learning most about one of the 40-45 kDal proteins, known as p42. This is a minor cell protein, estimated to comprise 0.002% of cell protein (about 100,000 molecules per fibroblast). It appears to be synthesized at the same rate in growing and resting cells. It is also found in cells that are not actively growing such as liver cells. Upon stimulation with mitogen, as much as 50% of p42 becomes phosphorylated. There are two forms of phosphorylated p42: pp42B, the more basic, contains phosphoserine and phosphotyrosine; pp42A, the more acidic, contains phosphoserine, phosphothreonine and phosphotyrosine. It is not yet known whether pp42B contains one phosphate per polypeptide chain and pp42A two, or whether the two forms are related by some other post-translational modification. This phosphorylation is complete within 5-15 min of mitogen addition (Figure 2). pp42B is also found in chick cells infected with retroviruses carrying genes for tyrosine protein kinases. This phosphorylation could in principle be catalyzed by any of several tyrosine protein kinases. Candidates include the retroviral tyrosine protein kinase itself, a cellular enzyme, or a growth factor receptor activated by factors secreted by the transformed cells. The latter may be tentatively excluded by the rapidity of p42 phosphorylation following renaturation of thermolabile v-<u>src</u> protein by decreasing the culture temperature: within 30 min of temperature shift p42 phosphorylation approaches the maximum (Figure 1). As expected for a phophoprotein whose phosphorylation state can rapidly reach a new equilibrium level, phosphate turnover on pp42 is very rapid. pp42 is dephosphorylated totally within 30 min of either inactivating the v-<u>src</u> kinase by temperature shift (Figure 1), or of inactivating the PDGF receptor kinase by removal of PDGF (Figure 2).

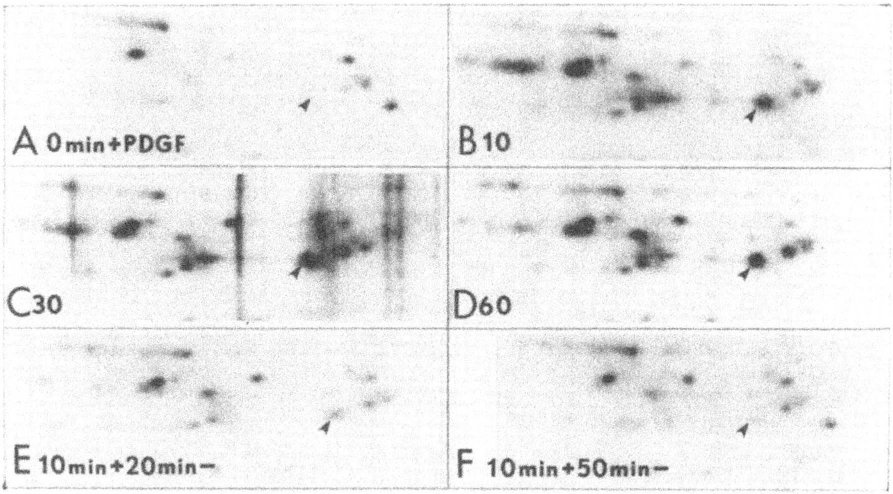

Figure 2. Phosphorylation and dephosphorylation of pp42B. Confluent cultures of NR6 3T3 cells were incubated for a total of 23 hr with 0.5 mCi of $^{32}P_i$ in 1 ml of Dulbecco medium having 3% the normal phosphate concentration, 1% calf serum and 10 mM Hepes buffer, pH 7.2. PDGF (0.66 pmol) and antiserum to PDGF (titrated to neutralize the mitogenic action of 0.66 pmol PDGF) were added directly to the labeling media at various times before samples were prepared and analyzed (27,42). Autoradiographs of alkali-treated two-dimensional gels are shown. Control sample (panel A); 10 min, 30 min or 60 min exposure to PDGF (panels B, C and D); 10 min exposure to PDGF followed by 20 min or 50 min with antiserum to PDGF also present (panels E and F). The arrowhead in each panel points to pp42B. Close inspection shows that other phosphotyrosine-containing proteins (viz pp41, pp42A, pp45A and pp45B) are phosphorylated and dephosphorylated with the same kinetics as pp42B, but some proteins that are phosphorylated only at serine and/or threonine in response to PDGF are not dephosphorylated in the time period studied.

We are attempting to purify p42 to raise specific antisera, for localization and microinjection studies. If phosphorylation of p42 is important for some aspect of the mitogenic response, it is possible that some mutations in the p42 gene may have a dominant effect on cell growth or metabolism. Potentially, replacement of the phosphorylated tyrosine with an acidic amino acid by genetic manipulation will drive cells to incessant replication.

Acknowledgements We thank Bart Sefton and Anthony Bretscher for discussions and practical advice. PDGF and antiserum to PDGF were the kind gifts of Elaine Raines and Russell Ross. Thrombin and diisopropyl phospho-fluoridate-inactivated thrombin were the kind gifts of George Wilner. This work was supported by Public Health Service grants CA14158, CA 17096 and CA 28458.

REFERENCES

1. Hunter T, Cooper JA: Adv Cyc Nuc Res Mol Biol (17):443-455, 1984.
2. Sefton BM, Hunter T: Adv Cyc Nuc Res Mol Biol (18):195-226, 1984.
3. Sefton BM, Hunter T, Beemon K, Eckhart W: Cell (20):807-816, 1980.
4. Yamamoto T, Nishida T, Miyajima N, Kawai S, Ooi T, Toyoshima K: Cell (34):225-232, 1983.
5. Privalsky M, Ralston R, Bishop MJ: Proc Natl Acad Sci USA (81) in press.
6. Hampe A, Gobet M, Sherr CJ, Galibert F: Proc Natl Acad Sci USA: (81):85-89, 1984.
7. Kan NC, Flordellis CS, Mark GE, Duesberg PH, Papas TA: Science (223):813-816, 1984.
8. Van Beveren C, Galleshaw JA, Jonas V, Berns AJM, Doolittle RF, Donoghue D, Verma IM: Nature (289):258-262, 1981.
9. Feldman RA, Wang L-H, Hanafusa H, Balduzzi PC: J Virol (42):228-236, 1982.
10. Hunter T, Sefton BM, Beemon K: in: Fields BN et al (eds): Animal Virus Genetics. Academic Press, New York, 1980, pp499-514.
11. Ushiro H, Cohen S: J Biol Chem (255):8363-8365, 1980.
12. Downward J, Yarden Y, Mayes E, Scrace G, Totty N, Stockwell P, Ullrich A, Schlessinger J, Waterfield MD: Nature (307):521-527, 1984.
13. Macara IG, Marinetti GV, Balduzzi PC: Proc Natl Acad Sci USA (81):2728-2732, 1984.
14. Sugimoto Y, Whitman M, Cantley L, Erikson RL: Proc Natl Acad Sci USA (81):2117-2122, 1984.
15. Martinez R, Nakamura KD, Weber MJ: Mol Cell Biol (2):653-665, 1982.
16. Beemon K, Ryden T, McNelly EA: J Virol (42):742-747, 1982.
17. Ross AH, Baltimore D, Eisen H: Nature (294):654-656, 1981.
18. Frackelton AR, Ross AH, Eisen HN: Mol Cell Biol 3:1343-1352, 1983.
19. Hunter T, Sefton BM: Proc Natl Acad Sci USA (77):1311-1315, 1980.
20. Brugge J, Yonemoto W, Darrow D: Mol Cell Biol (3):9-19, 1983.
21. Courtneidge S, Bishop JM: Proc Natl Acad Sci USA (79):7117-7121, 1982.
22. Sefton BM, Hunter T, Ball EH, Singer SJ: Cell (24):165-174, 1981.
23. Ito S, Richert N, Pastan I: Proc Natl Acad Sci USA (79):4628-4631, 1982.
24. Rohrschneider LR, Rosok M: Mol Cell Biol (3):731-746, 1983.
25. Hunter T, Cooper JA: Cell 24:741-752, 1981.
26. Ullrich A, Coussens L, Hayflick JS, Dull TJ, Gray A, Tam AW, Lee J, Yarden Y, Libermann TA, Schlessinger J, Downward J, Mayes ELV, Whittle N, Waterfield MD, Seeburg PH: Nature (309):418-425, 1984.
27. Cooper JA, Hunter T: Mol Cell Biol (1):165-178, 1981.
28. Radke K, Martin GS: Proc Natl Acad Sci USA (76):5212-5216, 1979.
29. Radke K, Gilmore T, Martin GS: Cell (21):821-828, 1980.

30. Erikson E, Erikson RL: Cell (21):829-836, 1980.
31. Decker S: Proc Natl Acad Sci USA (78):4112-4115, 1981.
32. Cooper JA, Reiss N, Schwartz RJ, Hunter T: Nature (302):218-223, 1983.
33. Cooper JA, Esch F, Taylor SS, Hunter T: J Biol Chem (259): in press.
34. Hunter T, Cooper JA: Prog Nucl Acid Res Mol Biol (29):221-233, 1983.
35. Cooper JA, Scolnick EM, Ozanne B, Hunter T: J Virol (48):752-764, 1983.
36. Bretscher A: J Cell Biol (97):425-432, 1983.
37. Nigg EA, Cooper JA, Hunter T: J Cell Biol (96):1601-1609, 1983.
38. Courtneidge SA, Ralston R, Alitalo K, Bishop JM: Mol Cell Biol 3:340-350, 1983.
39. Radke K, Carter VC, Moss P, Dehazya P, Schliwa M, Martin GS: J Cell Biol (97):1601-1611, 1983.
40. Lehto V-P, Virtanen I, Ralston R, Alitalo K: EMBO J (2):1701-1705, 1983.
41. Erikson E, Shealy DJ, Erikson RL: J Biol Chem (256):11381-11384, 1981.
42. Cooper JA, Bowen-Pope D, Raines E, Ross R, Hunter T: Cell (31):263-273, 1982.
43. Cooper JA, Sefton BM, Hunter T: Mol Cell Biol (4):30-37, 1984.
44. Nakamura KD, Martinez R, Weber MJ: Mol Cell Biol (3):380-389, 1983.
45. Bishop R, Martinez R, Nakamura KD, Weber MJ: Biochem Biophys Res Commun (115):536-543, 1983.
46. Gilmore T, Martin GS: Nature (306):487-490, 1983.

5

ACTIVATION OF A GENE CODING FOR A NORMAL HUMAN GROWTH FACTOR TO ONE WITH TRANSFORMING PROPERTIES

STUART A. AARONSON AND KEITH C. ROBBINS
National Cancer Institute, Building 37, Room 1A07, Bethesda, Maryland 20205

INTRODUCTION

One of the most intensely investigated areas in cancer research has evolved from studies of a small group of viruses, the acute transforming retroviruses. These agents have arisen in nature as apparently rare events resulting from recombination of replication competent type C retroviruses with a small set of evolutionarily highly conserved cellular genes termed proto-oncogenes. Such transduced cellular (onc) sequences confer new properties required for the rapid induction of malignancies by the viruses. Recent studies have indicated that proto-oncogenes can be activated as oncogenes directly within human cells in the absence of retrovirus involvement, and that such oncogenes may very well play a role in the development of the fully neoplastic cell. If so, understanding of the normal functions of proto-oncogenes as well as how alterations in their coding sequences or transcriptional control lead them to acquire transforming properties may be critical to the development of new and better approaches to cancer diagnosis and treatment. The present review summarizes how investigations of one transforming gene, sis, has led to fundamental insights concerning the normal functions of this small set of cellular genes which appear to be frequent targets for the genetic alterations that lead normal cells along the pathways to malignancy.

PROCEDURES

Nucleotide sequencing. Appropriate restriction fragments were labeled either at their 5' end by using [γ-^{32}P]ATP (Amersham, 3,000 Ci/mmol; 1 Ci=3.7 X 10^{10} becquerels) and polynucleotide kinase (P-L Biochemicals) or at their 3' end by using cordycepin 5'-[α^{32}P]triphosphate (Amersham, 3,000 Ci/mmol) and terminal deoxynucleotidyltransferase (P-L Biochemicals). End-labeled DNA fragments were digested with appropriate restriction endonucleases (New England BioLabs) and isolated by agarose or polyacrylamide gel electrophoresis. The nucleotide sequence was determined by the procedure of Maxam and Gilbert (1).

Peptide antibodies. We chose for synthesis pentadecapeptides derived from the 5' and 3' terminal regions of v-*sis*. Rabbits were immunized with 100 μg of the peptide either alone or after conjugation with thyroglobulin. Thereafter, 100 μg of peptide was administered intraperitoneally at 14-day intervals. Animals were bled 1 week after each injection. The effectiveness of the immune response was monitored by the ability of serum from sequential bleedings to precipitate ^{125}-I-labeled *sis* peptides.

Immunoprecipitation analysis. Subconfluent cultures (around 10^7 cells per 10-cm petri dish) were labeled for 3 hours at 37°C with 4 ml of methionine-free Dulbecco's modified Eagle's minimal essential medium containing 100 μCi of [^{35}S]cysteine (1,200 Ci/nmole; Amersham) per milliliter. Labeled cells were lysed with 1 ml of a buffer containing 10 mM sodium phosphate, pH 7.5, 100 mM NaCl, 1 percent Triton X-100, 0.5 percent sodium deoxycholate, 0.1% sodium dodecyl sulfate and 0.1 mM phenylmethyl-sulfonyl fluoride per petri dish, clarified at 100,000 g for 30 minutes and divided into four identical aliquots. Each aliquot was incubated with 4 μl of antiserum for 60 minutes at 4°C. Immunoprecipitates were recovered with the aid of *Staphylococcus aureus* protein A bound to Sepharose beads (Pharmacia) and analyzed by electrophoresis in sodium dodecyl sulfate-14 percent polyacrylamide gels (SDS-PAGE) (2).

RESULTS

The sis oncogene. The *sis* oncogene was initially identified as the transforming gene of simian sarcoma virus (SSV). SSV is the only primate-derived acutely transforming retrovirus (3). Like a number of other such viruses, SSV transforms cultured fibroblasts (4). However, it possesses a rather narrow spectrum of target cells for malignant transformation *in vivo* inducing only fibrosarcomas or glioblastomas in appropriate host animals (5, 6, Arnstein and Aaronson, unpublished observations).

The cloning of biologically active SSV DNA made possible a detailed analysis of this transforming viral genome (7). When the cloned 5.8 kbp

SSV genome was compared to the genome of its helper virus, simian sarcoma associated virus (SSAV), by restriction enzyme mapping and heteroduplexing analysis, we identified an approximately 1 kbp sequence towards the 3' end of the genome that was not detectably related to SSAV. In accordance with convention, this segment was designated *sis*.

In order to determine the origin of the *sis* sequence, retroviral DNAs and normal cellular DNAs were analyzed by Southern blotting using a molecularly cloned v-*sis* specific probe. Retroviral genomes failed to hybridize with *sis*; however, *sis*-related restriction fragments were found to be present at low copy number in the DNAs of species as diverse as human and quail. These findings suggested that recombination between SSAV and a normal cellular gene had led to the creation of SSV (7).

In order to determine the species of origin of *sis*, we measured the extent to which a v-*sis* probe could anneal to DNAs of various species. DNAs derived from New World primates annealed with this probe to a significantly greater degree than the DNAs isolated from any other species tested. Furthermore, hybrids formed between *sis* and woolly monkey cellular DNA exhibited the same thermal stability as that of the homologous v-*sis* DNA duplex. These results strongly implied that v-*sis* arose from the woolly monkey genome (8).

v-sis is required for SSV transforming activity. In order to determine the role of v-*sis* in SSV transforming activity, we constructed a series of deletion mutants from molecularly cloned SSV DNA. These DNAs were then tested for their ability to transform NIH/3T3 cells in transfection assays. All constructs that resulted in the deletion of *sis* sequences were unable to transform NIH/3T3 cells (9). For example, deletion of the 3' LTR had no effect on transforming efficiency. However, when the deletion was extended 82 base pairs into v-*sis*, the resulting clone was no longer biologically active. Similarly, a mutant that lacked 250 bp at the 5' end of v-*sis* also lost transforming function. By this approach, it was possible to establish that v-*sis* was required for SSV transforming activity.

Nucleotide sequence analysis of SSV. The potential coding capacity of v-*sis* was revealed by determination of the complete nucleotide sequence of SSV (10). An open reading frame of 271 codons encompassed v-*sis* and 254 nucleotides of upstream 5' helper viral sequences. A termination codon was identified within v-*sis* 347 bp upstream from its 3' terminus. By sequence comparison with Moloney MuLV and SSAV, the 5' end of the open reading frame was identified as the amino terminus of the SSAV *env* gene. The carboxy terminus of the SSAV *env* gene encoding p15E was found to flank v-*sis* at its 3' end. Thus, creation of SSV involved a large deletion of the SSAV *env* gene and substitution of v-*sis*. How might a *sis* gene product or products be synthesized? In addition to the first methionine of the open reading frame at position 3657, two methionines were predicted to occur prior to the start of v-*sis* (positions 3969 and 3792). RNA splice acceptor sites reside near each of these methionine codons. One of the ATG codons corresponds to that proposed as the initiator of the Moloney MuLV *env* gene product (11). Thus, one possibility is that the *sis* transforming gene uses the same sequences for the initiation of its transcription and translation as the *env* gene it replaced. In fact, the SSV genome codes for a 2.7 kb mRNA that contains LTR and v-*sis* sequences, but does not hybridize with *gag*-specific probes (Robbins et al., unpublished observations). A message of this size could accommodate sufficient information to encode proteins of around 33,000, 30,000, or 28,000 MW predicted to initiate from the first three methionines, respectively, in this open reading frame.

Identification of the SSV transforming protein. Efforts to identify a v-*sis* coded protein(s) utilized antiserum directed against synthetic peptides predicted by v-*sis* nucleotide sequence (8). One such antibody directed towards amino terminal sequences of the predicted *sis* protein specifically precipitated a 28,000 MW polypeptide from extracts of SSV-transformed cells. In contrast, antibodies against the SSAV *env* gene product did not precipitate this protein. Further confirmation that the 28,000 MW polypeptide ($p28^{sis}$) was encoded by the v-*sis* open reading frame was obtained by the demonstration that cyanogen bromide fragments predicted by sequence analysis could be detected with the anti-*sis* peptide serum. Additionally, antiserum prepared against a carboxy terminal *sis* peptide specifically precipitated $p28^{sis}$ from SSV-transformed cells. Some of the salient structural features of the SSV genome and its gene products are summarized in Fig. 1.

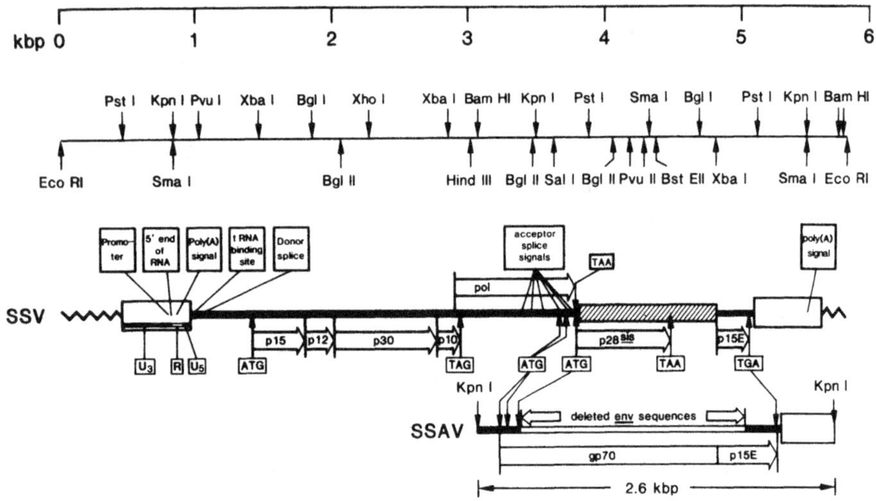

FIGURE 1. Summary of the major structural features of the SSV genome. The v-sis open reading frame, transcriptional and translational signals, as well as donor and acceptor splice signals are illustrated.

Having identified the SSV transforming protein, we endeavored to identify its function. Studies on the origin of oncogenes over the last few years have shown that related sequences are highly conserved among eucaryotic species. Mammalian v-onc probes have even been found to detect related genes in such evolutionarily distant species as flies and worms (12), and even in yeasts (13). This high degree of evolutionary conservation implies that proto-oncogenes must serve important functions in normal cellular growth and development.

Elucidation of the molecular structure of retroviral onc genes has led to the detection, in many instances, of their protein products. The prototype of one group of onc genes, the src gene of Rous sarcoma virus, was found to possess a protein kinase activity (14, 15), specific for tyrosine residues (16). Several other v-onc encoded proteins, also possess tyrosine kinase activity and also share partial amino acid sequence similarities with the src tyrosine kinases (for review see 17). Ras oncogenes represent another family which encodes proteins possessing GTP-binding activity (18), and appears to be distinct from the src family. Like src, ras genes appears to be localized to the inner surface of the cell membrane. Several other onc gene encoded proteins are believed to interact with substrates in the cell nucleus, due to their localization in this cell compartment (19, 20, 21). The transforming protein of SSV displayed none of the known structural or functional properties of any of these previously characterized transforming gene products.

The SSV transforming protein is related to human platelet-derived growth factor. The rapid proliferation of nucleotide sequence and, thus, of predicted amino acid sequence data, in combination with the development of sequence banks and programs for computer search for sequence similarities (22), has recently led to a number of important observations. By this approach a striking match was discovered between the partial amino acid sequence of a peptide chain of platelet-derived growth factor, PDGF, a potent human connective tissue cell mitogen, and the predicted v-sis sequence (23, 24). These findings pointed the way toward identification of the first normal function of a proto-oncogene.

In active PDGF preparations, two peptides designated PDGF-1 and PDGF-2, have been identified (25). At their amino terminal ends, these peptides were reported to share 8 of 19 residues without the introduction of gaps in their sequences. The predicted v-sis coding sequence, starting at residue 67, demonstrated an 84% match with PDGF-2 over this same stretch. Furthermore, in a total of 70 PDGF-2 residues identified, 87.1% corresponded to the predicted $p28^{sis}$ sequence. The observed amino acid differences between human PDGF-2 and v-sis could be accounted for by the known degree of divergence between the genomes of humans and cebids (26). Thus, we concluded that the v-sis transforming gene arose by recombination between the SSAV genome and a woolly monkey cellular gene for PDGF or a very closely related protein.

Efforts were undertaken to directly establish that the v-sis gene product and human PDGF shared structural, immunological, and biological properties (27). We utilized antibodies directed against peptides synthesized on the basis of the predicted amino and carboxy termini of $p28^{sis}$ (10) to study its biogenesis. Marmoset cells infected with SSV were pulse-labeled with ^{35}S-methionine for various times, extracted, and then immunoprecipitated with the appropriate antisera. The immunoprecipitates were then analyzed by pulse chase analysis on SDS-gels in the presence or absence of reducing agent. We observed a complex series of processing steps initiated by translation of the primary $p28^{\underline{sis}}$ product. This protein was shown to rapidly undergo disulfide-bond formation yielding a 56,000 dalton dimer. The 56,000 dalton species is then cleaved at its amino terminal end and then its carboxy terminus to yield progressively smaller but discrete polypeptides. These species were detected not only by anti-*sis* peptide sera but by using anti-PDGF serum as well. In addition, the PDGF antiserum detected a 24,000 dalton protein that was not recognized by the *sis* N- and C-terminal specific antisera. This species appeared to be the most stable processed form of the *sis* gene product.

The intracellular forms of the *sis* protein(s) bear striking similarities to biologically active PDGF. Thus, PDGF is comprised of a range of molecules from 28,000 to 35,000 daltons that upon reduction are converted to peptides ranging from 12,000 to 18,000 daltons (28, 29, 30, 31). In fact, there is a proteolytic cleavage signal (Lys-Arg) at residues 65-66 in the v-*sis* sequence with homology between v-*sis* and PDGF-2 commencing at the next residue. Cleavage here results in an approximately 20,000 dalton peptide corresponding closely in size to PDGF-2. In fact, we have observed this cleavage product of $p28^{\underline{sis}}$ by analysis of immunoprecipitates from SSV transformed cells under reducing conditions. All of these findings imply that the *sis* transforming protein represents a processed dimer, structurally and immunologically related to PDGF (27).

The human sis proto-oncogene. In order to characterize the human *sis* locus, we isolated v-*sis*-related sequences from a bacteriophage library of normal human DNA (32). These clones represented a continuous stretch of approximately 30 kbp. By Southern blotting analysis and hybridization with a v-*sis* probe, five v-*sis*-homologous restriction fragments were identified which could be localized within a 15 kbp region. Nucleotide sequence analysis of the v-*sis*-related regions demonstrated the existence of an open reading frame contained within v-*sis* related exons. The 5'-most exon lacked a translation initiation codon in its open reading frame (32, 33). Thus, c-*sis*, like v-*sis*, represented an incomplete gene, a conclusion further supported by observations that some human cells express a 4.2 kbp sis-related transcript, much larger than the 1.0 kbp v-sis open reading frame (34).

When the predicted c-sis (human) coding sequence was compared with that of known PDGF-2 peptides, we detected almost complete homology. The two amino acid differences in a total of 104 residues are very likely due to technical artificats in sequence determination or to polymorphism associated with PDGF polyeptides. These results made it possible to conclude that c-sis (human) was indeed the structural gene for PDGF-2 (32, 35, 36) (Fig. 2).

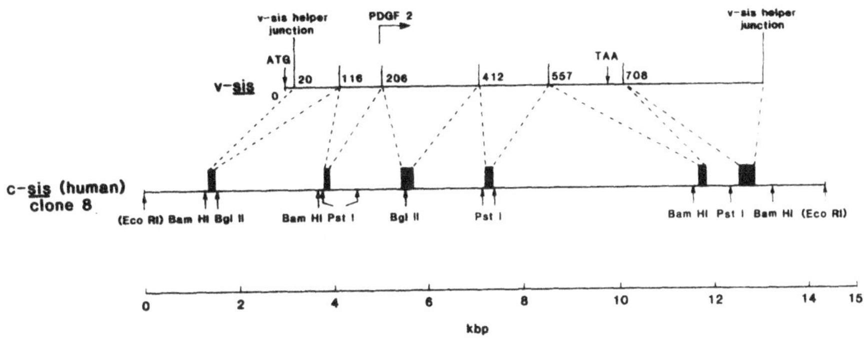

FIGURE 2. Relationship of v-sis to human c-sis/PDGF-2, as determined by nucleotide sequence analysis. Kpb, kilobase pairs.

Expression of the normal coding sequence for human PDGF-2/sis causes cellular transformation. There is as yet no information concerning the sequence of the normal woolly monkey homologue of v-sis or of its gene product. Thus, it is not known whether v-sis contains alterations in its coding sequence which contribute to the transforming properties of this PDGF-2 related gene. Knowledge that the normal human homologue of v-sis is the structural gene for PDGF-2 provided the opportunity for us to investigate whether expression of the normal PDGF-2 coding sequence would be sufficient to induce cellular transformation. Our efforts to activate human c-*sis*/PDGF-2 took into account the fact that v-*sis* derives both transcription and translation initiation signals from its helper viral sequences (10). Moreover, our human c-*sis* clone, which contained all of the coding information for PDGF-2, lacked transcription and translation initiation signals as well (32, 33).

We were able to activate this human sequence as a transforming gene by two *in vitro* manipulations, neither of which was alone sufficient. Placement of human c-*sis* under the control of a retroviral LTR led to its transcription but not to the synthesis of detectable *sis*-related translational products. We identified a putative upstream exon in a c-*sis* flanking genomic DNA clone isolated from a normal human library. Insertion of this region upstream from c-*sis* was ineffective in activating transforming properties. However, addition of an LTR to this construct led to acquisition of high titered transforming activity, comparable to that of SSV DNA (Fig. 3). Moreover, the foci induced were indistinguishable in their appearance from those induced by SSV. Our findings that PDGF-2 gene products were expressed in such transformants argued strongly that the putative upstream exon provided signals necessary for translation of these proteins. The extraordinary high efficiency at which the LTR human c-*sis* chimera induced transformed foci excludes the possibility of a minority population of altered DNA molecules accounting for this activity.

Transformants induced by the activated human *sis*/PDGF-2 coding sequence contained two major *sis*/PDGF-2 related protein species of 52,000 and 35,000 daltons, which were detected using anti-*sis* peptide serum and nonreducing assay conditions. In contrast, a 26,000 dalton species, presumed to be the primary translational product, was observed under reducing conditions. These findings implied that the putative upstream exon sequences served to initiate translation of a PDGF-2 precursor molecule, which underwent dimer formation and subsequent processing. In light of our knowledge that the human *sis* gene codes for PDGF-2 and our findings of highly efficient transforming activity by the construct, we conclude that normal PDGF-2 expressed in NIH/3T3 cells is sufficient to induce transformation.

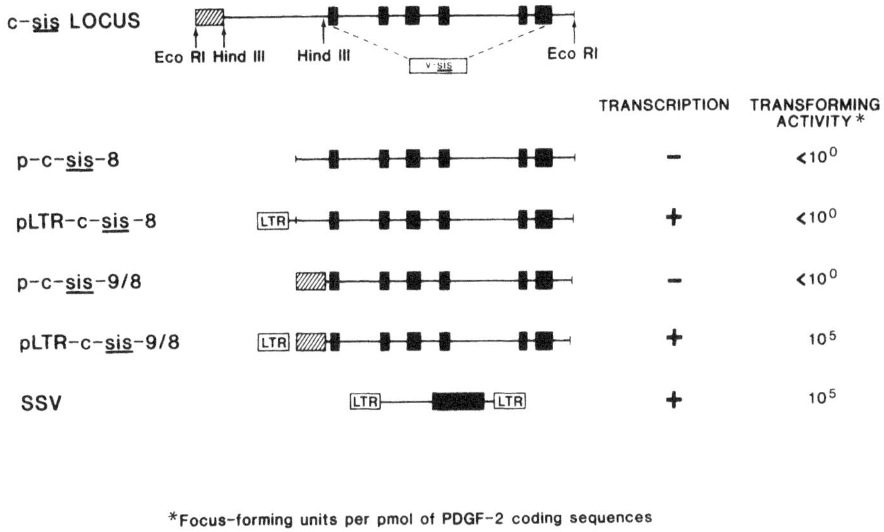

FIGURE 3. Expression of the normal PDGF-2 coding sequence induces morphologic transformation. Genomic DNA molecules cloned in plasmid vectors were transfected into NIH/3T3 cells and tested for transcriptional activation and transforming activity. Black boxes represent c-sis coding exons related to v-sis. Hatched box represents upstream c-sis exon not related to v-sis. LTR, retrovirus long terminal repeat.

DISCUSSION

It still remains to be determined whether the transforming PDGF-2 molecule functions exactly as does normal PDGF. Reduced forms of human PDGF contain another related polypeptide, PDGF-1 (25, 24). Thus, biologically active PDGF may be comprised of PDGF-1 and PDGF-2 homodimers, heterodimers or a mixture of the two. Efforts are underway to compare the structure and biologic properties of the processed forms of the human sis/PDGF-2 transforming gene product with that of dimers found in native PDGF preparations. Moreover, cloning of the human gene for PDGF-1 should allow direct investigation as to whether PDGF-1 may modulate PDGF-2 transforming activity or itself demonstrate transforming properties.

Our studies have potentially important implications concerning the role of normal genes coding for growth regulatory molecules in the neoplastic process. A number of growth promoting molecules have been shown to be released by a variety of tumor cells (37, 38, 39, 40). In some cases, such molecules have been postulated to play a role in the neoplastic state of these cells. However, the alternative possibility exists that the expression of such factors is a secondary result of the genetic instability and dedifferentiated state known to exist in tumor cells.

Our present findings establish that derepression of the coding sequence for a normal human growth factor can cause it to acquire transforming properties in an appropriate target cell. Moreover, when incorporated by a retrovirus, the v-*sis*/PDGF-2 transforming gene has been shown to induce fibrosarcomas and glioblastomas (5; our unpublished observations). Many human glioblastomas and fibrosarcomas express *sis*/PDGF-2 transcripts (34), whereas normal fibroblasts and glial cells so far analyzed do not (34; our unpublished observations). Thus, transcriptional activation of this gene could be involved in the induction of naturally occurring tumors of connective tissue origin. If so, it will be important to gain more detailed knowledge of the regulation of the human *sis* proto-oncogene in order to determine what mechanisms may lead to its transcriptional activation.

REFERENCES

1. Maxam AM, Gilbert W: A new method for sequencing DNA. Proc Natl Acad Sci USA (74): 560-564, 1977.
2. Barbacid M, Lauver AL, Devare SG: Biochemical and immunological characterization of polyproteins coded for by the McDonough, Gardner-Arnstein, and Snyder-Theilen strains of feline sarcoma virus. J Virol (33): 196-207, 1980.
3. Theilen GH, Gould D, Fowler M, Dungworth DL: C-type virus in tumor tissue of a woolly monkey (*Lagothrix spp*.) with fibrosarcoma. J Natl Cancer Inst (47): 881-899, 1971.
4. Aaronson SA: Biologic characterization of mammalian cells transformed by a primate sarcoma virus. Virol (52): 562-567, 1973.
5. Wolfe LG, Deinhardt F, Theilen GJ, Rabin H, Kawakami T, Bustad LK: Induction of tumors in marmoset monkeys by simian sarcoma virus, type 1 (*lagothrix*), a preliminary report. J Natl Cancer Inst (47): 1115-1120, 1971.

6. Wolfe LG, Smith RK, Dienhardt F: Simian sarcoma virus type 1 (lagothrix): Focus assay and demonstration of nontransforming associated virus. J Natl Cancer Inst (48): 1905-1907, 1972.
7. Robbins KC, Devare SG, Aaronson SA: Molecular cloning of integrated simian sarcoma virus: Genome organization of infectious DNA clones. Proc Natl Acad Sci USA (78): 2918-2922, 1981.
8. Robbins KC, Devare SG, Reddy EP, Aaronson SA: In vivo identification of the transforming gene product of simian sarcoma virus. Science (218): 1131-1133, 1982.
9. Robbins KC, Hill RL, Aaronson SA: Primate origin of the cell-derived sequences of simian sarcoma virus. J Virol (41): 721-725, 1982.
10. Devare SG, Reddy EP, Law JD, Robbins KC, Aaronson SA: Nucleotide sequence of the siman sarcoma virus genome: Demonstration that its acquired cellular sequences encode the transforming gene product, $p28^{sis}$. Proc Natl Acad Sci USA (80): 731-735, 1983.
11. Shinnick TM, Lerner RA, Sutcliffe JG: Nucleotide sequence of Moloney murine leukemia virus. Nature (293): 543-548, 1981.
12. Shilo BZ, Weinberg RA: DNA sequences homologous to vertebrate oncogenes are conserved in Drosophila melanogaster. Proc Natl Acad Sci USA (78): 6789-6792, 1981.
13. DeFeo-Jones D, Scolnick EM, Koller R, Dhar R: Ras-related gene sequences identified and isolated from Saccharomyces cerevisiae. Nature (306): 707-709, 1983.
14. Collet MS, Erickson RL: Protein kinase activity associated with the avian sarcoma virus src gene product. Proc Natl Acad Sci USA (75): 2021-2084, 1978.
15. Levinson AD, Opperman H, Levintow L, Varmus HE, Bishop JM: Evidence that the transforming gene of avian sarcoma virus encodes a protein kinase aasociated with a phosphoprotein. Cell (15): 561-572, 1978.
16. Hunter T, Sefton BM: Transforming gene product of Rous sarcoma virus phosphorylates tyrosine. Proc Natl Acad Sci USA (77): 1311-1315, 1980.
17. Bishop JM: In: Snell EE, Boyer PD, Meister A, Richardson CC (eds) Ann Rev Biochemistry 52. Academic Press, Palo Alto, 1983, pp 301-354.
18. Scolnick EM, Papageorge AG, Shih TY: Guanine nucleotide-binding activity as an assay for src protein of rat-derived murine sarcoma viruses. Proc Natl Acad Sci USA (76): 5355-5359, 1979.
19. Alitalo K, Ramsay G, Bishop JM, Pfeifer SO, Colby WW, Levinson AD: Identification of nuclear proteins encoded by viral and cellular myc oncogenes. Nature (306): 274-277, 1983.
20. Hann SR, Abrams HD, Rohrschneider LR, Eisenman RN: Proteins encoded by v-myc and c-myc oncogenes: Identification and localization in acute leukemia virus transformants and bursal lymphoma cell lines. Cell (34): 789-798, 1983.
21. Curran T, Miller AD, Zokas L, Verma IM: Viral and cellular fos proteins: A comparative analysis. Cell (36): 259-268, 1984.
22. Wilbur WJ, Lipman DJ: Rapid similarity searches of nucleic acid and protein data banks. Proc Natl Acad Sci USA (80): 726-730, 1983.
23. Doolittle RF, Hunkapiller MW, Hood LE, Devare SG, Robbins KC, Aaronson SA, Antoniades HN: Simian sarcoma virus onc gene, v-sis, is derived from the gene (or genes) encoding a platelet-derived growth factor. Science (221): 275-277, 1983.
24. Waterfield MD, Scrace GT, Whittle N, Stroobant P, Johnsson A, Wasteson A, Westermark B, Heldin CH, Huang JS, Deuel TF: Platelet-derived growth factor is structurally related to the putative transforming protein $p28^{sis}$ of simian sarcoma virus. Nature (304): 35-39, 1983.

25. Antoniades HN, Hunkapiller MW: Human platelet-derived growth factor (PDGF): Amino terminal amino acid sequence. Science (220): 963-965, 1983.
26. Wilson AC, Carlson SS, White TJ: Biochemical evolution. Ann Rev Biochem (46): 573-639, 1977.
27. Robbins KC, Antoniades HN, Devare SG, Hunkapiller MW, Aaronson SA: Structural and immunological similarities between simian sarcoma virus gene product(s) and human platelet-derived growth factor. Nature (305): 605-608, 1983.
28. Antoniades HN, Scher CD, Stiles CD: Purification of human platelet-derived growth factor. Proc Natl Acad Sci USA (76): 1809-1813, 1979.
29. Heldin CH, Westermark B, Wasteson A: Demonstration of antibody against platelet-derived growth factor. Exp Cell Res (136): 255-261, 1981.
30. Deuel TF, Huang JS, Proffit RT, Baenziger UU, Chang D, and Kennedey BB: Human platelet-derived growth factor. Purification and resolution into two active protein fractions. J Biol Chem (256): 8896-8899, 1981.
31. Raines EW, Ross R: Platelet-derived growth factor I. High yield purification and evidence for multiple forms. J Biol Chem (257): 5154-5160, 1981.
32. Chiu I-M, Reddy EP, Givol D, Robbins KC, Tronick SR, Aaronson SA: Nucleotide sequence analysis identifies the human c-sis proto-oncogene as a structural gene for platelet-derived growth factor. Cell (37): 123-129, 1984.
33. Josephs SF, Dalla Favera R, Gelmann EP, Gallo RC, Wong-Staal F: 5' viral and human cellular sequences corresponding to the transforming gene of simian sarcoma virus. Science (219): 503-505, 1983.
34. Eva A, Robbins KC, Andersen PR, Srinivasan A, Tronick SR, Reddy EP, Ellmore NW, Galen AT, Lautenberger JA, Papas TS, Westin EH, Wong-Staal F, Gallo RC, Aaronson SA: Cellular genes analogous to retroviral onc genes are transcribed in human tumor cells. Nature (295): 116-119, 1982.
35. Josephs SF, Guo C, Ratner L, Wong-Staal F: Human proto-oncogene nucleotide sequences corresponding to the transforming region of simian sarcoma virus. Science (223): 487-491, 1984.
36. Johnsson A, Heldin, C-H, Wasteson, A, Westermark, B, Deuel, TF, Huang, JS, Seeburg, PH, Gray, A, Ullrich, A, Scrace, G, Stroobant, H, Waterfield, MD: The c-sis gene encodes a precursor of the B chain of platelet-derived growth factor. EMBO J (3): 921-928, 1984.
37. De Larco JE, Todaro GJ: Growth factors from murine sarcoma virus-transformed cells. Proc Natl Acad Sci USA (75): 4001-4005, 1978.
38. Heldin CH, Westermark B, Wasteson A: Chemical and biological properties of a growth factor from human-cultured osteosarcoma cells: Resemblance with platelet-derived growth factor. J Cell Phys (105): 235-246, 1980.
39. Nister M, Heldin CH, Wateson A, Westermark B: A platelet-derived growth factor analog produced by a human clonal glioma cell line. Ann NY Acad Sci (397): 25-33, 1982.
40. Graves DT, Owen AJ, Antoniades HN: Evidence that a human osteosarcoma cell line which secretes a mitogen similar to platelet-derived growth factor requires growth factors present in platelet-poor plasma. Cancer Res (43): 83-87, 1983.

6

CELL CYCLE CONTROL OF C-MYC EXPRESSION

KATHLEEN KELLY, BRENT COCHRAN, CHARLES STILES AND PHILIP LEDER

Immunology Branch, National Cancer Institute, Bethesda, Maryland
Harvard Medical School, Boston, Massachusetts

1. ABSTRACT

c-myc mRNA is a cell-cycle associated transcript whose induction is regulated by agents that initiate the first phase of a proliferative response. Specifically, c-myc mRNA levels are increased between 10 and 40 fold within one to three hours after incubation of lymphocytes with lipopolysaccharide or Concanavalin A or fibroblasts with platelet-derived growth factor (PDGF). This induction of c-myc does not require the synthesis of new protein species and therefore is regulated directly by the biochemical events that immediately follow PDGF binding in fibroblasts and mitogen binding in lymphocytes. Thus, the c-myc oncogene encodes a product which may function as an intracellular mediator of the growth response to mitogens. PDGF is the putative translation product of the sis gene. The product of the v-sis gene, obtained as a supernatant from v-sis transfected NRK cells, induces c-myc expression in quiescent BALB/c 3T3 cells. Also, v-sis transfected BALB/c 3T3 cells display induced levels of c-myc mRNA following prolonged incubation in platelet poor plasma. Thus, oncogenes may be linked in functional hierarchies: the product of one oncogene, sis, regulates the expression of a cellular proto-oncogene, c-myc.

2. INTRODUCTION

Viral oncogenes act as dominant growth transforming agents, and in some cases, somatically-altered cellular proto-oncogenes also transform certain cells to tumorigenicity (1,2). It seems likely that some oncogenes may deregulate normal proliferation by acting at control points in the cell cycle. Growth control is governed by growth factors that exert their effect in the G1 phase of the cell cycle (3). In fibroblasts, two control points have been defined that are regulated by either platelet derived growth factor (PDGF) or epidermal growth factor (EGF) and the somatomedins.

PDGF has been shown to act in the initial competence phase of G1, while EGF and somatomedins are required for the progression of cells through a later stage in G1 (4,5), see Table I. Thus, the identification of two oncogenes, sis and erb B, as the structural gene for PDGF II (6,7) and a truncated EGF receptor-like gene (8), respectively, lends strong support to the idea that at least some oncogenes mediate their effects by deregulating control of the cell cycle.

The metabolic pathway(s) regulated by growth signals are of significance in considering the physiological action of oncogenes. In this paper we consider the c-myc gene, identified originally as the cellular homolog of the transforming determinant carried by avian MC 29 virus. We asked whether normal c-myc expression is regulated in relation to the cell cycle as a function of growth signals. In order to test such a possibility, we analyzed the temporal expression of c-myc mRNA in three types of quiescent cells that can be stimulated to growth by mitogens.

The three systems that we have utilized are lipopolysaccharide (LPS) activated B cells, Concanavalin A (Con A) activated T cells and PDGF stimulated fibroblasts. By analogy to the previously discussed growth requirements of fibroblasts, lymphocytes also appear to require two temporally separated signals in order to transit from a quiescent state to DNA synthesis (Table I). The first signal is mediated in T cells via

Table I. Cell cycle progression requires multiple signals

	Signal 1 (Competence)	Signal 2 (Progression)
Fibroblasts	Platelet-derived growth factor	Epidermal growth factor
	Fibroblast growth factor	Somatomedins/Insulin
	Phorbol esters	Platelet-poor plasma
T Lymphocytes	Concanavalin A	Interleukin 2
	Phytohemmaglutinin	
B Lymphocytes	Anti-immunoglobulins	B cell stimulating factors
	LPS	

a lectin-receptor interaction (9,10), and the second signal can be replaced by the T cell-specific growth factor, interleukin 2 (11). Although LPS activation of B cells does not require any additional comitogens, indirect evidence suggests that LPS stimulates proliferation by the delivery of two separate signals to B cells (12, 13). In addition, it has been shown in B lymphocytes primed with anti-immunoglobulin reagents that T cell-derived, B cell stimulating factors are subsequently required for entry into S phase (14).

Our results show that c-myc mRNA is strongly induced in several different cells by agents that initiate the first phase of a proliferative response. Enhanced c-myc expression occurs very soon following the activation of T lymphocytes with Con A, B lymphocytes with LPS and 3T3 cells with PDGF. By contrast, c-myc mRNA is not induced following EGF or insulin/somatomedin treatment of quiescent 3T3 cells. Thus, c-myc is an inducible gene that is shown to be modulated by a specific type of growth signal and expressed in a cell cycle dependent manner.

3. RESULTS

3.1. Transient Induction of c-myc mRNA in B Lymphocytes

In order to investigate the role of c-myc in normal lymphocyte proliferation, resting spleen cells were stimulated with the B cell specific mitogen, LPS, or the T cell specific mitogen, Con A. To look at the possible cell cycle associated expression of c-myc, aliquots of splenic lymphocytes were harvested at various times following the addition of polyclonal mitogens. A constant amount of total RNA, extracted from the various cell aliquots, was analyzed for c-myc RNA by an S1 nuclease assay.

A representative experiment showing the temporal expression of c-myc mRNA following LPS stimulation of B cells is seen in Figure 1A. c-myc mRNA is induced approximately 20-fold between one and two hours after addition of LPS to lymphocyte cultures. As shown by the incorporation of tritiated uridine and tritiated thymidine, the increase in c-myc expression precedes by 6 hours general increases in RNA synthesis associated with cell enlargement and precedes by 13 hours the onset of replicative DNA synthesis (15). c-myc mRNA levels peak between 2 and 9 hours, remain at an induced level for approximately 48 hours, and subsequently drop to near background levels. Qualitatively and quantitatively similar results for c-myc induction have been found following the stimulation of spleen cells by the T cell-specific mitogen, Con A (15). The asynchrony of mitogen-stimulated lymphocytes in the late G1 phase of the cell cycle (16) precludes any conclusions concerning the subsequent relative levels of c-myc mRNA following early G1 induction.

To control for the relative amount of mRNA in each sample, aliquots of total RNA were analyzed for beta-2 microglobulin mRNA by the S1 nuclease assay. As shown in Figure 1B, beta-2 microblobulin mRNA remains nearly constant relative to total RNA throughout the course of LPS-induced proliferation.

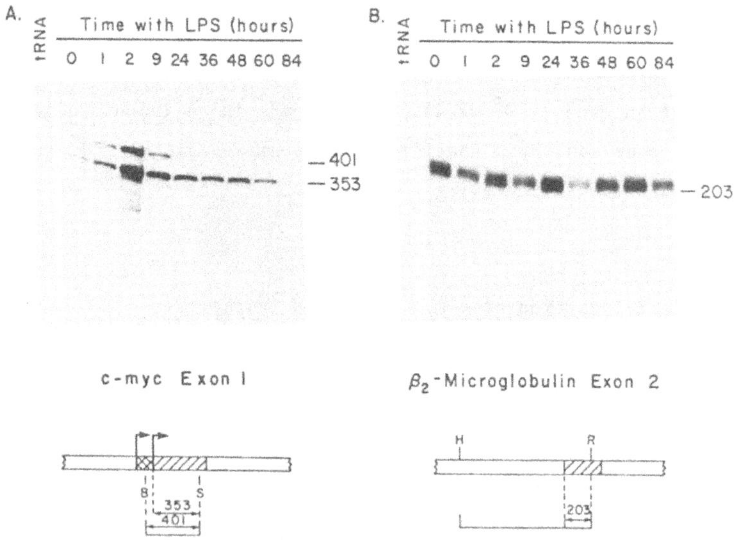

FIGURE 1. c-myc mRNA expression is enhanced in LPS-treated B cells. A. S1 nuclease analyses were performed on RNA samples extracted from spleen cell cultures stimulated for the indicated times with LPS. A uniformly-labeled, single-stranded c-myc probe was utilized. Ten micrograms of total RNA from each sample were analyzed. The expected S1-nuclease resistant DNA products are shown in the diagram below the figure. The map position of the 5' boundary of the c-myc clone, relative to the two promotor regions, is indicated. The S1-resistant products are displayed on a 5% denaturing polyacrylamide gel. Size determinations were made relative to radioactive phosphate-end labeled molecular weight markers (HinfI-digested pBR327). The control tRNA lane shows the result when the appropriate amount of probe is incubated with 10 micrograms of tRNA and digested with S1 nuclease. Unstimulated spleen cells cultured for various lengths of time (up to 84 hours) showed no variation in the amount of c-myc mRNA that was expressed. B. The amounts of beta-2 microglobulin mRNA contained in parallel identical samples relative to those shown in panel A were determined by S1 nuclease protection of a uniformly-labeled beta-2 microglobulin probe. The differing GC contents of the c-myc and beta-2 microglobulin probes preclude their hybridization in a single sample. The expected S1-nuclease resistant DNA product is shown in the diagram below the figure. All other experimental details are identical to those described in part A.

3.2. PDGF-Mediated Induction of c-myc mRNA in 3T3 cells

The observation that c-myc mRNA levels dramatically increase promptly after the delivery of a proliferation signal to resting lymphocytes suggests that c-myc expression may be an important component in controlling the transit of cells through the cell cycle. Since there are parallels between the proliferative response of resting lymphocytes to mitogens and quiescent fibroblasts to growth factors, we have analyzed c-myc expression in quiescent and growth factor-treated 3T3 cells.

Density arrested monolayers of BALB/c 3T3 cells were incubated overnight in medium supplemented with platelet-poor plasma which lacks PDGF. The cultures were then exposed to PDGF, EGF, insulin or platelet poor plasma. High concentrations of insulin will substitute for somatomedins in promoting 3T3 cell growth, and platelet poor plasma contains both EGF-like and somatomedin-like growth factors (4). Total RNA was extracted from cell monolayers harvested after 3 hours in the presence of growth factors. The amount of c-myc mRNA detected by S1 nuclease analyses of a constant amount of RNA from the various samples is shown in Figure 2A. Quiescent fibroblasts have almost undetectable levels of c-myc mRNA. c-myc mRNA is induced approximately 40-fold after 3 hours in fibroblasts treated with either crude or electrophoretically homogeneous PDGF. Consistent with the role of growth factors required late rather than early in a mitogenic response, EGF, and insulin alone have virtually no effect on the induction of c-myc mRNA (Fig. 2A). Agents such as fibroblast growth factor (FGF) and TPA that mimic PDGF action (4) also stimulate c-myc mRNA expression (Figs. 2A and 2B). In contrast to the variability of c-myc mRNA detected in samples from growth factor treated cells, the amount of beta-2 microglobulin mRNA in parallel samples remains relatively constant (Fig. 2C).

As discussed earlier, PDGF II is the translation product of the sis gene (6,7). Therefore, we have assayed in two ways the effect of the v-sis gene product on c-myc expression of fibroblasts. Firstly, supernatants from v-sis transfected NRK cells (17) were substituted for PDGF in the protocol described for Fig. 2. Secondly, v-sis transfected BALB/c 3T3 cells were grown to confluence, incubated overnight in 5% platelet poor plasma and subsequently assayed for c-myc expression.

In both experiments, c-myc mRNA levels were found to be comparable to those found after a 3 hour incubation of quiescent BALB/c 3T3 cells with optimum concentrations of PDGF (data not shown). Therefore, we have directly shown that the product of one oncogene, v-sis, regulates the expression of a cellular proto-oncogene, c-myc.

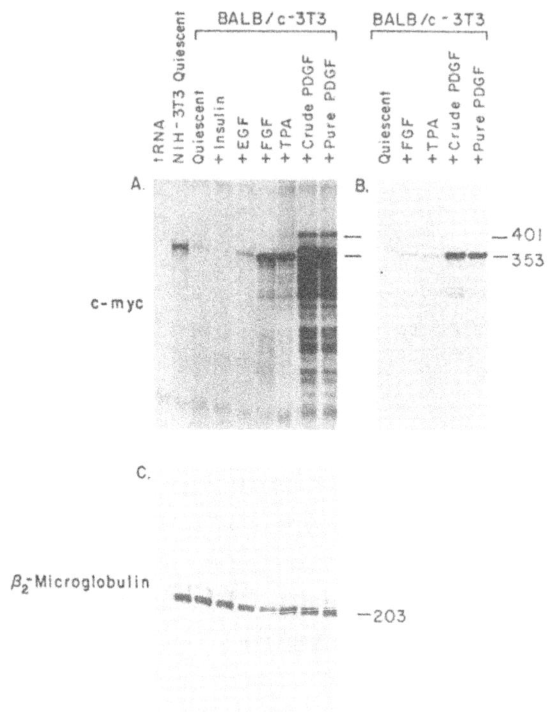

FIGURE 2. c-myc mRNA is induced in quiescent 3T3 cells by PDGF, FGF, and TPA. A. S1 nuclease analyses were performed on RNA samples extracted from quiescent BALB/c-3T3 cells, quiescent NIH-3T3 cells, and quiescent BALB/c-3T3 cells treated for 3 hours with partially-purified PDGF, 38 ng/ml electrophoretically pure PDGF, 100 ng/ml EGF, 10 microgram/ml insulin, 100 ng/ml FGF, 250 ng/ml TPA and 5% platelet poor plasma. The c-myc probe utilized is as described in the legend to Fig. 1A. No induction of c-myc mRNA was observed in the legend to Fig. 1A. No induction of c-myc mRNA was observed with 5% platelet poor plasma (not shown). The control tRNA lane displays the nonspecific background following S1 nuclease digestion of the labeled c-myc probe which is observed in the absence of homologous c-myc mRNA. B. Panel B is an approximately ten-fold shorter exposure of the indicated lanes from panel A. C. Parallel samples to those shown in Fig. 2A were analyzed for beta-2 microglobulin mRNA as previously described.

4. DISCUSSION

The induction of c-myc mRNA is regulated in fibroblasts by agents (PDGF, TPA, FGF) which induce competence, the initial priming step for progression through G1. Thus c-myc mRNA increases very early in G0/G1 after incubation of quiescent fibroblasts with PDGF. By analogy, c-myc mRNA is induced within 2 hours after the treatment of lymphocytes with Con A or LPS. Polyclonal mitogens are known to either directly or indirectly mediate more than one growth signal (see Introduction). However, the kinetics of c-myc induction in lymphocytes implies that the myc gene is regulated by the first signal of mitogen binding, a signal which is likely to be comparable to antigen binding to its matching receptor. In addition, c-myc mRNA is induced in the presence of protein synthesis inhibitors (15). Thus, the c-myc gene appears to be regulated directly by those biochemical events which immediately follow PDGF binding in fibroblasts and mitogen binding in lymphocytes. The product encoded by c-myc is a nuclear protein (18). Perhaps the c-myc protein is required as a nuclear mediator of the mitogenic response.

How is c-myc regulated with the cell cycle in continuously-proliferating cells? In fibroblasts that have been synchronized with respect to the cell cycle by a short incubation in PDGF, c-myc mRNA levels are maximal in early G0/G1 and diminish to a quiescent level by the time the cells enter S phase (19). Cells pulsed with PDGF, however, will not undergo a subsequent round of proliferation. By contrast, continuously-proliferating IL-2 dependent normal T lymphocytes, separated by centrifugal elutriation into fractions of cells within early G1, late G1, or S+G2+M show virtually identical steady-state levels of c-myc throughout the cell cycle (K. Kelly, manuscript in preparation). In addition, it has been demonstrated in a variety of cell types, that induction of differentiation and accompanying inhibition of proliferation is associated with decreases in steady-state levels of c-myc mRNA (20,21). Diminished c-myc mRNA levels preceed decreases in the number of cells in the S+G2+M phase of the cell cycle. Thus, the presence of c-myc mRNA is not required for progression through the S phase. It becomes important to determine the fluctuation of c-myc protein levels relative to the cell cycle. An interesting possibility is that the level of c-myc mRNA expressed during S phase is an important signal for determining subsequent entry into the quiescent G0 state or the active cycling G1 state. Perhaps temporal deregulation of c-myc expression may be important in considering the role of c-myc in malignant transformation.

The fundamental role of growth factors in regulating the control of normal proliferation is well established. Although the physiological consequences of growth factor-receptor interactions are largely unknown, the identification of the sis and erb B genes as a growth factor and an altered growth factor receptor, respectively, suggests a mechanism of action associated with normal cell cycle restriction or control points. This idea is further strengthened by the identification of the c-myc gene as a cell cycle associated transcript whose expression is regulated by competence factors. Importantly, this work then links the action of two oncogenes, sis and myc. It is tempting to speculate that yet another class of oncogenes may be added to his hierarchy that disrupts normal proliferation control by acting upon those physiological pathways which mediate the signals between cell surface growth factor receptors and the expression of genes required for cell cycle progression.

5. REFERENCES

1. Bishop JM: Cellular oncogenes and retroviruses. Ann Rev Biochem (52):301-354. 1983.
2. Cooper GM: Cellular transforming genes. Science (217):801-806. 1982.
3. Pardee AB, Dubrow R, Hamlin JL, Kletzien RF: Animal cell cycle. Ann Rev Biochem (47):715-750. 1978.
4. Stiles CD, Capone GT, Scher CD, Antoniades HN, Van Wyk JJ, Pledger WJ: Dual control of cell growth by somatomedins and platelet-derived growth factor. Proc Natl Acad Sci USA (76):1279-1283. 1979.
5. Leof EB, Wharton W, Van Why JJ, Pledger WJ: Epidermal drowth factor and somatomedin C regulate G1 progression in competent BALB/c-3T3 cells. Exp Cell Res (141):107-115. 1982.
6. Doolitte RF, Hunkapiller MW, Hood, LE Devare SG, Robbins KC, Aaronson SA, Antoniades HN: Simian sarcoma virus onc gene, v-sis, is derived from the gene (or genes) encoding a platelet-derived growth factor. Science (221):275-277. 1983.
7. Waterfield, MD, Scrace GT, Whittle N, Stroobant P, Johnson A, Wasteson A, Westermark B, Heldin CH, Huang JS, Deuel TF. Platelet-derived growth factor is structurally related to the putative transforming protein $p28^{sis}$ of simian sarcoma virus. Nature (304): 35-39. 1983.
8. Downward J, Yarden Y, Mayes E, Scrace G, Fotty N, Stockwell G, Ullrich A, Schlessinger J, Waterfield MD: Close similarity of epidermal growth factor receptor and v-erbB oncogenic protein sequences. Nature (307):521-527. 1984.

9. Larsson EL, Coutinho A: The role of mitogenic lectins in T cell triggering. Nature (304):596-602. 1979.
10. Hall DJ, O'Leary JJ, Sand TT, Rosenberg A: Commitment and proliferation kinetics of human lymphocytes stimulated in vitro: effects of alpha-MM addition and suboptimal dose on concanavalin A response. J Cell Physiol (108):25-34. 1981.
11. Maizel AL, Mehta SR, Hauft S, Franzini D, Lachman L, Ford RJ. Human T lymphocyte/monocytic interaction in response to lectin: kinetics of entry into the S-phase. J Immunol (127):1058-1064. 1981.
12. Bretscher PA: The two signal-model for B-cell induction. Transpl Rev (23):37-48. 1975.
13. DeFranco AL, Kung JT, Paul WE: Regulation of growth and proliferation in B cell populations. Immunological Rev (64):161-182. 1982.
14. Howard M, Nakanishi K, Paul W: B cell growth and differentiation factors. Immunol Rev (78):185-210. 1984.
15. Kelly K, Cochran BH, Stiles CD, Leder P: Cell-specific regulation of the c-myc gene by lymphocyte mitogens and platelet-derived growth factor. Cell (35):603-610. 1983.
16. Cantrell DA, Smith KA: Transient expression of interleukin 2 receptors: consequences for T cell growth. J Exp Med (158):1895-1911. 1983.
17. Devare SG, Reddy EP, Law KD, Robbins KC, Aaronson SA: Nucleotide sequence of the simian sarcoma virus genome: demonstration that its acquired cellular sequences encode the transforming gene product $p28^{sis}$. Proc Natl Acad Sci USA (80):731-735. 1983.
18. Hann SR, Abrams HD, Rohrschneider LR, Eisenman RN: Proteins encoded by v-myc and c-myc oncogenes: identification and localization in acute leukemia virus transformants and bursal lymphoma cell lines. Cell (34):789-798. 1983.
19. Kelly K, Cochran B, Stiles C, Leder P: The regulation of c-myc by growth signals. In: Melchers F and Potter M (eds) Second NCI International Workshop of B cell Neoplasia. Springer-Verlag. 1984 (in press).
20. Reitsma PH, Rothberg PG, Astrin SM, Trial J, Bar-Shavit Z, Hall A, Teitelbaum SL, Kahn AJ: Regulation of myc gene expression in HL-60 leukemia cells by a vitamin D metabolite. Nature (306): 492-494. 1983.
21. Jonak GJ, Knight, Jr. E: Selective reduction of c-myc mRNA in Daudi cells by human B interferon. Proc Natl Acad Sci USA (81): 1747-1750. 1984.

7

A NEW CLASS OF HUMAN ENDOGENOUS RETROVIRAL GENES

Robert Callahan, Ing-Ming Chiu, Toby Horn, Igbal Ali, Joan Robbins, Stuart Aaronson and Jeffrey Schlom

National Cancer Institute, Bethesda, Maryland

1. INTRODUCTION

Several factors have been implicated in the etiology of human breast cancer. The potential involvement of members of the Retroviridae family of viruses has represented a major focus of investigation (1 for review). This is primarily a result of studies of mammary cancer in laboratory mice, where infectious type-B oncoviruses (mouse mammary tumor virus, MMTV) have been shown to be associated with a high incidence of mammary tumors. With the exception of species of the genus *Mus* (2,3) and *Rattus* (4), attempts to identify DNA sequences related to the MMTV genome in DNAs of all other mammalian species tested have not been consistently successful (5,6). Other studies (7,8), using liquid hybridization and MMTV cDNA probes, reported the presence of RNA species, in human mammary tumors, related to the viral genome. The lack of uniform probes, the potential for contamination of cDNA preparations with cellular DNA or RNA, and the relative lack of sensitivity of liquid hybridization techniques made these findings difficult to interpret.

The availability of molecularly cloned MMTV genomic DNA and the increased sensitivity of the blot-hybridization technique for analysis of restriction endonuclease digests of DNA led us to reexamine the possibility of MMTV related sequences in human cellular DNA. We found that by lowering the stringency of blot-hybridization, molecularly cloned MMTV proviral DNA reacts with restriction fragments of human cellular DNA. Using this approach, we isolated several recombinant clones from a library of human cellular DNA which hybridize to the MMTV genome (9). Recently, it has been possible to demonstrate that within some of these human recombinant clones the MMTV related sequences are organized in a manner consistent with genetically transmitted (or endogenous) proviral genomes (Callahan et al., manuscript in preparation).

In recent years, efforts have been made to ascertain the evolutionary relationships among different oncovirus genera. One of the most useful approaches has involved the demonstration of shared antigenic determinants in their translational products. The detection of immunological relatedness between the major structural proteins of type B and D viruses, as well as between mammalian type C and D viruses, has suggested that evolutionary links may exist among these three major oncovirus genera (10). Using low stringency blot hybridization and nucleotide sequence analysis, we have established the existence of two major *pol* gene families in the evolution of oncoviruses (11). One family consists of mammalian type C viruses. Two laboratories have recently demonstrated human endogenous oncoviral sequences which are related to known mammalian type C viruses (12,13). The second *pol* gene family consists of type A, B,D and avian type C viruses. In this article we review the evidence for MMTV related sequences in human cellular DNA and summarize our results which establish this class of human oncoviral genomes as members of the second *pol* gene family.

2. RESULTS AND DISCUSSION

2.1 Identification of MMTV related sequences in human cellular DNA

Previous attempts to identify MMTV related sequences in human cellular DNA have been hampered by the lack of sensitivity of the techniques used, and by the potential for contamination of the viral cDNA probe with non-viral sequences. We have sought to circumvent these problems by using the more sensitive blot-hybridization technique, and cloned MMTV proviral DNA as a probe. Preliminary attempts to detect MMTV related sequences in *PstI*, *EcoRI*, and *BamHI* restricted human cellular DNA using stringent conditions for blot-hybridization were unsuccessful. Using less stringent hybridization conditions, labeled MMTV Rep probe detected four major bands (3.7, 3.5, 2.9, and 1.9kbp), as well as other less intense bands (2.1, 1.8, 1.6, and 1.4kbp) in *EcoRI* restricted human breast tumor and normal cellular DNAs (Figure 1A, lanes a and d). *EcoRI* res-

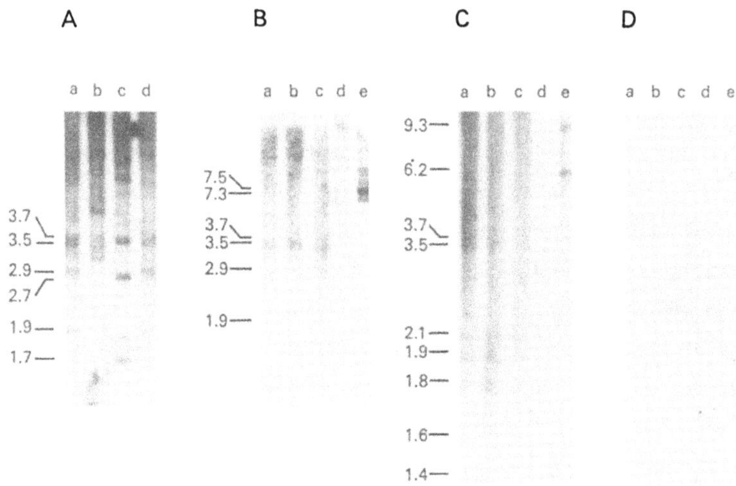

FIGURE 1. Identification and characterization of type-B proviral sequences in EcoRI restricted human cellular DNAs. 10 μg. of EcoRI restricted DNA from normal or neoplastic cells was separated on 1% agarose gels, transferred to nitrocellulose filters, and hybridized at 54°C to the indicated ^{32}P-labeled probe. Panel A: Hybridization of cellular DNA to 5 x 10^7 cpm of MMTV 'Rep' DNA. Autoradiography was for 72 hrs. The cellular DNA was from: lane a, normal human spleen; lane b, mink lung tissue culture cells; lane c, rat kidney tissue culture cells; lane d, human mammary adenocarcinoma. Panel B: Hybridization of cellular DNA to 2 x 10^7 cpm of MMTV gag-pol DNA. Autoradiography was for 72 hrs. Cellular DNA was from: lane a, human mammary adenocarcinoma; lane b, human mammary adenocarcinoma metastatic to the liver; lane c, human spleen; lane d, salmon sperm; lane e, MMTV(C3H) infected feline CrFK cells; Panel C: Hybridization of cellular DNA with 2 x 10^7 cpm of MTV env DNA. Autoradiography was for 72 hrs. Cellular DNA was from: lane a, human mammary adenocarcinoma; lane b, human mammary adenocarcinoma metastatic to the liver; lane c, human placenta; lane d, salmon sperm; lane e, normal Balb/c liver. Panel D: The nitrocellulose filter used for the autoradiograph in Panel C was incubated for three 15 min rinses with 3XSSC at 65°C. Autoradiography was for 96 hrs. The DNA samples within each Panel (A-D) were run on the same gel.

tricted cellular DNAs, from rat kidney and mink lung tissue culture cells, each contained a unique pattern of MMTV related bands (Figure 1A, lanes b and c).

The specific regions of the MMTV provirus represented in the discrete EcoRI human bands were evaluated using subgenomic fragments, corresponding to the gag-pol, and env regions of the viral genome, as probes. The gag-pol probe reacts primarily with the 3.7 and 3.5kbp bands, and to a lesser extent with the 2.9 and 1.9kbp bands (Figure 1B, lanes a to c). The env probe (Fig. 1C, lanes a-c) reacts with five (2.1, 1.9, 1.8, 1.6 and 1.4kbp) restriction bands. Neither of the subgenomic MMTV probes reacts with salmon sperm DNA (Fig 1B, lane d; Fig. 1C, lane d).

In addition to the discrete restriction fragments detected with each of the subgenomic probes, a smear pattern of sequences (greater than 4kbp) reacting with the gag-pol and env probes was observed in high molecular weight human cellular DNA (lanes a to c of Fig. 1B and 1C). The thermal stability of the hybrids formed with the MMTV env probe was assessed to determine whether the MMTV probe could be selectively eluted off the unresolved high molecular weight DNA. The filter used for Figure 1C was washed in 3XSSC at higher temperatures. A 60°C wash eluted much of the hybridized MMTV env probe: however, there was no evidence that the unresolved hybrids in the high molecular weight DNA were selectively removed (data not shown). After a 65°C wash in 3XSSC, all of the env probe reacting with human cellular DNA was removed (Figure 1D, anes a to c), while the intensity of the Balb/c EcoRI bands were not significantly altered (Fig. 1D, lane e). Similar results were obtained using the MMTV Rep and MMTV gag-pol probes. This suggests that the Tm of the MMTV proviral - human DNA hybrids is between 54 and 60°C in 3XSSC.

These observations have been confirmed by Westin and May (14) and Sweet et al. (personal communication) using similar blot hybridization conditions. Recently, we (unpublished observations) and May et al. (14) have also detected sequences related to the long terminal repeat region (LTR) of the MMTV genome in restricted human cellular DNA. This is of particular interest since the MMTV LTR contains sequences which bind the glucocorticoid receptor protein making expression of the viral genome hormone dependent. The significance of this observation and its relevance to the known hormone responsiveness of many human breast tumors must await further analysis of human recombinant clones containing these sequences.

2.2 Isolation and characterization of recombinant clones containing MMTV related human DNA sequences.

A library of human fetal liver cellular DNA (15) in lambda Charon 4A (16), was screened for the presence of MMTV related sequences. The use of low stringency hybridization conditions led to the identification of 55 plaques, out of 5 x 10^5 plaques screened, which reacted specifically with labeled MMTV proviral DNA. One of these clones, designated HLM-2, was chosen for further study. A partial restriction map of HLM-2 DNA is shown in Figure 2. EcoRI restriction fragments of HLM-2 DNA were hybridized with labeled DNA probes representing the *gag*, *pol*, *env* and LTR regions of the MMTV genome. Most striking was the intensity with which the MMTV *pol* probe hybridized with the 3.7 kbp *EcoRI* fragment (Figure 3; lane b). Upon longer exposure, sequence homology is detectable between the MMTV *gag* probe and the 3.7 kbp *EcoRI* fragment (Figure 3, lane a), and between the MMTV *env* probe and the 8.0 and 1.8 kbp *EcoRI* fragments (Figure 3, lane c). The MMTV LTR probe did not hybridize specifically with HLM-2 DNA, nor with several other recombinant clones which did hybridize with MMTV proviral DNA.

The organization of the MMTV related sequences in HLM-2 DNA has been defined by additional restriction enzyme mapping using the MMTV *gag*, *pol*, and *env* probes, and is summarized in Figure 2. Two unexpected observations emerged from this analysis. First, two regions at the opposite ends of the HLM-2 DNA contain MMTV env related sequences. Second, the MMTV *pol* and *env* related sequences (on the right hand side of the map, Figure 2) are interrupted by non-MMTV related sequences which are repeated between map position 4 and 5 in the HLM-2 DNA.

Recently, we have analyzed several more MMTV related human recombinant clones by restriction enzyme and heteroduplex analysis (Callahan et al., manuscript in preparation). Two relevant observations emerged from this study. First, the human MMTV related sequences defined in HLM-2 are members of a highly diverged family of retroviral related sequences in human cellular DNA. This was demonstrated by the large number of restriction site polymorphisms observed between different clones and by heteroduplex analysis. Under stringent spreading conditions several combinations of recombinant clones showed no homology. As the spreading conditions were relaxed long stretches of homology were observed. In some cases deletion or insertion loops could be observed within a heteroduplex. Second, each of the recombinant clones contained

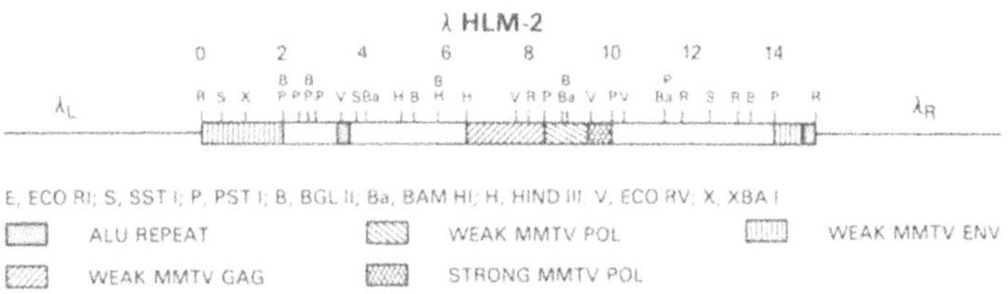

FIGURE 2. A partial restriction enzyme map of human recombinant clone HLM-2. The symbol λ_L and λ_R designate respectively the long and short arms of lambda Charon 4A. The restriction sites and regions of HLM-2 which contain MMTV related sequences are indicated.

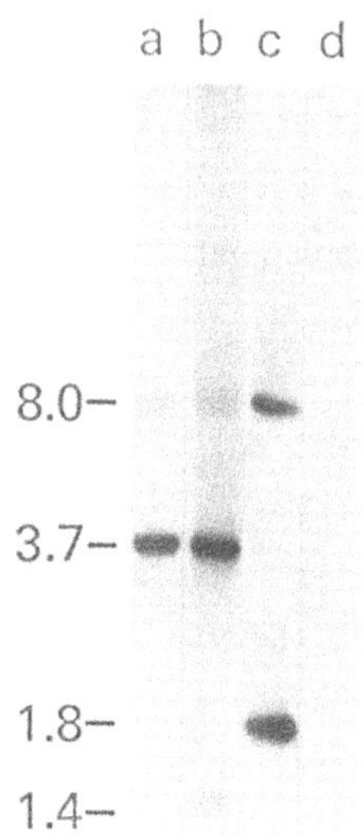

FIGURE 3. Identification of MMTV related sequences in EcoRI restricted human recombinant HLM-2 DNA. 0.3 μg of an equal molar mixture of EcoRI fragments (purified away from the λ arms) of HLM-2 was electrophoresed on a 0.8% agarose gel transferred to nitrocellulose filters, and blot hybridized using low stringency conditions with 2 x 10^7 cpm of ^{32}P labeled: a) MMTV *gag*; b) MMTV *pol*; c) MMTV *env*; and MMTV LTR proviral DNA. All lanes were blotted from the same gel. The filters were washed using low stringency conditions. Autoradiography for lanes a, c and d was 5 days and for lane b one day.

the repeat sequence observed in HLM-2. The sequence shares no homology with the *alu* family of repetitive sequences and was always found flanking the MMTV *gag-pol* related sequences. Based on these and other results we have speculated that the MMTV *gag* and *pol* related sequences in the human recombinant clones represent genetically transmitted or endogenous proviral genomes. The repeat sequences found in HLM-2 and the other MMTV related recombinant clones correspond to long terminal repeat sequences. Nucleotide sequence analysis of the HLM-2 repeats has shown that they are 88 percent related and contain transcription regulatory signal sequences (Callahan et al., manuscript in preparation). The large sequence diversity of the different recombinant clones suggests that in evolutionary terms, this family of oncoviral genes was not recently introduced into the human cellular genome.

2.3 Evolutionary relationships between different classes of oncoviruses

Oncoviruses (17) have been classified on the basis of their morphological properties (18,19). While four different genera are recognized (Table 1), viruses within the type A, B, and D virus genera share certain morphogenic and biochemical properties. Initially, defective intracisternal type A viral particles were observed in early mouse embryos and in certain murine tumors (20-24). Later studies revealed the existence of infectious retroviruses containing extensive homology to the A particle genome (25). Type C viruses, which are widely distributed among birds and mammals, have been shown to cause leukemia and other tumors. The most recently described type D oncoviruses appear limited to primate species, and their oncogenicity remains to be established (26). Earlier studies have shown that the major structural proteins encoded within the _gag_ gene of type C and D oncoviruses share antigenic determinants, as do the major proteins of type B, and D oncoviruses (10). Moreover, certain mammalian type C, and type D oncoviruses share common determinants in the _env_ coded gp70 protein (41-42), as well as sequence homology in their p15E coding region (43). These patterns of homology indicate that the evolution of present oncovirus groups involved genetic interactions among their progenitors.

We have analyzed the genetic relatedness of oncoviruses using low stringency blot hybridization conditions. The cloned viral DNAs studied include recombinant type A virus M432 (25); a type B virus (MMTV) (27); the mammalian type C viruses, Rauscher murine leukemia virus (R-MuLV) (28), Moloney murine leukemia virus (M-MuLV) (29,30), simian sarcoma associated virus (SSAV) (31,32), and baboon endogenous virus (BaEV) (33); avian type C viruses, Rous sarcoma virus (RSV) (34) and avian myeloblastosis associated virus (MAV) (35), and the type D Squirrel Monkey Retrovirus (SMRV) (36). As summarized in

Table 1. Comparative Morphological and Biochemical Properties of Infectious Type A, B, C, and D Oncoviruses

Characteristic	Type A	Type B	Type C		Type D
			avian	mammalian	
Prototypes	M432*	MMTV	RSV, MAV	MuLV, SSAV, BaEV	SMRV
Intracytoplasmic A-particles	-	+	-	-	+
Complete budding nucleoid	+	+	-	-	+
DNA Polymerase preferred cation	Mg++	Mg++	Mg++	Mn++	Mg++
Mature particle					
Nucleoid morphology	centric	eccentric	centric	centric	eccentric
Envelope spikes	NA	long with knobs	short	short	short
Hormone responsiveness of virus	no	yes	no	no	no

*M432 is an endogenous virus from *M. cervicolor* containing extensive sequence homology with type A intracisternal A particle (IAP) genes (25). There is no extracellular form of the IAP, with budding seen into endoplasmic reticulum.

Figure 4, reciprocal relationships were observed among each class of oncoviruses. A major region of homology could be demonstrated in the *pol* genes of type A, B, D and avian type C oncoviruses. These findings strongly imply genetic relatedness between the *pol* genes of representatives of the four major oncovirus genera. In contrast, when analogous studies were performed using mammalian type C viral DNAs, no *pol* gene homologies were observed. The relatedness of SMRV to other sequences in the mammalian type C oncoviral DNAs will be described below. In order to precisely assess the extent of homology between the *pol* genes of these oncoviruses, we undertook comparative nucleotide sequence analysis. The complete nucleotide sequences of RSV (37) and M-MuLV (38) *pol* genes, as well as the 3' terminal region of the MMTV *pol* (39) and SMRV *pol* genes (36), have been reported. The predicted amino acid sequences for the respective *pol* gene products were aligned by the PRTALN computer program of Wilbur and Lipman (40). As shown in Figure 5 within the region encompassing bp. 193 to bp. 303, 69% homology between SMRV and MMTV was observed. This probably accounts for the hybridization detected between SMRV and MMTV (Fig. 4). The predicted amino acid sequence homology in this region was as high as 70%. In the total of 540 bp displayed, there was 55% homology (296/540) between SMRV and MMTV <u>pol</u> genes without introducing any insertions or deletions. Nucleotide homology between SMRV and RSV, as well as between MMTV and RSV was about 46%. At the amino acid level, the homologies between SMRV and MMTV, MMTV and RSV, as well as SMRV and RSV were 52% and 38%, and 38% respectively.

A retrovirus designated human T-cell leukemia virus (HTLV) has been isolated from patients with certain forms of adult T-cell leukemia (44,45). Epidemiologic studies have implicated this agent in the etiology of such tumors (46). The functional characteristics of the HTLV polymerase have been reported to resemble those of A, B and D oncovirus, rather than mammalian type C

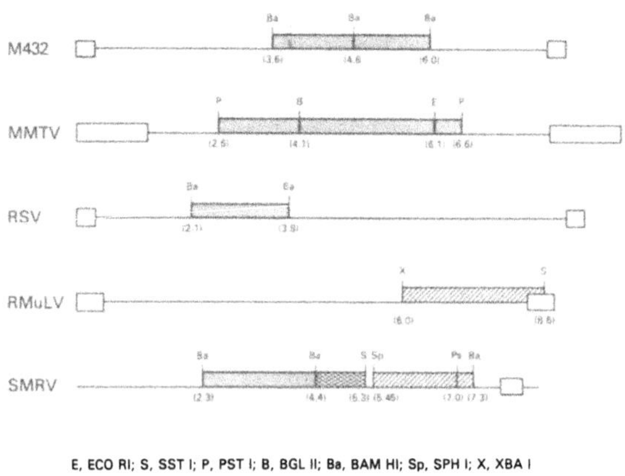

FIGURE 4. Regions of homology between prototypes of different oncovirus genera. Type A, B, D and avian type C <u>pol</u> related sequences as well as mammalian type C and D <u>env</u> related sequences were determined by reciprocal low stringency blot hybridization of restricted recombinant proviral DNA. The open boxes represent long terminal repeat sequences. The shaded boxes represent regions of homology between type A (M432), B (MMTV),(SMRV), and avian type C (RSV) oncoviruses. The cross hatched box represents type A, and B oncoviral related sequences in the SMRV (type D) viral genome. The hatched boxes represent related sequences in the <u>env</u> regions of the mammalian type C (RMuLV) and type D (SMRV) viral genomes.

viruses (47). Recently, the HTLV genome has been completely sequenced (48), making it possible to perform direct comparisons of its sequence to the corresponding regions of SMRV, MMTV and RSV pol genes. HTLV was found to possess significant homology with these sequences in the region between amino acids #57 and #171 (Fig. 5). The degrees of homology were 46%, 38%, and 39%, respectively, without introducing insertions or deletions. These studies establish, by both molecular hybridization analysis and nucleotide sequence comparison, that the pol genes of prototype type A, type B, avian type C, and type D oncovirus genera are all genetically related. These findings correlate well with the known functional similarities in the reverse transcriptases coded for by their pol genes. These enzymes exhibit similar template and cation preferences which differ markedly from those of mammalian type C viruses (49-51). In contrast, this analysis detected no comparable homology at either the nucleotide or amino acid sequence levels between any of these pol genes and that of M-MuLV (data not shown). Thus, our studies provide strong support for the concept of two major pol gene progenitors, one for mammalian type C viruses and the other for types A, B, D, avian C, and HTLV oncoviruses.

Previous studies have indicated that mammalian type C and D viruses possess related sequences that could be localized to their env genes (41-43). These results were confirmed and extended by low stringency blot hybridization and are summarized in Figure 4. The region of homology between SMRV and R-MuLV, as well as SSAV (not shown) corresponded to their env genes. Under stringent hybridization conditions the region of homology between BaEV and SMRV (not shown) was reduced to a 0.3 kbp stretch. Heteroduplex analysis localized the region to the p15E coding segment of BaEV. These findings indicate that type D and mammalian type C env genes diverged from a common progenitor, but that SMRV and BaEV became evolutionarily linked by a more recent recombinational event involving their p15E regions.

2.4 The organization of type A,B, and D oncoviral related sequences in the human recombinant clone HLM-2

Since infectious type B oncoviruses (MMTV) have only been isolated

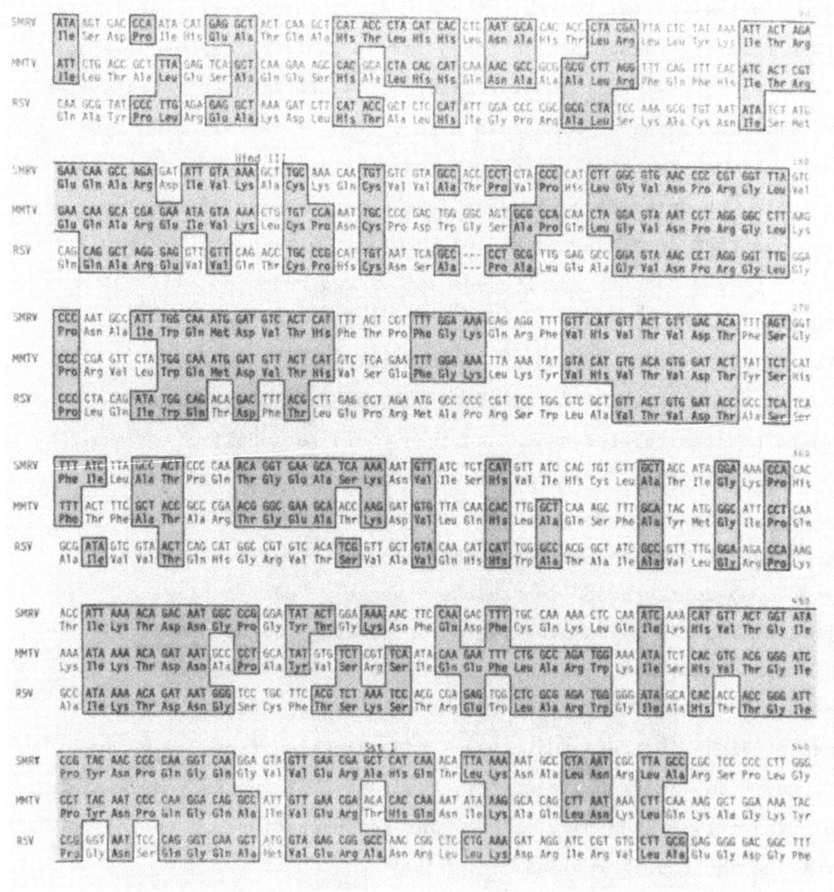

FIGURE 5. Comparative nucleotide sequence analysis of the pol gene segments of SMRV, MMTV, and RSV (11) and translation into amino acids. The predicted amino acid sequences were aligned by using Lipman and Wilbur's PRTALN computer program (40). The shaded areas represent regions of amino acid sequence identity.

from murine species, we have explored the possibility that infectious members of other classes of oncoviruses might also share homology with the human recombinant clone HLM-2 (Callahan et al., manuscript in preparation). The results of recipirocal low stringency blot hybridization experiments using recombinant proviral DNA corresponding to prototypes of the different oncoviral genera is illustrated in Figure 6. The major region of homology between the type A, B, and D oncoviral genomes and HLM-2 DNA corresponds to their respective pol genes. In the case of SMRV (type D oncovirus) the homology spans the 3' half of the gag gene through the entire pol gene. The SMRV LTR also hybridizes weakly with the HLM-2 LTR. The M432 viral genome (Type A oncovirus) also hybrides to a region of HLM-2 immediately adjacent to the 3' LTR. No homology was detected with a number of different mammalian type C proviral genomes.

In order to more precisely identify the conserved regions of the HLM-2 pol gene, the nucleotide sequence of the 3.6 kbp EcoRI fragment (8.0 to 11.6 HLM-2 map units, Figure 1 and 6) was determined (unpublished data). A comparison of a portion of this nucleotide sequence (9.5 to 10.0 HLM-2 map units) with those of pol genes from other infectious retroviruses revealed regions of significant homology between HLM-2 and MMTV (51%), SMRV (50%), RSV (44%) and HTLV (37%). Similar results were obtained by comparing the translated amino acid sequence of this region (45,38,33, and 27%, respectively). No comparable nucleotide or amino acid sequence homology could be detected between this region of HLM-2 and the MuLV pol gene. These findings show that the HLM-2 pol gene probably arose from the same progenitor that gave rise to pol genes of the infectious Type A,B,D, and avian type C oncovirus genera. There is accumulating evidence, described in earlier sections, that genetic interactions between oncoviruses have played an important role in their evolution. As shown here, the HLM-2 genome represents a mosaic of sequences characteristic of different oncovirus genera.

2.5 The organization of MMTV related sequences in human cellular DNA

We have begun to assess the organization of HLM-2 proviral related sequences in human cellular DNA. Since the HLM-2 3.7 kbp

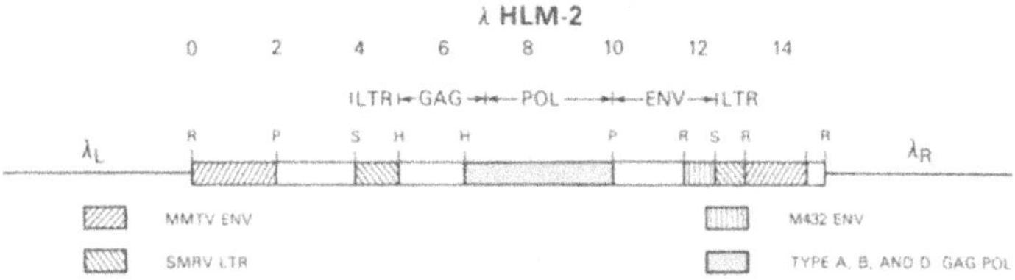

FIGURE 6. Homology regions between human recombinant HLM-2 and prototypes of different oncoviral genera. The regions of homology were determined by reciprocal low stringency blot hybridization of restricted HLM-2 and proviral DNA (Callahan et al. manuscript in preparation).

EcoRI fragment shares the greatest homology with several different classes of oncoviruses we used this fragment to probe restricted cellular DNA from the MCF-7 human mammary tumor cell line using stringent blot hybridization conditions. As shown in Figure 7, families of discrete restriction fragments containing sequences related to the HLM-2 3.7 kbp EcoRI fragment were detected. Significantly, the pattern of major EcoRI related fragments (3.7, 3.5, 2.9 and 1.9 kbp, lane c) is similar to that observed using the MMTV Rep probe under low stringency blot hybridization conditions (Figure 1A, lanes a and d). Moreover, SST-I, HindIII and BamHI restricted MCF-7 cellular DNA each contain, in addition to a 8.0-8.2 kbp major band (or doublet), major bands which correspond in size to HLM-2 fragments obtained with the respective enzymes.

The organization of MMTV gag and pol related sequences in HLM-2 is probably representative of the major families of MMTV related restriction fragments detected in human cellular DNA. We have begun to screen cellular DNA from normal and breast tumor tissue to determine whether there are tumor specific amplifications of the HLM-2 proviral sequences and how conserved these sequences are between individuals. Our results to date provide no evidence for the amplification of proviral sequences in primary breast tumor DNA. This may reflect the limited number of tumors tested or the variability in the fraction of the material which are tumor cells. In this connection May et al. (14) have shown that the MCF-7 human breast tumor cell line contains two

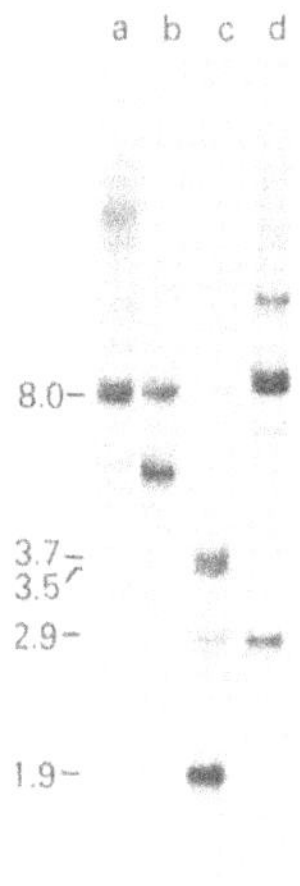

FIGURE 7. Identification of sequences related to the HLM-2 3.7 kbp EcoRI fragment in restricted human cellular DNA using stringent hybridization conditions. 10 μg of cellular DNA from the MCF-7 human mammary tumor cell line was restricted with: a) SST-I; b) HindIII; c) EcoRI; d) BamHI. The restricted DNAs were electrophoresed on a 0.8% agarose gel, transferred to nitrocellulose filters and hybridized with 2 x 10^7 cpm of ^{32}P labeled HLM-2 3.7 kbp EcoRI DNA using stringent hybridization conditions (9). After hybridization the filters were washed using stringent conditions. Autoradiography was for 1 day.

EcoRI restriction fragments not seen in a normal human placenta cellular DNA. The significance of this finding is difficult to assess since the karyotype of the MCF-7 cell line is very different from normal cells indicating several rearrangements which may have been incurred during passage in tissue culture. In addition, we have observed several restriction site polymorphisms in cellular DNA from normal human tissues. Whether these polymorphisms reflect the presence or absence of specific proviral genomes in individual cellular DNAs or the highly diverged nature of this family of proviral genomes will require further study.

In conclusion, we have identified and molecularly cloned a new class of human endogenous oncoviral genomes. This class is characterized by the following features: 1) extensive sequence homology with type A, B, D and avian type C oncoviral *pol* genes, 2) Weak homology with the type A oncoviral *env* gene and type D oncoviral LTR sequences, and 3) no detectable homology with mammalian type C oncoviral genomes. This unusual pattern of sequence homology suggests that genetic interactions between different oncoviral genera contributed significantly to the evolution of the progenitor of this class of human oncoviral genomes. The relationship of MMTV *env* and LTR related sequences in human cellular DNA to this family of human oncoviral genomes remains unresolved. One would suspect that human proviral genomes containing these sequences represent a subclass of this family. The role which these proviral genomes play in the etiology of human neoplasia is unknown, however, the reagents are now available to unambiguously approach this question.

REFERENCES

1. Sarkar, N. (1980) in The Role of Viruses in Human Cancer, eds. Giraldo, G. and Beth, E. (Elsevier North Holland, New York) pp. 207-235.

2. Morris, V.L., Medeiros, E., Ringold, G.M., Bishop, J.M. and Varmus, H.E. (1977) J. Mol. Biol. 114, 73-91.

3. Schlom, J., Drohan, W., Teramoto, Y.A., Hand, P., Colcher, D., Callahan, R., Todaro, C., Kufe, D., Howard, D., Gautsch, J., Lerner, R. and Schidlovsky, C. (1978) in Origins of Inbred Mice, ed. Morse, C.M., III (Academic Press, New York) pp. 343-368.

4. Drohan, W. and Schlom, J. (1979) J. Natl. Cancer Inst. 62, 1279-1286.

5. Das, M.R., and Mink, M.M. (1979) Cancer Research 39, 5106-5113.

6. Bishop, J.M., Quintrell, N., Medeiros, E., and Varmus, H.E. (1974) Cancer 34, 1421-1426.

7. Axel, R., Schlom, J. and Spiegelman, S. (1972) Nature 235, 32-36.

8. Vaidya, A.B., Black, M.M., Dion, A.S., and Moore, D. (1974) Nature 249, 565-567.

9. Callahan, R., Drohan, W., Tronick, S., Schlom, J. (1982) Proc. Natl. Acad. Sci (USA) 79, 5503-5507.

10. Barbacid M., Long, L.K., Aaronson, S.A. (1980) Proc. Natl. Acad. Sci. (USA) 77, 72-76.

11. Chiu, I.M., Callahan, R., Tronick, S.R., Schlom, J., Aaronson, S.A. (1984) Science 223, 364-370.

12. Martin, M.A., Bryan, T., Rasheed, S. and Khan, A.S. (1981) Proc. Natl. Acad. Sci. (USA) 78, 4892-4896.

13. Bonner, T.I., O'Connell, C. and Cohen, M., (1982) Proc. Natl. Acad. Sci. (USA) 79, 4709-4713.

14. May, F.E.B., Westley, B.R., Rochefort, H., Buetti, E., Diggelman, H. (1983) Nucl. Acids Res. 11, 4127-4139.

15. Lawn, R.M., Fritsch, E.F., Parker, R.C., Blake, G., and Maniatis, T. (1978) Cell 15, 1157-1174.

16. Williams, B. and Blattner, F.R. (1979) J. Virol. 29, 555-575.

17. Fenner, F. (1976) Virology 71, 371-376.

18. Schidlovsky, G. in Cancer Research: Cell Biology, Molecular Biology and Tumor Virology, Gallo, R. Ed., CRC, Cleveland, OH (1977), pp. 189-245.

19. Dalton, A. (1972) J. Natl. Cancer Inst. 49, 323-330.

20. Biczysko, W., Pienkowski, M., Solter, D., Koprowski, H.J. (1973) J. Natl. Cancer Inst. 51, 1041.

21. Callarco, P.G., and Szollosi (1973) Nature 243, 91-93.

22. Chase, P.G., Piko, L. (1973) J. Natl. Cancer Inst. 51, 1971-1976.

23. Dalton, A.J., Potter, M., Merwin, R.M. (1961) J. Natl. Cancer Inst. 26, 1221-1226.

24. Perk, K., Dahlberg, J.E. (1974) J. Virol. 14, 1304-1309.

25. Callahan, R., Kuff, E.L., Lueders, K.K., Birkenmeir, E. (1981) J. Virol. 40, 901-908.

26. Herberling, R.L., Barker, S.T., Kalter, S.S., Smith, G.C. Helmke, R.J. (1977) Science 195, 289-294.

27. Majors, J.E., Varmus, H.E. (1981) Nature 289, 253-254.

28. Habara, A., Reddy, E.P., Aaronson, S.A. (1982) J. Virol. 44, 731-737.

29. Reddy, E.P., Smith, M.J., Canaani, E., Robbins, K.C., Tronick, S.R., Zain, S., Aaronson, S.A. (1981) Proc. Natl. Acad. Sci. (USA) 77, 5234-5239.

30. Srinivasan, A., Reddy, E., Aaronson, S.A. (1981) Proc. Natl. Acad. Sci. (USA) 78, 2077-2081.

31. Devare, S.G., Reddy, E.P., Robbins, K.C., Andersen, P.R., Tronick, S.R., Aaronson, S.A. (1982) Proc. Natl. Acad. Sci. (USA) 79, 3179-3183.

32. Gelmann, R., Wong-Staal, F., Kramer, R.A., Gallo, R.C. (1981) Proc. Natl. Acad. Sci. (USA) 78, 3373-3377.

33. Battula, N., Hager, G., Todaro, G.J. (1982) J. Virol. 41, 583-589.

34. Shalloway, D., Zelentz, A.P., Cooper, G.M. (1981) Cell 24, 531-540.

35. Souza, L.M., Strommer, J.N., Hillyard, R.L., Komaromy, M.C., Baluda, M.A. (1980) Proc. Natl. Acad. Sci. (USA) 77, 5177-5182.

36. Chiu, I.M., Andersen, P., Aaronson, S.A., Tronick, S. (1983) J. Virol. 47, 434-441.

37. Schwartz, D.E., Tizard, R., Gilbert, W. (1983) Cell 32, 853-860.

38. Shinnick, T.M., Lerner, R.A., Sutcliff, J.G. (1983) Nature 253, 543-545.

39. Redmond, S.M.S. and Dickson, C. (1983) EMBO Journal 2, 125-130.

40. Wilbur, W.J. and Lipman, D.J. (1983) Proc. Natl. Acad. Sci. (USA) 80, 726-730.

41. Stephenson, J.R., Hino, S., Garrett, E.W., Aaronson, S.A. (1976) Nature 261, 609-612.

42. Devare, J.G., Hanson, R.E., Stephenson, J.R. (1978) J. Virol. 26, 316-323.

43. Cohen, M., Rice, N., Stephens, R., O'Connell, C. (1982) J. Virol. 41, 801-808.

44. Polesz, B.J., Ruscetti, F.W., Gazdar, A.F., Bunn, P.A., Minna, J.D., Gallo, R.C. (1980) Proc. Natl. Acad. Sci. (USA) 77, 7415-7419.

45. Yoshida, M., Miyoshi, I., Hinuma, Y. (1982) Proc. Natl. Acad. Sci. (USA) 79, 2031-2035.

46. Blattner, W.A., Blayney, D.W., Robert-Guroff, M., Sarngadharan, M.G., Kalyanaraman, V.S., Sarin, P.S., Jaffe, E.S., Gallo, R.C. (1980) J. Infect. Dis. 147, 406-413.

47. Rho, H.M., Poiesz, B., Ruscetti, F.W., Gallo, R.C. (1981) Virology 112, 355-364.

48. Seiki, M., Hattori, S., Hirayama, Y., Yoshida, M. (1983) Proc. Natl. Acad. Sci. (USA) 80, 3618-3622.

49. Schlom, J. in Molecular Biology of RNA Tumor Viruses, Stephenson, J. Ed., Academic Press, Inc., New York, 1980, pp. 447-484.

50. Wilson, S.H., Kuff, E.L. (1972) Proc. Natl. Acad. Sci. (USA) 69, 1531-1535.

51. Scolnick, E., Rands, E., Aaronson, S.A., Todaro, G.J. (1970) Proc. Natl. Acad. Sci. (USA) 67, 1789-1793.

8

STRUCTURE AND FUNCTION OF HUMAN ENDOGENOUS TYPE C RETROVIRAL DNAS

A. B. RABSON, P. E. STEELE, R. REPASKE, M. A. MARTIN

Laboratory of Molecular Microbiology, National Institute of Allergy and Infectious Diseases, National Institutes of Health, Bethesda, MD 20205.

INTRODUCTION

A unique feature of infection with retroviruses is the synthesis of a DNA copy of the viral RNA genome, a reaction catalyzed by reverse transcriptase. The newly synthesized retroviral DNA is subsequently integrated into the chromosome of the infected cell and is the template that is transcribed by RNA polymerase II to generate viral genomic and mRNAs. When mammalian reproductive tissues are infected with retroviruses, copies of viral DNA may become incorporated into and become "endogenous" to the germline. Some endogenous retroviral DNA sequences (proviruses) may be spontaneously expressed as complete, infectious virions such as the ecotropic and xenotropic murine leukemia viruses (MuLVs) (1-3) or the baboon endogenous virus (BaEV) (4). Other endogenous proviruses may be involved in the generation of novel recombinant retroviruses with altered biological and disease-causing properties such as the leukemogenic murine mink cell focus-forming (MCF) viruses. The latter represent the product of a recombinational event involving ecotropic MuLVs and endogenous MuLV sequences (5,6). Incomplete retroviral DNA segments may also be expressed at the mRNA and protein levels (7-10). Such retroviral gene products may be abundant constituents of a variety of mammalian cells and, in some instances, be detected in the serum (e.g., the MuLV envelope [*env*] glycoprotein identified in several strains of inbred mice) (7,11). In some mice an incomplete MuLV provirus containing polymerase (*pol*) and *env* sequences is expressed in the form of gp70 related polypeptide that apparently confers resistance to exogenous infection by competing for cellular binding sites.

During the molecular characterization of MuLV proviruses and study of their role in the genesis of spontaneous murine lymphomas and leukemias, we began an analysis of endogenous MuLV-related DNAs in a variety of mammalian species. Such experiments led, first, to the molecular cloning of endogenous type C retroviral sequences from African green monkey (AGM) DNA and, subsequently, from human DNA. It should be noted that no infectious retroviruses have been induced from either of these two primate species.

CHARACTERIZATION OF CLONED HUMAN ENDOGENOUS RETROVIRAL SEQUENCES

Human endogenous retroviral structures were first identified and selected from a genomic recombinant phage library using two cross-species, low-stringency DNA hybridizations: the first, using a subclone of a MuLV to screen an AGM genomic library (12); the second, using a subclone of an endogenous AGM retroviral segment to probe a human genomic library (13,14). Two human retroviral clones were isolated and characterized following the initial screening of the human DNA library (14). Four additional screenings of human DNA libraries have been undertaken using subgenomic probes derived from various regions of the human retroviral segments and have resulted in the isolation of more than 50 different human clones.

As shown in Figure 1, two classes of endogenous retroviral sequences, exemplified by clones λ4-1 and λ51, were identified (15). Both contained gag and pol regions that shared polynucleotide sequence

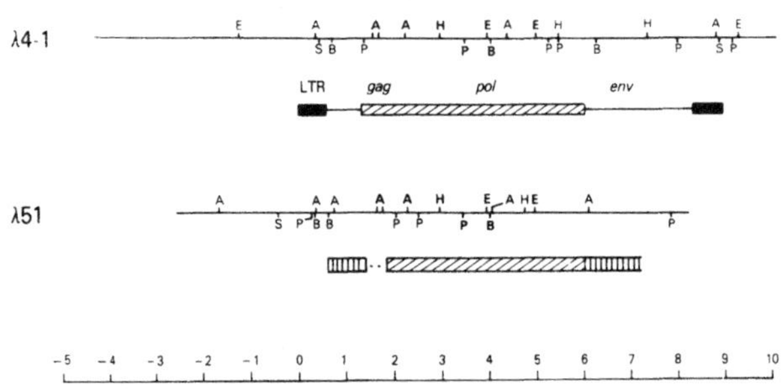

FIGURE 1. Structure of Two Classes of Human Endogenous Retroviral Clones. The restriction enzyme maps of λ4-1 and λ51 are drawn in alignment with each other; A = AccI; B = BamHI; E = EcoRI; H = HindIII; P = PvuII; S = SacI. A schematic representation of the retroviral sequences in each clone is shown below the restriction map. The hatched region corresponds to sequences homologous to MuLV (16). The black boxes are the LTRs of λ4-1 and the vertical lines denote the 72-76 bp repeat units of λ51.

homology with Moloney MuLV (16,17) indicated by the cross-hatched segments in Figure 1. In this conserved region, the nucleotide sequence of the two classes was very similar as evidenced by the presence of several common restriction enzyme sites (e.g., the EcoRI sites at 3.9 and 4.9 kb, the HindIII site at 2.8 kb and the BamHI site at 4.0 kb). λ4-1 exhibits many of the features of a typical full-length endogenous provirus. Paired AccI and SacI sites (at 0.4 and 8.8 kb) lie within cross-hybridizing, 500 bp long terminal repeat (LTR) elements that flank an 8.8 kb provirus. Sequences exhibiting colinear deduced amino acid homology with the gag and pol regions of Moloney MuLV span a region from 1.0-6.2 kb on the map shown in Figure 1 including the splice acceptor sequence for the MuLV env mRNA (16). A long open reading frame located 3' to the potential env mRNA splice acceptor at 5.9 kb is the appropriate length to encode putative retroviral env proteins. No homology between the deduced amino acid sequence of this "env" region and the env gene of other type C retroviruses has yet been demonstrated (R. Repaske, in preparation).

In contrast to full-length proviral DNAs typified by clone λ4-1, the human genome also contains a second family of retroviral sequences that are truncated relative to clone λ4-1. This family, represented by clone λ51 shown in Figure 1, contains 4.1 kb of gag and pol sequences that are very similar to those present in λ4-1. However, the retroviral segment present in clone λ51 or in related clones is not bounded by LTRs nor does it contain any env sequences. Instead, the retroviral sequences present are flanked by a tandem array of imperfect repeats 72-76 bp in length. Nucleotide sequence analysis of the terminal repeating structure associated with the different members of this truncated class of retroviral sequences has indicated the existence of at least eight 72-76 bp tandem repeats at the 5' terminus and at least 13 repeats at the 3' terminus. The 5' and 3' repeat unit clusters are sufficiently homologous to cross-hybridize under standard conditions yet individual 72-76 bp units show considerable variation in their nucleotide sequence (P. Steele, in preparation). The tandem repeats associated with the truncated retroviral family are not homologous to sequences in the Los Alamos nucleotide sequence library.

The complete nucleotide sequence of the retroviral DNA present in clone 4-1 has recently been determined (R. Repaske, in preparation). A comparison of its deduced amino acid sequence with Moloney MuLV by dot matrix analysis is presented in Figure 2. Amino acid homology begins within the p15 region of the <u>gag</u> gene but is essentially absent within the p12 <u>gag</u> segment, a region of considerable sequence variability even between closely related retroviruses. Amino acid homology is again observed in the p30 <u>gag</u> region and continues through p10 and the entire <u>pol</u> region, including the <u>env</u> splice acceptor site. No significant amino acid or nucleotide homology is demonstrable between the human retroviral <u>env</u>, LTR or pre-<u>gag</u> regions and comparable segments of Moloney MuLV.

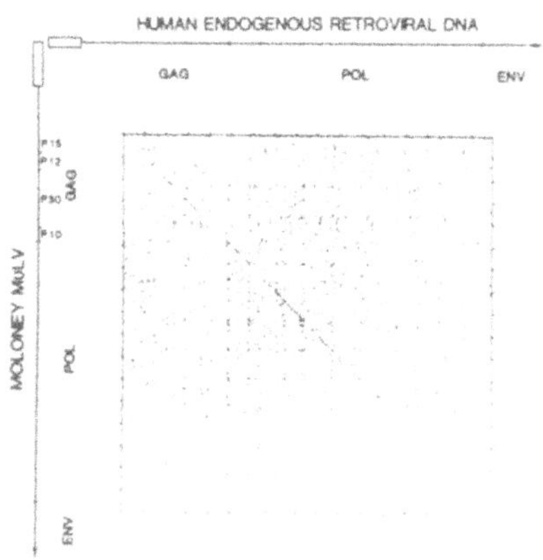

FIGURE 2. Homology Between Human Retroviral DNA and MuLV. Comparison of the amino acid sequence of λ4-1 and Moloney MuLV is illustrated by a dot matrix analysis (performed with the assistance of Drs. J. Maizel and J. Owens, NICHD). A diagonal line indicates regions of colinear amino acid homology.

Although the LTRs of clone λ4-1 show no sequence homology to those of other type C retroviruses including MuLV (16), BaEV (18) and human T-cell leukemia virus-I (19), the human endogenous LTRs do possess the structural features described for other LTR elements (20,21). The 5' and 3' LTRs of λ4-1 are 495 and 499 bp, respectively, and are 95% homologous to one another. The major structural and regulatory features of the human endogenous LTRs are compared with those of Moloney MuLV in Figure 3. An imperfect inverted complementary repeat (6 of 10 match) is present at the ends of the LTRs. A putative TATA box and polyadenylation signal are present at positions 374 and 446, respectively, and a possible CCAAT sequence is located at position 330.

		U3				R		U5		
Retroviral DNA	Plus Strand Primer	Inverted Repeat	Length BP	CCAAT	TATAA	Poly A Signal	Length BP	Length BP	Inverted Repeat	tRNA Binding Site
Mo MuLV	AGAAAAAGGGGGG	AATGAAAGACCC	371-442	CCAAT (46)	AATAAAAG (74)	AATAAA	70	75	GGGGTCTTTCATT	TGGGGGCTCGTCCGGGAT
Human Endogenous	AAAGGGGGGGAAA	TATGGTAGGA	385	ACAAT (43)	TTAAAAG (64)	AATAAA	67-70	44	TCCTGCTACA	TCTTGGTTCCCTGACCTGGAA

FIGURE 3. Comparison of the Human Endogenous LTR with the MoMuLV LTR. The positions of important structural and regulatory DNA sequences in the LTRs of MoMuLV (16) are compared with those of the λ4-1 human LTRs.

These segments allow the subdivision of the λ4-1 LTRs into U3, R and U5 regions of approximately 380, 70 and 44 bp, respectively. The U3 and R lengths are typical of type C LTRs; the U5 region, however, is significantly shorter (44 bp vs. 75 bp) (20). The nucleotide sequence of five different human endogenous LTRs has been determined (P. Steele, in press). As is the case for the LTRs of other species, the greatest homology between different human LTRs exists within the R and U5 regions with significantly less polynucleotide sequence homology within the U3. A 13 bp polypurine tract (the proposed site of the initiation of plus-strand DNA synthesis during reverse transcription) precedes the 3' LTR and a potential tRNA primer binding site follows the 5' LTR. Interestingly, this 18 bp sequence is not homologous to tRNA ^{pro}, the primer for all known infectious mammalian type C retroviruses; it is a 16/18 or a 17/18 match with the 3' end of a rat glutamic acid tRNA in the two 5' human LTRs examined (22).

GENOMIC ORGANIZATION OF HUMAN ENDOGENOUS RETROVIRAL SEQUENCES

The results of molecular cloning experiments indicate that human DNA contains multiple copies of the two families of type C endogenous retroviral sequences. Semi-quantitative DNA dot-blot hybridizations of genomic DNA (data not shown) suggest that 35-50 copies of both the truncated and full-length retroviral familes are present in the human genome. LTR sequences are represented about 200 times per haploid human genome. Southern blot analyses of restricted human DNA is in agreement with these findings. Figure 4 shows the results obtained when three human DNA preparations were cleaved with SacI, an enzyme which cleaves within the LTRs of many of the full-length clones, and hybridized to human pol, env and LTR probes. Multiple bands of varying intensity are seen, suggesting the existence of endogenous human retroviral DNAs with conserved restriction sites. Some of the reactive bands would therefore represent recruited viral DNA segments.

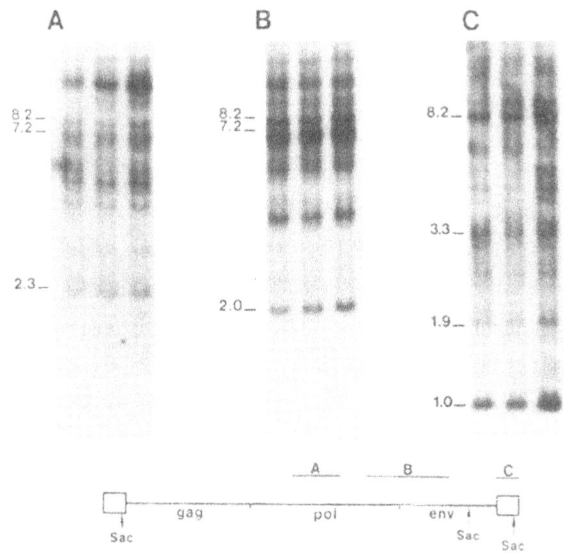

FIGURE 4. Hybridizations of Human genomic DNAs with Human Endogenous Retroviral Probes. Three human DNA preparations were cleaved with SacI and subjected to blot hybridization as previously described (42) with the P^{32}-labeled subgenomic probes indicated at the bottom of the figure.

Full-length proviruses containing only the LTR SacI sites would be cleaved to generate a recruited 8.2 kb band in genomic DNA that would anneal to the LTR, pol and env probes. A subset of full-length proviruses contains an additional SacI site (indicated by the dashed arrow, Figure 4) within the envelope gene region. Hybridization of this subset of retroviral DNAs with the LTR probe would generate a recruited 1.0 kb band (seen in panel C of Figure 4); pol or env probes would react with a recruited 7.2 kb band visualized in panels A and B.

The results presented in Figure 4, panel C, suggest that human DNA contains many more LTR sequences than can be accounted for by those associated with full-length endogenous proviruses (see Figure 4, panel B for comparison). Using an LTR probe to screen a human DNA library, we have molecularly cloned a number of unaffiliated LTRs that are not associated with retroviral gag, pol or env sequences. DNA sequence analysis of one of these solitary LTRs (Steele et al., in press) has shown that it is virtually identical to the LTR present in clone 4-1 and is flanked by the 4 bp direct repeat, ACAG. This LTR element could represent the product of homologous recombination between the LTRs of a full-length provirus attending the elimination of 8.2 kb of retroviral DNA from the human genome (23). Alternatively, it could reflect transposition of an individual LTR element.

A comparison of the three restricted human DNA samples analyzed in Figure 4 reveals striking consistency in the hybridization pattern seen with each of the preparations. A similar lack of polymorphism has been noted using different subgenomic human retroviral DNA probes and a variety of restriction enzymes for the analysis of more than ten different human DNA samples. Considering the large number of reactive bands, the structural stability of endogenous retroviral sequences in man is quite striking. An interesting feature of this study has been the observation of numerous, intensely reacting and presumably recruited bands of sizes significantly larger (12-20 kb) than type C proviral DNA, suggesting the association of retroviral sequences with "conserved" flanking cellular DNA. Employing a cloned, radiolabeled 500 bp segment isolated from such a "conserved" region of human DNA in Southern blot analyses, we have obtained results (data not shown) consistent with the amplification of large blocks of human DNA containing both retroviral and cellular components. This suggests that the copy number (35-50) of retroviral segments in present-day human chromosomal DNA as determined by dot blot hybridization experiments may far exceed the number of primary retroviral integration events attending their introduction into the germline.

EXPRESSION OF HUMAN ENDOGENOUS RETROVIRAL SEQUENCES

Although no human endogenous retrovirus has been induced from human cells, the presence of multiple copies of type C proviral DNA in the human genome raises the possibility that some may be expressed in the form of RNA or polypeptide products. Initial experiments using the RNA dot blot hybridization technique suggested the presence of retroviral RNA in a variety of human tissues and cell lines. Northern blot analysis has confirmed that a wide range of human cell types are expressing defined species of retroviral RNA (15). Figure 5 shows a Northern blot analysis of polyadenylated RNAs from four different human cell types that were hybridized to subgenomic probes from the LTR, gag, pol and env regions of the full-length human clone λ4-1. Full-term human placenta contains two prominent LTR and env-reactive mRNAs 3.0 and 1.7 kb in size. The 3.0 kb RNA comigrates with the "21S" LTR-env-reactive mRNA present in MuLV-infected cells and thus appears to be an authentic spliced retroviral env message. More detailed hybridization analysis as well as cDNA cloning has indicated that the 1.7 kb mRNA is missing sequences mapping to the 3' portion of the env region (data not shown), making it analogous to a 1.8 kb LTR and env-reactive mRNA present in mouse lymphoid tissues (24). These latter MuLV RNAs are missing the p15E membrane anchoring region encoded by the env gene and thus could generate a secreted env gene product. Both the 3.0 and

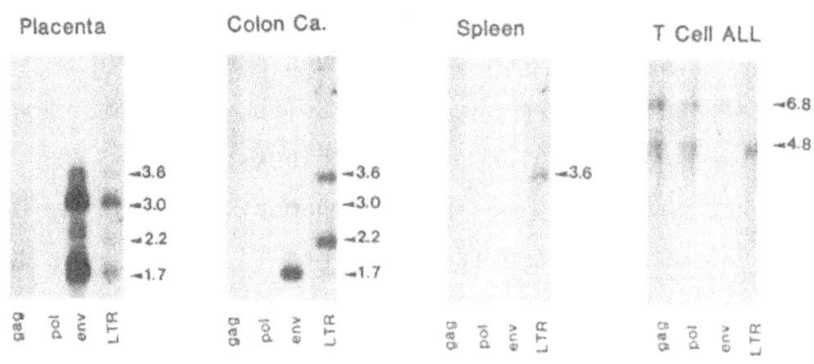

FIGURE 5. Hybridization of Human mRNA with Human Endogenous Retroviral DNA. Poly A+ RNA was isolated from human placenta, spleen, colon carcinoma line SW1116 and the T-cell leukemia line 8402, and was subjected to Northern blot hybridization with LTR, gag, pol and env probes as previously described (15).

1.7 kb env reactive mRNAs are present in colon carcinoma cells (Figure 5). Prominent 3.6 and 2.2 kb LTR reactive mRNAs that do not hybridize to other retroviral probes are also present in colon carcinoma cells. Normal spleen also contains the 3.6 kb "LTR-only" mRNA. Several hematopoietic cell lines have been found to contain gag and pol retroviral mRNAs (Figure 5 and Table 1); the acute T cell lymphocytic leukemia line 8402 contains a 6.8 kb mRNA that hybridizes to gag, pol and env probes, but not with the LTR segments (Figure 5), suggesting that it either contains no reactive LTR sequences or contains its own unique LTR element.

A summary of the results of a number of Northern blot hybridizations is presented in Table 1. These results demonstrate that a wide variety of human cells are synthesizing retroviral RNA. The abundance of LTR-containing transcripts suggests that human endogenous LTRs might function as enhancers and/or promoters of RNA synthesis. Retroviral env-reactive mRNAs seem to be particularly prevalent in secretory epithelial cells and some hematopoietic cells while gag and pol mRNAs seem to be limited to the latter cell type.

DISCUSSION

Human cells, like those of other mammals, contain multiple copies of endogenous type C retroviral DNA sequences. Some of these exist as full-length proviruses containing LTRs, gag, pol and env sequences. Others have a truncated structure containing only gag and pol sequences flanked by non-LTR repeat units. While no infectious human endogenous retrovirus has been isolated to date, the fact that these sequences are present within the genome raises the possibility that such a virus might exist. The observation that human placenta contains abundant LTR and env-reactive mRNAs is of particular interest in light of the numerous reports of the electron microscopic detection of C-type particles in normal human placenta (25) and the reported induction of retroviral partcles from human teratocarcinoma cells (26).

Even though no infectious retrovirus has been induced from human cells, it is clear that the type C retroviral sequences are expressed as polyadenylated RNA in a wide variety of tissues. It is possible that "captured" retroviral genes have been evolutionarily adapted to

Table 1. Detection of poly A^+ retroviral mRNA in human cells

Tissue	No. analyzed	LTR	*gag*	*pol*	*env*
Placenta	2	+	-	-	+
Spleen	2	+/-	-	-	-
Brain	1	+	-	-	-
Liver	1	-	-	-	-
Appendiceal carcinoma	1	+	-	-	-
Cell lines					
Hematopoietic					
T cell leukemia	2	+	+	+	+
Promyelocytic leukemia	1	+	-	-	+
Erythroleukemia	1	+	+	+	+
Null cell leukemia	1	+	-	-	-
Burkitt lymphoma	2	-	-	-	-
EBV-transformed B cell	2	+	+/-	+/-	+
Carcinoma					
Breast	1	+	-	-	+
Colon	1	+	-	-	+
Pancreas	1	+	-	-	+
Lung	1	-	-	-	-
Cervix	1	-	-	-	-
Prostate	1	+	-	-	-
Choriocarcinoma	1	+	-	-	+
Bladder	1	+	-	-	-
Sarcoma					
Rhabdomyosarcoma	2	+	-	-	-
Neural					
Neuroblastoma	2	+	-	-	-
Retinoblastoma	1	+	-	-	-
Glioblastoma	1	-	-	-	-
Melanoma	2	+	-	-	-

Note: a "+/-" designation means that only 1 of the 2 samples hybridized to the probe.

encode products vital to mammalian cells. In this regard, expression of endogenous retroviral sequences as RNA and protein, even in the absence of viral production, has been previously reported in mice (7-11) and primates (27). The mouse epididymis and the primate placenta (28) have been shown to be prime sites of retroviral protein expression, suggesting a specific functional role of such gene products in reproductive tissue. Retrovirus-related *env* glycoproteins on the surface of germ cells or placental tissue could block the binding of infectious retroviruses to cell receptors during the initial phase of virus infection. This would prevent efficient infection and the accompanying integration of new proviruses into the germline, thus reducing the potential for insertional mutagenesis (29). An alternative role of the *env* glycoprotein might be in the formation of syncytiotrophoblast. The gp70 molecule is involved in the fusion of virions to cell membranes (30) as exemplified by XC syncytial formation (31). A gp70-like protein might be responsible for fusion of cytotrophoblastic cells during the generation of syncytial cells in the placenta. Recently, an immune-inhibitory effect of the MuLV p15E envelope protein has been reported and a similar protein has been identified in human cells (32). Perhaps a human retroviral *env* protein plays a role in allowing the placenta to escape allograft rejection.

Evidence for the existence of a functional mammalian reverse transcriptase can be inferred from studies describing processed pseudogenes. The latter appear to have arisen as a product of reverse transcription of spliced and polyadenylated mRNAs (33). Reverse transcription has also been invoked to explain the apparent mobility of highly repetitive DNAs. Even apart from such indirect evidence, there have been a number of reports of reverse transcriptase activities in various human cells, particularly leukemic cells (34-36), retinoblastoma (37), and normal placenta (38). It is interesting to note that *pol*-reactive mRNAs have been detected only in leukemic cell lines and an EBV-transformed B lymphocyte line (Rabson *et al.*, in preparation).

Clearly, human endogenous LTRs are functional enhancers and promoters as shown by the frequency with which LTR-containing mRNA species are observed. Particularly intriguing is the frequent occurrence of "LTR-only" mRNAs. These messages could contain LTR sequences associated with a different class of retroviral sequences that are not related to *gag*, *pol* or *env* segments of clone 4-1 or with cellular genes adjacent to one of the unaffiliated LTRs present in the human genome. The fact that human LTR elements are components of polyadenylated mRNAs in normal human cells and tumor cell lines raises the possibility that they might have a role in oncogene activation. This could occur through the translocation of oncogenes adjacent to active LTR enhancers in a manner analogous to *myc* activation by immunoglobulin enhancer elements (39,40). Alternatively, the transposition or reintegration of LTRs adjacent to oncogenes could also result in their activation such is seen in the activation of c-*mos* by an A particle LTR in a mouse plasmacytoma (41).

REFERENCES

1. Chattopadhyay SK, Rowe WP, Teich NM, Lowy DR: Definitive Evidence that the murine C-type virus inducing locus AKV-1 is viral genetic material. Proc Natl Acad Sci USA (72): 906-910, 1975.

2. Rowe WP: Leukemia virus genomes in the chromosomal DNA of the mouse. Harvey Lect Ser (71): 173-192, 1978.

3. Risser R, Horowitz JM: Endogenous mouse leukemia viruses. Ann Rev Genet (17): 85-121, 1983.

4. Benveniste RE, Todaro GJ: Multiple divergent copies of endogenous C-type virogenes in mammalian cells. Nature (London) (252): 170-173, 1974.

5. Chattopadhyay SK, Clpyd MW, Linemeyer DL, Lander MR, Rands E, Lowy DR: Cellular origin and role of mink cell focus-forming viruses in murine thymic lymphomas. Nature (London) 295: 25-31, 1982.

6. Khan AS, Rowe WP, Martin MA: Cloning of endogenous murine leukemia virus-related sequences from chromosomal DNA of BALB/c and AKR/J mice: identification of an *env* progenitor of AKR-247 mink cell focus-forming proviral DNA. J Virol (44): 625-636, 1982

7. Lerner RA, Wilson CB, DelVillano BC, McConahey PJ, Dixon FJ: Endogenous oncoviral gene expression in adult and fetal mice: quantitative, histologic and physiologic studies of the major viral glycoprotein. J Exp Med (143): 151-166, 1976.

8. Morse HC, Chused TM, Boehm-Truitt M, Mathieson BJ, Sharrow SO, Hartley JW: XenCSA: cell surface antigens related to the major glycoproteins (gp70) of xenotropic murine leukemia viruses. J Immunol (122): 443-454, 1979.

9. Tung JS, Vitetta ES, Fleissner E, Boyse EA: Biochemical evidence linking the G IX thymocyte surface antigen to the gp69/71 envelope glycoprotein of murine leukemia virus. J Exp Med (140): 198-205, 1975.

10. Levy DE, Lerner RA, Wilson MC: A genetic locus regulates the expression of tissue-specific mRNAs from multiple transcription units. Proc Natl Acad Sci USA (79): 5823-5327, 1982.

11. Elder JH, Jensen FC, Bryant ML, Lerner RA: Polymorphism of the major envelope glycoprotein (gp70) of murine C-type viruses: virion associated and differentiation antigens encoded by a multi-gene family. Nature (London) (267): 23-28, 1977.

12. Martin MA, Bryan T, McCutchan TF, Chan HW: Detection and cloning of murine leukemia virus-related sequences from African green monkey liver DNA. J Virol (39): 835-844, 1981.

13. Maniatis T., Hardison RC, Lacy E, Lauer U, O'Connell C, Quon D, Sim GK, Efstratiadis A: The isolation of structural genes from libraries of eucaryotic DNA. Cell (15): 687-701, 1978.

14. Martin MA, Bryan T, Rasheed S, Khan AS: Identification and cloning of endogenous retroviral sequences present in human DNA. Proc Natl Acad Sci USA (78): 4892-4896, 1981.

15. Rabson AB, Steele PE, Garon CF, Martin MA: mRNA transcripts related to full-length endogenous retroviral DNA in human cells. Nature (London) (306): 604-607, 1983.

16. Shinnick TM, Lerner RA, Sutcliffe JG: Nucleotide sequence of Moloney murine leukemia virus. Nature (London) (293): 543-548, 1981.

17. Repaske R, O'Neill RR, Steele PE, Martin MA: Characterization and partial nucleotide sequence of endogenous type C retrovirus segments in human chromosomal DNA. Proc Natl Acad Sci USA (80): 678-682, 1983.

18. Tamura T, Noda M, Takano T: Structure of the baboon endogenous virus genome: nucleotide sequences of the long terminal repeat. Nucl Acids Res (9): 6615-6626, 1981.

19. Seiki M, Hattori S, Hirayama Y, Yoshida M: Human adult T cell leukemia virus: complete nucleotide sequence of the provirus genome integrated in leukemia cell DNA. Proc Natl Acad Sci USA (80): 3618-3622, 1983.

20. Temin HM: Structure, variation and synthesis of retrovirus long terminal repeat. Cell (27): 1-3, 1981.

21. Varmus HE: Form and function of retroviral proviruses. Science (216): 812-820, 1982.

22. Sekiya T, Kuchino Y, Nishimura S: Mammalian tRNA genes: nucleotide sequence of rat genes for $tRNA^{Asp}$, $tRNA^{Gly}$, and $tRNA^{Glu}$. Nucl Acids Res (9): 2239-2250, 1981.

23. Hughes SH, Toyoshima K, Bishop JM, Varmus HE: Organization of the endogenous proviruses of chicken: implications for origin and expression. Virology (108) 189-207, 1981.

24. Boccara M, Souyri M, Magarian C, Stavnezer E, Fleissner E: Evidence for a new form of retroviral env transcript in leukemic and normal mouse lymphoid cells. J Virol (48): 102-109, 1983.

25. Kalter SS, Helmke RJ, Heberling RL, Panigel M, Fowler AK, Strickland JE, Hellman A: C-type partcles in normal human placentas. J Natl Cancer Inst (50): 1081-1084, 1973.

26. Harzman R, Löwer J, Löwer R, Biehler KH, Kurth R: Synthesis of retrovirus-like particles in testicular teratocarcinomas. J Virol (128): 1055-1059, 1982.

27. Sherr CJ, Benveniste RE, Todaro GJ: Type C viral expression in primate tissues. Proc Natl Acad Sci USA (71): 3721-3725, 1974.

28. Stromberg K, Huot RI: Preferential expression of endogenous type C viral antigen in Rhesus placenta during ontogenesis. Virology (112): 365-369, 1981.

29. Jaenisch R, Harbers K, Schnieke A, Löhler J, Chumakov I, Jähner D, Grotkopp D, Hoffmann E: Germline integration of Moloney murine leukemia virus at the Mov13 locus leads to recessive lethal mutation and early embryonic death. Cell (32): 209-216, 1983.

30. DeLarzo J, Todaro GJ: Membrane receptors for murine leukemia viruses: characterization using the purified viral envelope glycoprotein, gp71. Cell (8): 365-371, 1976.

31. Rowe WP, Pugh WE, Hartley JW: Plaque assay techniques for murine leukemia viruses. Virology (42): 1136-1139, 1970.

32. Ciancolo GJ, Phipps D, Snyderman RJ: Human malignant and mitogen-transformed cells contain retroviral p15E-related antigen. J Exp Med (159): 964-969, 1984.

33. Sharp PA: Conversion of RNA to DNA in mammals: Alu-like elements and pseudogenes. Nature (London) (301): 471-472, 1983.

34. Gallo RC, Yang SS, Ting RC: RNA dependent DNA polymerase of human acute leukemic cells. Nature (London) (228): 927-929, 1970.

35. Witkin SS, Ohno T, Spiegelman S: Purification of RNA-instructed DNA polymerase from human leukemic spleens. Proc Natl Acad Sci USA (72): 4133-4136, 1975.

36. Van Muijen GNP, Velde JT, den Ottolander FJ, Brand A, Koopman-Broekhuyzen N, Schaberg A, Warnaar SO: On the presence of reverse transcriptase in myelo- and lymphoproliferative disorders. Cancer (43): 1682-1688, 1979.

37. Reid TW, Albert DM, Rabson AS, Russell P, Craft J, Chu EW, Tralka TS, Wilcox SL: Characteristics of an established cell line of retinoblastoma. J Natl Cancer Inst (53): 347-360, 1971.

38. Nelson J, Leong JA, Levy JA: Normal human placentas contain RNA-directed DNA polymerase activity like that in viruses. Proc Natl Acad Sci USA (75): 6263-6267, 1978.

39. Dalla-Favera R, Bregni M, Erikson J: Human c-myc oncogene is located on the region of chromosome 8 that is translocated in Burkitt lymphoma cells. Proc Natl Acad Sci USA (79): 7824-7827, 1982.

40. Taub R, Kirsch I, Morton C: Translocation of the c-myc gene into the immunoglobulin heavy chain locus in human Burkitt lymphoma and murine plasmacytoma cells. Proc Natl Acad Sci USA (79): 7837-7841, 1982.

41. Kuff EL, Feenstra A, Lueders K, Rechavi G, Givol D, Canaani E: Homology between an endogenous viral LTR and sequences inserted in an activated cellular oncogene. Nature (London) (302): 547-548, 1983.

42. Israel MA, Vanderryn DF, Meltzer ML, Martin, MA: Characterization of polyoma viral DNA sequences in polyoma-induced hamster tumor cell lines. J Biol Chem (255): 3798-3805, 1980.

9

ERV3, A FULL-LENGTH HUMAN ENDOGENOUS PROVIRUS: SEQUENCE ANALYSIS AND EVOLUTIONARY RELATIONSHIPS

CATHERINE D. O'CONNELL AND MAURICE COHEN

National Cancer Institute, Frederick Cancer Research Facility, Frederick, Maryland

Introduction

The question of whether or not the human genome contains retroviral sequences is interesting in terms of both evolution and potential expression of these sequences. We have isolated baboon endogenous virus (BaEV) related sequences from a human DNA library (1) in order to address these questions (2,3). Hybridization and DNA sequence analyses of clones containing the human locus, ERV3, reveals that this region contains an apparent full length integrated retroviral genome (3,4). Significant homology was found between the gag and pol DNA sequences of this provirus and those of other mammalian type C retroviruses including: BaEV (5), Moloney murine murine leukemia virus (M-MuLV) (6), human T-cell leukemia virus (HTLV) (7) and two previously characterized human proviruses, ERV1 (2) and 51-1 (8). The complete nucleotide sequence has been obtained for both ERV3 long terminal repeats (LTRs). These elements contain known transcriptional control sequences within the LTRs in positions characteristic of mammalian type C retroviruses. In contrast, the nucleotide sequence immediately following the U5 region of the 5' LTR (that region commonly containing the primer binding site) is complementary not to the $tRNA^{pro}$ utilized in the replication of type C mammalian retroviruses (9), but to a $tRNA^{arg}$ (10). This difference may define a new group of human retroviruses.

Materials and Methods

$5X10^5$ phage from a recombinant library of human fetal liver DNA cloned into λ-Charon 4A (1) were screened by low stringency hybridization. Duplicate nitrocellulose filters containing DNA from individual λ phage plaques were separately hybridized with two retroviral probes. The probes were: a) a 0.75 kb RI-BamHI restriction fragment from the 3' end of the pol gene of the endogenous chimpanzee retroviral clone CH2 (2) (this fragment displays homology to the BaEV pol gene); and b) the BaEV LTR isolated from a subcloned fragment of the BaEV isolate, M7 (11). The hybridization and wash conditions were: 0.9 M Na+, pH 7, 1X Denhardt's solution, 0.1% sodium dodecyl sulfate (SDS), 60°C. DNAs were labeled by nick translation using [^{32}P] dCTP of specific activity 400 Ci/mMole. Solutions contained $8X10^4$ cpm/ml for hybridization to phage DNAs or $2X10^6$ cpm/ml for hybridization to DNA restriction fragments. Hybridizations to genomic blots were in 1 M Na+, 0.1% SDS, pH 7, 68°C; washes were 0.02 M Na+, 0.1% SDS, pH 7, 68°C for high stringency and 0.2 M Na+, 0.1% SDS, pH 7, 68°C for low stringency. Nucleotide sequences were derived both by the dideoxy (12) and chemical cleavage (13) methods.

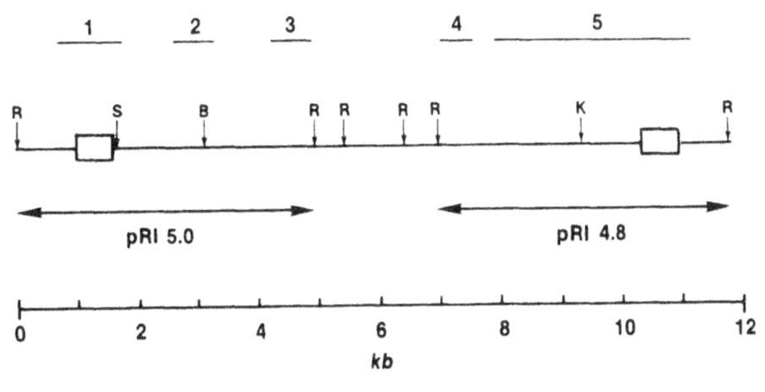

FIGURE 1. A restriction map of the human endogenous retroviral locus ERV3. B = BglII, K = KpnI, R = EcoRI, S= SmaI. Boxed regions contain the sequenced LTRs. 2 EcoRI subclones, pRI 5.0 and pRI 4.8 hybridized to the BaEV LTR; pRI 4.8 also hybridized to the pol-env probe. Regions 1-5 were sequenced.

Results

We initially characterized the ERV3-containing clone by Southern transfers (14) of clone restriction digests hybridized to the two probes used in its isolation. We detected two regions of homology to the BaEV LTR spaced about 9 kb apart, with the *pol*-*env* sequence detected in a region between them (Fig. 1). The probable 5' to 3' orientation in the provirus was determined by hybridization with a *gag*-*pol* subclone of the human provirus, ERV1 (2). The termini of the ERV3 genome were located by DNA sequence analysis of the LTRs (4), thus revealing a proviral length of 9.9 kb.

Table 1. Nucleotide and amino acid homologies in *gag* and *pol*

Gag

	M-MuLV nt	M-MuLV aa	BaEV nt	BaEV aa	51-1 nt	51-1 aa
ERV3	40%	31%	43%	35%	62%	56%
51-1	47%	35%	52%	37%		
BaEV	60%	64%				

Pol

	ERV1 nt	ERV1 aa	M-MuLV nt	M-MuLV aa	BaEV nt	BaEV aa	HTLV nt	HTLV aa
BaEV							56%	38%
M-MuLV					75%	72%	63%	37%
ERV1			60%	52%	72%	48%	65%	33%
ERV3	72%	60%	58%	44%	68%	45%	60%	27%

gag ERV3 sequences were aligned with those of M-MuLV between M-MuLV nucleotides 1245 and 1613. The same region was used for the BaEV alignments. 51-1 sequences were compared to ERV3, M-MuLV and BaEV between M-MuLV nucleotides 1329 and 1499. Small deletions and insertions were made for best fit. A 33 nucleotide insertion at M-MuLV nucleotide 1496 was seen relative to M-MuLV and BaEV in the two human sequences, ERV3 and 51-1.

pol ERV3 sequences were aligned with: the human endogenous provirus termed ERV1, M-MuLV, BaEV and HTLV. The sequences aligned corresponded to M-MuLV nucleotides 4980 thru 5129. The computer program ALIGN (19) was used in the comparisons of the ERV3 sequences with those of other retroviruses.

The partial nucleotide sequence of the ERV3 locus was determined for five separate regions illustrated in Fig. 1. The sequences obtained from regions 3 and 4 show homology to the pol gene of M-MuLV and other sequenced retroviruses. These sequences were separated in ERV3 by the same distance as the homologous regions in M-MuLV, showing that the two maps are colinear in this region. Region 2 contains homologies to the gag genes of other retroviruses. The gag and pol sequences were compared by computer assisted alignments to the published DNA sequences of M-MuLV, BaEV, HTLV, ERV1 and 51-1. Table 1 summarizes the results of these comparisons. It is evident from the data derived from these short comparisons of the genomes that these human endogenous proviruses are more highly related to one another than they are to either HTLV, the only known infectious human retrovirus, or M-MuLV and BaEV, two typical type C retroviruses. The reading frame of both the gag and pol genes contain stop codons, precluding production of normal gag and pol proteins.

The two ERV3 LTRs were completely sequenced in order to determine whether the necessary signals for promotion of viral and/or cellular genes (15) were present in these elements. The two ERV3 EcoRl restriction fragments hybridizing to the BaEV LTR were sublconed into pBR322 for sequence analysis (Fig. 1). A comparison of the sequences from the two LTR-hybridizing regions revealed a region of 593 nucleotides in one sequence that was 91.2% homologous to 590 nucleotides in the other. Two features common to proviruses further suggested that the ERV3 clone contains intact, full-length LTRs: 1) The presence of TG...CA termini surrounding each LTR, and 2) the presence of duplicated host sequences at the viral/host junctions (15). The inverted, complementary repeats characteristic of retroviral LTRs range in length from 2 to 16 nucleotides. As shown in Figure 2, those of ERV3 are only 2 nucleotides long, as are those HTLV (7). Also shown in Figure 2 are the directly repeated host DNA sequences at the site of ERV3 integration: TATA.

In addition, examination of the sequences immediately 3' of the LTR for complementarity to the $tRNA^{pro}$ used in

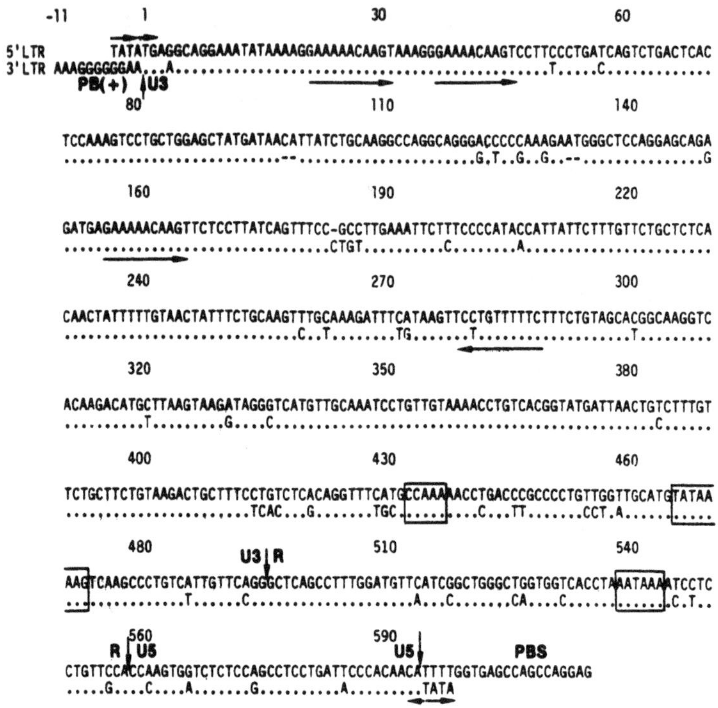

FIGURE 2. The nucleotide sequence of the 5' and 3' LTRs and immediate flanking sequences. Dots represent identities between the two sequences. Vertical arrows separate LTR regions. Horizontal arrows indicate repeated sequences: TATA, duplication of human sequences upon provirus integration; TG-CA, inverted termini of LTRs; and -GAAAAACAAGT- repeated sequences within U3. Boxed regions indicate transcriptional regulatory sequences. PBS-primer binding site for (-) strand synthesis. PB(+) primer binding site for second strand synthesis.

replication by mammalian type C retroviruses, revealed only a 10 out of 18 nucleotide match. However, this region was complementary to 17 out of 18 nucleotides of a mouse $tRNA^{arg}$. Since tRNAs have been highly conserved in evolution, the human equivalent of this $tRNA^{arg}$ gene may well be identical. The proviral sequences at the end of the genome immediately upstream of the 3' LTR are also characteristic of retroviruses. This region contains the putative primer binding site for second strand synthesis, usually consisting of a short stretch of purine nucleotides (9). As seen in Fig. 2, an 11 nucleotide stretch of purines precedes the ERV3 3' LTR.

These LTRs also contain characteristic eucaryotic transcriptional control signals, located in positions characteristic of the type C mammalian retroviruses (15) (Fig. 2, boxed sequences). Long, direct repeats characteristic of enhancer elements (16) are not found in the ERV3 LTRs. These repeats are also absent from the LTRs of the two HTLV isolates (7,17) and an isolate of the related bovine leukemia virus (18), although these retroviruses are certainly expressed. The two HTLV isolates do contain a shorter 21 base pair sequence repeated three times in the U3 region of each genome. Shimotohno *et al.* (17) postulate that these repeats may be equivalent to the enhancer sequences of other retroviruses. As shown underlined in Fig. 2, the ERV3 LTRs also contain short, repeated sequences in the U3 regions. The characteristic LTR features have been maintained despite a divergence between the two LTRs of 8.8%. The maintenance of these features suggests that the LTRs may be capable of expression.

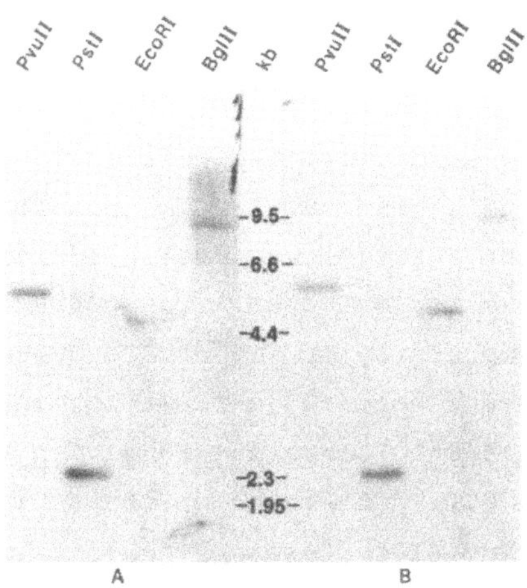

FIGURE 3. Detection of ERV3 proviral sequences in human DNA. 12.5 g of human placental DNA was digested with the indicated restriction enzyme, electrophoresed in a 1% agarose gel and transferred to a nitrocellulose filter (Southern, 1975). ERV3 sequences were detected by hybridization with a ^{32}P-labeled ERV3 envelope subclone and autoradiography. A, low stringency hybridization wash and B, high stringency hybridization wash (see Materials and Methods).

The *env* region of a retrovirus is highly specific for a given genome. For this reason, a subclone from this region was obtained for hybridization to human DNA. The results (Fig. 3) reveal that at high stringency, a single intense fragment corresponding to that expected from the ERV3 restriction map is detected. These results indicate that ERV3 is present in the human genome at a single locus. In another study this locus has been shown to reside on human chromosome 7 (3).

Discussion

A clone isolated from a human recombinant DNA library was found to contain a full-length provirus of 9.9 kb. DNA sequence comparisons indicate that the ERV3 provirus retains the typical LTR-*gag*-*pol*-*env*-LTR gene order of retroviruses. Although proviruses related to ERV3 are present in the human genome, as revealed by sequence homology in the more highly conserved regions of the retroviral genome, ERV3 is present at a single chromosomal locus on human chromosome 7. DNA sequence comparisons reveal a higher degree of homology among three human endogneous proviruses than between these proviruses and other mammalian type C retroviruses. The human endogenous proviruses are even more distantly related to the infectious exogenous retrovirus of man, HTLV. The possible use of a $tRNA^{arg}$ primer by ERV3 suggests a distinct lineage for ERV3 from all other known retroviruses. Our current studies focus on the potential expression of the ERV3 provirus. Although both *gag* and *pol* genes contain in-frame termination stop codons, the *env* region appears to contain a long open reading frame. Additionally, both LTRs contain known transcriptional control sequence. The potential for expression of an *env* protein or a human gene downstream from the provirus is under investigation.

References

1. Lawn RM, Fritsch EM, Parker RC, Blake G, Maniatis T: The isolation and characterization of linked δ- and β-globin genes from a cloned library of human DNA. Cell (15):1157-1174. 1978.
2. Bonner TI, O'Connell C, Cohen M: Cloned endogenous retroviral sequences from human DNA. Proc Nat Acad Sci USA (79): 4709-4713. 1982.

3. O'Connell C, O'Brien S, Nash WG, Cohen M: ERV3, a full-length human endogenous provirus: chromosomal and evolutionary relationships. Virology, in press.
4. O'Connell C, Cohen M: The LTR sequences of a novel human endogenous retrovirus. Science, in press.
5. Tamura TA: Provirus of M7 baboon endogenous virus: Nucleotide sequence of the gag-pol region. J Virol (47):137-145. 1983.
6. Shinnick TM, Lerner RA, Sutcliff JG: Nucleotide sequence of Moloney murine leukemia virus. Nature (293):543-548. 1981.
7. Seiki M, Hattori S, Hirayama Y, Yoshida M: Human adult T-cell leukemia virus: complete nucleotide sequence of the provirus genome integrated in leukemia cell DNA. Proc Nat Acad Sci USA (80):3618-3622. 1983.
8. Repaske R, O'Neill RR, Steele PE, Martin MA: Characterization and partial nucleotide sequence of endogenous type C retrovirus segments in human chromosomal DNA. Proc Nat Acad Sci USA (80):678-682. 1983.
9. Chen HR, Barker WC: Nucleotide sequences of the retroviral long terminal repeats and their adjacent regions. Nucl Acids Res (12):1767-1778. 1984.
10. Sprinzl M, Gauss DH: Compilation of tRNA sequences. Nucl Acids Res (12):r1. 1984.
11. Battula N, Hager G, Todaro GJ: Organization of type C viral DNA sequences endogenous to baboons: analysis with cloned viral DNA. J Virol (41):583-592. 1982.
12. Sanger F, Nicklen S, Coulson AR: DNA sequencing with chain-terminating inhibitors. Proc Nat Acad Sci USA (74): 5463-5467. 1977.
13. Maxam A, Gilbert W: Sequencing end-labeled DNA with base-specific chemical cleavages. In: Grossman L, Moldane K, (eds) Methods in Enzymology. Academic Press, New York, 1980, pp 499-559.
14. Southern EM: Detection of specific sequences among DNA fragments separated by gel electrophoresis. J Mol Biol (98):503-517. 1975.
15. Temin HM: Structure, variation and synthesis of retrovirus long terminal repeat. Cell (27):1-3. 1981.
16. Gluzman Y, Shenk T: Enhancers and eukaryotic gene expression. Cold Spring Harbor Laboratory, Cold Spring Harbor, New York, 1981.
17. Shimotohno K, Golde DW, Miwa M, Sugimura T, Chen ISY: Nucleotide sequence analysis of the long terminal repeat of human T-cell leukemia virus type II. Proc Nat Acad Sci USA (81):1079-1083. 1984.
18. Couez D, Deschamps J, Kettmann R, Stephens RM, Gilden RV Burny A: Nucleotide sequence analysis of the long terminal repeat of integrated bovine leukemia proviral DNA and of adjacent viral and host sequences. J Virol (49):615-620. 1984.
19. Dayhoff MD: In: Atlas of Protein Sequence and Structure. National Biomedical Research Foundation, Washington, D.C., 1976.

10

MOLECULAR BASIS OF HUMAN B CELL NEOPLASIA

CARLO M. CROCE* AND PETER C. NOWELL+

*The Wistar Institute of Anatomy and Biology, Philadelphia, Pennsylvania
+Department of Pathology and Laboratory Medicine, University of Pennsylvania School of Medicine, Philadelphia, Pennsylvania

INTRODUCTION

Consistent karyotypic changes have been observed in several human malignancies of the hematopoietic system (1-4). Many of these somatic changes involve reciprocal chromosomal translocations.

In Burkitt's lymphoma, a neoplastic condition involving B cells and affecting predominantly children, three different reciprocal chromosomal translocations have been detected (5-7). In 75% of cases the distal end of the long arm of chromosome 8 (q24→qter) translocates to the long arm of chromosome 14 at band q32 (5-6). In the remaining 25% of cases the small segment of chromosome 8 translocates either to the long arm of chromosome 22 at band q11 (16% of cases) or to the short arm of chromosome 2 at band p11.2 (7-8). Thus the translocation of the segment q24→qter of human chromosome 8 is the common feature of Burkitt lymphoma (Fig. 1).

Supported in part by grants from the National Cancer Institute and the National Foundation-March of Dimes.

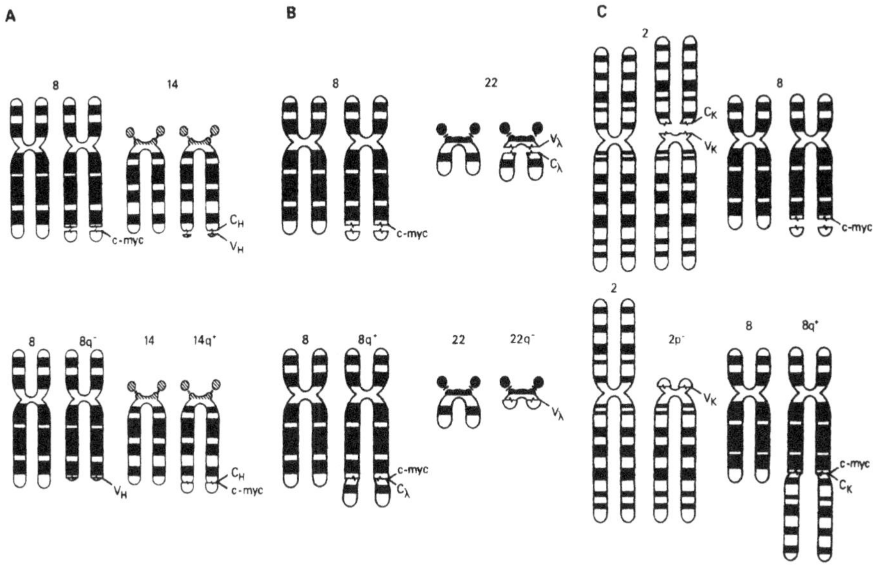

FIGURE 1. Chromosome translocations in Burkitt lymphoma. In Burkitt lymphomas with the t(8;14) translocation the c-myc oncogene translocates to the heavy chain locus (A). In some cases the translocated oncogene is in its germ line configuration, while in others it is rearranged head-to-head with one of the constant region (C_H) genes of heavy chains (predominantly $C\mu$) on the 14q+ chromosome. In Burkitt lymphomas with the variants t(8;22) (B) and t(2;8) (C) translocations, the c-myc oncogene remains on the involved chromosome 8, but the genes for immunoglobulin light chains ($C\kappa$ and $C\lambda$) translocate to a region 3' (distal) to the c-myc oncogene on the involved chromosome 8 (8q+).

Interestingly the loci for human heavy, lambda and kappa immunoglobulin chains are located on human chromosome 14 (9), 22 (10) and 2 (11-12) respectively, strongly suggesting a relationship between human immunoglobulin genes, chromosome rearrangements and neoplasia in Burkitt tumors (10).

The Chromosomal Breakpoints Directly Involve the Ig Genes

We have used somatic cell hybridization techniques to determine whether the chromosomal breakpoints in Burkitt's lymphoma with t(8;14) translocation involve directly the heavy chain locus (13). Since mouse x Burkitt lymphoma hybrids containing the 8q- chromosomes contained the human immunoglobulin heavy chain variable region (V_H) genes, while hybrids with the 14q+ chromosome retained the human heavy chain constant region (C_H) genes, we conclude that in Burkitt lymphoma with the t(8;14) translocation the chromosomal break directly involves the heavy chain locus, and that the variable region genes are distal and the constant region genes are proximal on band q32 of chromosome 14 (13-14) (Fig. 1). The chromosomal breakpoints within the heavy chain locus are, however, variable from case to case (13-14).

We have used the same approach to study the variant t(8;22) and t(2;8) translocations. By examining mouse x human hybrids with Burkitt cells carrying the t(8;22) translocation we found that hybrids with the 22q- chromosome retained the C genes (15). Thus, we conclude that the chromosomal breakpoints in the t(8;22) variant translocation split the lambda chain locus, and that the orientation of the V and C genes on chromosome 22 is opposite to the orientation of the heavy chain genes on chromosome 14 (15) (Fig. 1).

Similar results were obtained by analyzing Burkitt lymphomas with the t(2;8) translocation, where the breakpoint separates the V_κ and C_κ genes and C_κ translocates to the involved chromosome 8 (16) (Fig. 1). Again, the breakpoints within the light chain genes are variable from case to case.

Involvement of the c-myc Gene in Burkitt's Lymphoma

The human homologue of the avian myelocytomatosis virus oncogene, c-*myc*, is located on the segment of chromosome 8 that is translocated to chromosome 14 in Burkitt's lymphoma with the t(8;14) translocation (17). In some cases the translocated c-*myc* gene is in its germ line configuration, in others it is rearranged head-to-head (5' to 5") with one of the heavy chain constant region genes, predominantly $C\mu$ (17-18).

In the variant t(8;22) and t(2;8) translocations, the c-*myc* gene does not translocate, and remains in its germ line configuration on the involved chromosome 8 (8q+), while the light chain loci translocate to a region 3' (distal) to the c-*myc* oncogene (15-16) (Fig. 1). The breakpoint on chromosome 8 is also variable from case to case in the variant translocations.

Structure and Expression of the c-myc gene

The human c-*myc* gene is formed by three separated exons, the first of which contains termination codons on all three reading frames and therefore represents a non-coding leder sequence (19-20). The first

ATG (methionine) signal for protein synthesis is at the beginning of the second exon (19). A single open reading frame is present in the combined second and third exons coding for a protein of 439 amino acids (19). The c-myc gene has two promoters which are separated by approximately 160 nucleotides and which are utilized to different extents in different cells (21). When the chromosomal breakpoints occur in the first exon or the first intron, the c-myc gene loses its promoters, and the myc transcripts are initiated from cryptic sites within the first intron (21). Since the first intron is also non-coding, it can be concluded that the myc protein is the same in the cases in which the gene has been rearranged or not (22).

We have examined the levels of myc transcripts in different Burkitt lymphoma cell lines and found that these levels are variable from case to case, but are consistently elevated (23). These levels were higher than in non-tumorigenic Epstein-Barr virus transformed human lymphoblastoid cell lines (29). Such control cell lines do not carry specific chromosome translocations. Analysis of the myc transcripts in Burkitt lymphomas with the t(8;14) translocation containing a decapitated c-myc gene indicate that only the translocated c-myc gene is expressed at high levels while the c-myc gene on the normal chromosome 8 is either silent or expressed at extremely low levels in Burkitt lymphoma cells (21).

Regulation of the Expression of the c-myc Gene in Differentiated B Cells

We have introduced either the normal human chromosome 8 or the 14q+ chromosome derived from Burkitt's lymphoma cells with the t(8;14) translocation into mouse plasmacytoma cells and have measured the expression of the human c-myc gene in the hybrids. We found that all the hybrids containing the 14q+ chromosome derived from Burkitt's lymphoma expressed high levels of myc transcripts while the hybrids containing the normal 8 did not (29) (Fig. 2).

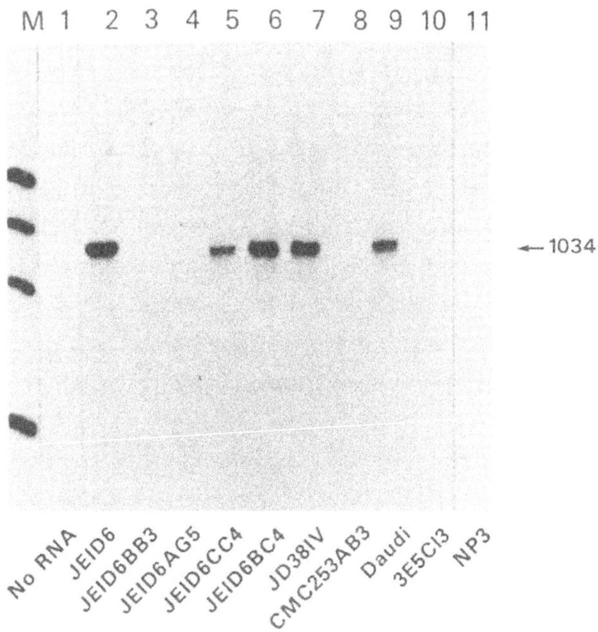

FIGURE 2. Expression of the c-*myc* oncogene on the normal chromosome 8 and on the 14q+ in hybrids with mouse myeloma. An S_1 nuclease protection assay was used to quantitate the expression of the human c-*myc* transcripts in the hybrids (23). By this method a human c-*myc* cDNA clone can be protected only by human *myc* RNA and not by mouse *myc* RNA. The NP3 mouse myeloma parental cells express high levels of mouse *myc* transcripts (23) As shown in lane 11, the RNA derived from NP3 does not protect the human *myc* cDNA clone. On the contrary we detect the expression (the protected fragment in 1034 nucleotides in length) of high levels of human *myc* transcripts in two lymphomas, JD38IV and Daudi, carrying the t(8;14) translocation (lanes 7 and 9). In lane 2 is the result of the protection experiment using the RNA of an NP3 x Burkitt Hybrid JE1D6) that contains both the normal chromosome 8 and the 14q+. As shown in lane 2

high levels of human myc transcripts are expressed in this hybrid. The hybrid JE1D6 was subcloned and hybrid subclones carrying chromosome 8 but not 14q+ (JE1D6BB3 and JE1D6AG5) (lanes 3 and 4) and hybrid subclones carrying chromosome 14q+ but not the normal 8 (JE1D6CC4 and JE1D6BC4) were analyzed. As shown in Fig. 2, the two hybrid subclones with only chromosome 8 did not express myc transcripts (lanes 3-4), while the two hybrid subclones with the 14q+ chromosome expressed high levels of human myc transcripts (lanes 5 and 6). In lane 8 is a hybrid between JD38IV and NP3 cells which has retained the normal chromosome 8 and lost the 14q+ chromosome.

Then we examined hybrids between the same mouse plasmacytoma cells and non-neoplastic human lymphoblastoid cells expressing moderate levels of myc transcripts. We found that hybrids containing human chromosome 8 derived from the lymphoblastoid parent did not express human myc transcripts (23). Thus we concluded that while the germ line c-myc gene on the normal chromosome 8 is capable of responding to normal transcriptional control and is shut off in plasma cells, the translocated c-myc gene fails to respond to transcriptional control and is transcribed constitutively at high levels (23). The failure of the translocated c-myc gene to respond to transcriptional control is independent of whether the translocated c-myc gene is in its germ line configuration or is rearranged.

We have also examined hybrids between a mouse plasmacytoma and Burkitt lymphoma cells with the variant chromosome translocations for the expression of human myc transcripts and found that while the myc gene on normal chromosome 8 is transcriptionally silent, the c-myc gene on the involved chromosome 8 (8q+) is transcribed constitutively at high levels (15-16). These findings indicate that in the variant translocations, the involved c-myc gene is also deregulated. Therefore, the biologic consequences of these different chromosomal rearrangements are the same: a transcriptional deregulation of the c-myc gene involved in the translocation leading to constitutive expression of the c-myc gene at elevated levels.

Role of Cellular Differentiation in the Regulation of the Transcribed c-myc Gene

Human immunoglobulin genes are expressed in somatic cell hybrids between mouse and human B cells if the productively rearranged human immunoglobulin genes are retained by the hybrids (9). On the contrary productively rearranged human immunoglobulin genes are not transcribed in hybrids between NIH-3T3 mouse fibroblasts and human B cells (24). Such hybrids retain the fibroblast phenotype. These results indicate that a B cell environment is necessary for the transcription of productively rearranged immunoglobulin genes (24).

We have also examined the expression of the translocated c-*myc* gene of Burkitt's lymphoma in hybrids between mouse fibroblasts and Burkitt lymphoma cells and found that in such hybrids the levels of *myc* transcripts are dramatically reduced. These results suggest that the transcription of the translocated c-*myc* gene requires a differentiated B cell environment (23-24).

Recently Leder *et al*. (31) and Rabbitts *et al*. (32) have proposed that decapitation of the c-*myc* gene or alteration in its 5' exon results in the failure of the involved c-*myc* gene to respond to a repressor, thus leading to *myc* deregulation. If this were true the altered c-*myc* gene should also be deregulated in fibroblasts, but this is not the case (24).

Molecular Basis of myc Deregulation

To determine whether the expression of the translocated c-*myc* gene depends on the stage of differentiation of the B cells carrying the chromosomal translocation, we have hybridized human lymphoblastoid cells with Burkitt lymphoma cells in which a decapitated c-*myc* gene is translocated to the 14q+ chromosome and found that the hybrids express immunoglobulin chains of both parent, but are phenotypically identical to the lymphoblastoid parent (27). Such hybrids expressed only the c-*myc* gene on normal chromosome 8 and did not express the translocated c-*myc* gene (27).

Since the translocated c-*myc* gene is expressed in Burkitt's lymphoma cells and in hybrids with plasma cells, these results indicate that the activation of the translocated c-*myc* gene depends on the stage of differentiation of the involved B cells. Therefore the activation of the translocated c-*myc* oncogene appears to involve a specific "window" of differentiation within the B cell lineage (27), suggesting that the involved c-*myc* locus has to interact with stage specific differentiation factors in order to be activated and transcribed constitutively at high level.

We speculate that *myc* activation depends on genetic elements present in all three immunoglobulin loci that are capable of activating gene transcription in *cis* following the interaction with transacting factors expressed or active in Burkitt lymphoma and plasma cells but not in less differentiated B cells (lymphoblastoid cells). Such interaction may result in an open chromatin configuration of the involved c-*myc* locus and consequent gene activation. Since the involved c-*myc* gene is activated even if it is located more than 50 kb from the involved immunoglobulin genes, we have called these putative differentiation stage-specific enhancer elements "long range enhancers" to distinguish them from the enhancer located between the J_H and the switch region of the heavy chain locus which is functional in lymphoblastoid cells and can activate transcription only over a shorter range. While the enhancers described to date activate transcription independently of their orientation, activation of c-*myc* transcription appears to occur only when the 5' end of a rearranged immunoglobulin constant region gene is looking at either the 5' end or the 3' end of the c-*myc* oncogene (27).

Genetics of B Cell Neoplasia of Adults

Chromosome translocations involving either human chromosome 11 (band q13) or chromosome 18 (band q21) and q32 of chromosome 14 are common in human B cell lymphomas of adults (4,8), in a fraction of human chronic B cell leukemias (29) and in multiple myeloma (28). We have used neoplastic cells derived from patients with B cell tumors with either the t(11;14) (q13;q32) or the t(14;18) (q32;q21) translocation to clone the breakpoints involved (29,30). DNA probes flanking the breakpoints on either chromosome 11 or 18 were then used to detect rearrangements of the homologous sequences in B cell lymphomas and leukemias carrying these translocations. Interestingly, we have found that the breakpoints in these cases are clustered within short DNA segments (5-10 kb) on chromosome 11 (30) and 18, and that the breakpoint on chromosome 14 is consistently 5' of the enhancer located between the switch and the J_H region of the involved heavy chain gene (29). Thus, it seems likely that this enhancer may have an important role in activating the transcription of the genes flanking the breakpoint on the involved chromosome 11 and 18. The characterization of these two genes and the study of their expression in normal and neoplastic cells and in B cells in different stages of differentiation may provide important insights into the genetic mechanisms of malignant transformation in B cells.

CONCLUSIONS

The studies with the Burkitt tumor and preliminary results with other lymphomas just described indicate how valuable are the tools of modern molecular genetics in probing the fundamentals of tumor biology and the genes important in tumorigenesis. Several caveats are in order, however. For the most part, the products and functions of genes critically involved in human hematopoietic neoplasia remain undefined, as well as how derangement of these genes influence adversely the complex intracellular and extracellular pathways that regulate proliferation and differentiation within the hematopoietic system. Much remains to be done before it is clear just how a cell may escape from normal growth controls.

It must also be recognized that the development of a clinical neoplasm frequently depends on the effects of multiple factors (for example, the role of Epstein-Barr virus and of other chronic infections in the pathogenesis of Burkitt's lymphoma in Africa), and these aspects must also be clarified. Recent developments in the recognition and characterization of human oncogenes are clearly providing major advances in our understanding of neoplasia, but the gap that remains between such basic knowledge and practical applications in prevention or treatment should not be underestimated.

REFERENCES

1. Nowell PC, Hungerford DA: Chromosome of normal and leukemic human leukocytes. Science (132) 1497, 1960.
2. Rowley JD: A new consistent chromosomal abnormality in chronic myelogenous leukaemia identified by quinacrine fluorescence and Giemsa staining. Nature (London) (243) 290, 1973.
3. Rowley JD: Identification of the constant chromosome regions involved in human hematologic malignant disease. Science (216) 749, 1983.
4. Yunis, J: The chromosomal basis of human neoplasia. Science (221) 227, 1983.
5. Manolov G, Manolova Y: Marker bank in one chromosome 14 from Burkitt lymphoma. Nature (London) (237) 33, 1972.
6. Zech L, Haglund V, Nilsson N, Klein G: Characteristic chromosomal abnormalities in biopsies and lymphoid-cell lines from patients with Burkitt and non-Burkitt lymphomas. Int J Cancer (17) 47, 1976.
7. Lenoir GM, Preud'Homme JL, Bernheim A, Berger R: Correlation between immunoglobulin light chain expression and variant translocation in Burkitt's lymphoma. Nature (London) (298) 474, 1982.
8. Emanuel BS, Selden JR, Chaganti RSK, Jhanwar S, Nowell PC, Croce CM: The 2p breakpoing of a 2;8 translocation in Burkitt lymphoma interrupts

the V_γ locus. Proc Natl Acad Sci USA (81) 2444, 1984.

9. Croce CM, Shander M, Martinis J, Cicurel L, D'Ancona GG, Dolby TW, Koprowski H: Chromosomal location of the human immunoglobulin heavy chain genes. Proc Natl Acad Sci USA 76: 3416, 1979.
10. Erikson J, Martinis J, Croce CM: Assignment of the human genes for immunoglobulin chains to chromosome 22. Nature (London) (294) 173, 1981.
11. McBride OW, Heiter PA, Hollis GF, Swan D, Otey MC, Leder P: Chromosomal location of human kappa and lambda immunoglobulin light chain constant region genes. J Exp Med (155) 1480, 1982.
12. Malcolm S, Barton P, Murphy C, Ferguson-Smith MA, Bently DL, Rabbitts TH: Localization of human immunoglobulin light chain variable region genes to the short arm of chromosome 2 by in situ hybridization. Proc Natl Acad Sci USA (79) 4957, 1982.
13. Erikson J, Finan J, Nowell PC, Croce CM: Translocation of immunoglobulin VH gene in Burkitt lymphoma. Proc Natl Acad Sci USA (79) 5611, 1982.
14. Erikson J, ar-Rushdi A, Drwinga HL, Nowell PC, Croce CM: Transcriptional activation of the c-myc oncogene in Burkitt lymphoma. Proc Natl Acad Sci USA (80) 820, 1983.
15. Croce CM, Theirfelder W, Erikson J, Nishikura K, Finan J, Lenoir G, Nowell PC: Transcriptional activation of an unrearranged and untranslocated c-myc oncogene by translocation of a C_λ locus in Burkitt lymphoma. Proc Natl Acad Sci USA (80) 6922, 1983.
16. Erikson J, Nishikura K, ar-Rushdi A, Finan J, Emanuel B, Lenoir G, Nowell PC, Croce CM: Translocation of an immunoglobulin locus to a region 3' of an unrearranged c-myc oncogene enhances c-myc transcription. Proc Natl Acad Sci USA (80) 7581, 1983.
17. Dalla Favera R, Bregni M, Erikson J, Patterson D, Gallo RC, Croce CM: Human c-myc onc gene is located in the region of chromosome 8 that is translocated in Burkitt lymphoma cells. Proc Natl Acad Sci USA (79) 7824, 1982.
18. Taub R, Kirsch I, Morton C, Lenoir G, Swan D, Tronick S, Aaronson S, Leder P: Translocation of the c-myc gene into the immunoglobulin heavy chain locus in human Burkitt lymphoma and murine plasmacytoma cells. Proc Natl Acad Sci USA (79) 7837, 1982.
19. Watt R, Stanton LW, Marcu KB, Gallo RC, Croce CM, Rovera G: Nucleotide sequence of cloned cDNA of the human c-myc gene. Nature (London) (303) 725, 1983.
20. Watt R, Nishikura K, Sorrentino J, ar-Rushdi A, Croce CM, Rovera G: The structure and nucleotide sequence of the 5' end of the human c-myc gene. Proc Natl Acad Sci USA (80) 6302, 1983.
21. ar-Rushdi A, Nishikura K, Erikson J, Watt R, Rovera G, Croce CM: Differentiation expression of the translocated and of the untranslocated c-myc gene in Burkitt lymphoma. Science (222) 390, 1983.
22. Colby W, Chen E, Smith D, Levinson A: Identification and nucleotide sequence of a human locus homologous to the v-myc oncogene of avian myelocytomatosis virus MC29. Nature (London) (303) 722, 1983.
23. Nishikura K, ar-Rushdi A, Erikson J, Watt R, Rovera G, Croce CM: Differential expression of the normal and of the translocated human c-myc oncogenes in B cells. Proc Natl Acad Sci USA (80) 4822, 1983.
24. Nishikura K, ar-Rushdi A, Erikson J, DeJesus E, Dugan D, Croce, CM: Repression of recombinant u gene and translocated c-myc in mouse 3T3 cells x Burkitt lymphoma cell hybrids. Science (224) 399, 1984.
25. Leder P, Battey J, Lenoir G, Moulding C, Murphy W, Potter H, Stewart T, Taub R: Translocations among antibody genes in human cancer.

Science (222) 765, 1983.

26. Rabbitts, TH, Foster A, Hamlyn P, Baer R: Effect of somatic mutation within translocated c-myc genes in Burkitt's lymphoma. Nature (London) (309) 592, 1984.
27. Croce CM, Erikson J, ar-Rushdi A, Aden D, Nishikura K: The translocated c-myc oncogene of Burkitt lymphoma is transcribed in plasma cells and repressed in lymphoblastoid cells. Proc Natl Acad Sci USA (81) 3170, 1984.
28. Van den Berghe H, Vermaelen K, Louwagie A, Criel A, Mecucci C, Vaerman JP: High incidence of chromosome abnormalities in IgG3 myeloma. Cancer Genetics Cytogenetics (11) 381, 1984.
29. Erikson J, Finan J, Tsujimoto Y, Nowell PC, Croce CM: The chromosome 14 breakpoint in neoplastic B cells with the t(11;14) translocation involves the immunoglobulin heavy chain locus. Proc Natl Acad Sci USA (In Press).
30. Tsujimoto, Y., Yunis J, Onorato-Showe L, Erikson J, Nowell PC, Croce CM: Molecular cloning of the chromosomal breakpoint of B-cell lymphomas and leukemias with the t(11;14) chromosome translocation. Science (224) 1403, 1984.

11

STAGE SPECIFIC TRANSFORMING GENES IN LYMPHOID NEOPLASMS

M.A. LANE, [1,2]H.A.F. STEPHENS; [1,2]M.B. TOBIN[1] AND KEVIN DOHERTY[1]
[1]LABORATORY OF MOLECULAR IMMUNOBIOLOGY
DANA-FARBER CANCER INSTITUTE AND
[2]DEPARTMENT OF PATHOLOGY
HARVARD MEDICAL SCHOOL

Identification of activated cellular transforming genes in a variety of neoplasms has been greatly facilitated by the use of the NIH 3T3 transfection assay. A unique property of the NIH 3T3 cells is that they have the ability to undergo transformation following integration of dominantly acting genes, possibly because they have already progressed some way down the path toward overt malignancy. The cells have the ability to be transformed by a variety of transforming genes and therefore may represent a multi potential cell capable of responding to many different growth stimulatory signals.

Utilizing the transfection assay, members of the ras, ras^H, ras^K, ras^N family have been found to be activated in 10-20% of all neoplasms assayed. Because ras genes are transcribed in all cells at all stages of differentiation, it is likely that these genes may be "at risk" to an activating event in all cells at some statistically low level. This finding may or may not imply a mechanism of protection for ras genes which prevents them from being activated in all tumors. Following exposure to chemical carcinogens however, ras gene activation in particular cell systems seems to increase but it is not yet clear from analysis of these systems whether the carcinogens utilized interact specifically with the genes encoding ras proteins (reviewed in Cooper and Lane, 1984).

Stage specific transforming genes, in contrast to ras genes, appear to be activated quite discreetly in cells of a particular lineage, representative of a particular stage of differentiation. The lymphoid system, in which cell lineages and differentiative pathways have been best characterized has provided the most useful system for analysis of stage specific transforming genes. As we previously reported, a common gene is activated in multiple isolates of pre B tumors of both humans and mice (Lane et al 1982). This gene differs both from the gene found to be activated in multiple intermediate B cell neoplasms and from that activated in mature B neoplasms. Blym1, the first of the B-lineage stage specific transforming genes to be isolated and characterized was initially identified in chicken Bursal lymphomas. Cloning and sequencing of this gene indicated that it encoded a small protein of 8kd which shared homology with the amino terminal domains of transferrin family molecules (Goubin et al 1983). Chicken Blym1 was utilized as a probe to isolate Human B-lym1 from Burkitts lymphomas and it was determined that human Blym1 gene also shared homology with the transferrins. Blym1, the gene activated in a variety of intermediate B-cell tumors, is therefore, well conserved evolutionarily, and is expressed in multiple tumor isolates from several different species including humans, but differs by restriction endonuclease inactivation patterns from genes activated in pre B or mature B tumors. Blym1 activation has not been detected in tumors of other cell lineages or B cell tumors at different stages of differentiation and therefore unlike ras genes represents a uniquely stage and lineage specific gene (Diamond et al 1983).

Within the T-lymphoid lineage two different stage specific genes have been found to be activated in neoplasms of rodent and human species. T-Lym I was isolated from a BALB/c T lymphoma and is representative of the gene activated in multiple isolates a pre T and intermediate T tumors. T-lymI differs from the gene activated mature T neoplasms as the two genes have differing patterns of susceptibility to restriction endonuclease inactivation.

Tlym-I was isolated by sib selection and transfection of a transforming gene - enriched λ Charon 30 library containing cell DNA inserts in the 8kb range. A single phage was isolated containing cell DNA inserts in the 8kb range. A single phage was isolated containing a cellular insert of 8.7kb which was biologically active. To facilitate further mapping a 4.7kb

Hind-Bam fragment containing an EcoRl site was subcloned into PBR322. This fragment which contains the transforming region of the gene was chosen because digestion with EcoRl was previously shown to inactivate the transforming activity of Tlym-I (Lane, 1982, 1984).

Hybridization of a flanking sequence probe to BALB/c liver DNA and to S49 tumor DNA indicated that activation of this gene did not occur as a result of gross rearrangements or deletions in cell DNA. Hybridization of coding sequence probe to human DNA under conditions of slightly relaxed stringency indicated that this sequence was conserved between mouse and human species (Lane, 1984).

Hybridization of the 4.7kb fragment containing the transforming region to lymphoid cellular RNA detected major message species of 0.6, 0.7 and 1.6kb in both T and B cells and in addition, a message of 1.8kb in RNA from a T-suppressor clone. These message sizes were of interest to us because of a report by Peter Rigby and his colleagues concerning their isolation of cDNA clones by subtractive RNA hybridization from SV40 transformed cells. One group of genes referred to as Set 1 genes shared extensive sequence homology with MHC 1 genes from the TL/QA region. Set 1 genes used as probes detected messenger RNAs of 0.6, o.7 and 1.6kb, and appeared to possess a novel repeat element having a structure similar to transposon, as it was flanked by direct repeat sequences (Brickell, 1983).

Because of the similarity of RNA messenger sizes identified by both Tlym-1 and Set 1 genes, and because Tlym-1 had been isolated from a thymic lymphoma it was of interest to determine whether Tlym-I did encode a gene within the MHC I region and it was of particular interest to determine whether our gene encoded an altered TL or QA product.

Tlym-I was found to hybridize to pMHCl (Evans, 1982) described by Seidman and coworkers as a probe crossreactive with most MHC I region genes; to 64-c, reported by Rigby's group to contain exons four, five and six of the Set 1 gene; and to 64-E which contained their Set 1 sequence (Brickell et al, 1983). The results of these experiments indicate that Tlym-I shares homology with Class 1 MHC genes.

As Tlym-1 contained a ClaI site, some further analysis was possible based upon the report by Steinmetz (1981) defining thirteen clusters containing 36 genes within the BALB/c MHC I region. From their reported analysis of ClaI sites within the gene clusters, we have been able to rule out all but nine genes mapping to four clusters. Clusters one and six map to QA regions, while clusters three and five map to TL regions as determined by these authors. If the genes contained in the thirteen clusters constitute all of the genes encoded within the MHC I region then this retrospective analysis further localizes Tlym-I to the QA/TL region of the MHC I complex, provided the cosmid clusters contain all of the MHC region genes.

An antisera crossreactive with all MHC I products was used to immunoprecipitate Tlym I protein products from ^{35}S labeled cell extracts and supernates. This antisera precipitated a 44kd. protein from the supernates of multiple T-lymI transformants which was not present in supernates from untransformed NIH 3T3 cells, NIH 3T3 cells transformed by ras genes or NIH 3T3 cells transformed by a mouse B-lym 1 gene. These findings further confirm that T LymI is an MHC I product and demonstrates that this gene encodes a secreted protein product. Use of TLymI transformant supernates in a soft agar colony growth factor assay indicated that these supernates had the ability to stimulate NIH 3T3 cells to form large numbers of colonies while control supernates from normal NIH 3T3 cells stimulated very few cells to produce colonies after 14 days culture.

Genes in the TL/QA region encode cell surface expressed proteins in the range of 40-45 thousand daltons, which have been found to be associated with Beta-2 microglobulin. TL antigens are expressed in a highly stage specific manner and have been found only on thymus cells. TL negative strains in which thymic leukemias develop often express a novel TL on their surface. At present, the biological role of the TL antigens is unclear.

QA1 antigens have been detected on approximately two thirds of all Thyl+ cells and are found on one class of helper T cells as well as a feedback suppressor cell. QA2 is also found on a majority of Thyl+ cells and is expressed on some but not all T-cell leukemias. Proliferation to the mitogens ConA and PhA can be blocked if T cells are pretreated with antiserum directed against the QA2 antigen. QA3 is also expressed predominantly on Th-1 positive cells and behaves as does QA2 in mitogen studies.

The antigens QA4 and QA5 have a different tissue distribution and appear not to be present on thymic cells. These antigens are present on Ig-cells from spleen and lymph nodes and are additionally expressed on B cell blasts following lipopolysaccharide stimulation (reviewed in Flaherty, 1980.)

At the nucleic acid level, the sequences encoding TL and QA do not exhibit extensive polymorphism and in some cases share homology of 80% or more, while the genes encoding H-2 seem to be more extensively polymorphic. For these reasons it will be of use to distinguish TL products from QA products utilizing specific serologic reagents.

In summary, TLymI is the first of the cellular transforming genes found to encode a secreted protein product and it appears that this gene shares substantial homology to genes encoded within the TL/Qa region of the major histocompatibility complex. It is therefore attractive to speculate that this gene functions in T-cell lymphomas by producing a secreted product which may associate with the T-cell receptor to provide an autologous growth stimulus. When this gene is integrated into NIH 3T3 cells the secreted protein product may function with a somewhat lower affinity by associating with other receptors involved with the initiation of proliferation.

The authors thank J. Seidman, Dept. of Genetics, Harvard Medical School for pMHCI and for MHCI Crossreactive Antisera; P.W.J. Rigby Imperial College, London, for 64-C and 64-E. The authors also wish to thank L. Hood and S. Hunt, California Institute of Technology, H. Cantor and G. Freeman, Dana-Farber Cancer Institute, and T. Boyse and F.W. Shen, Sloane-Kettering

Memorial Laboratory, for useful and productive discussions. This work was supported by CA33108. M.A. Lane is a Scholar of the Leukemia Society of America.

REFERENCES

1. Cooper, G.M. and Lane, M.A. (1984) Cellular transforming genes and Oncogenesis. Biochem., Biophys. ACTA (in press)
2. Lane MA, Sainten A, Cooper GM (1982) Stage-specific transforming genes of human and mouse B- and T- lymphocyte neoplasms. Cell 28:873-880
3. Goubin G, Goldman DS, Luce J, Neiman PE, Cooper GM (1983) Molecular cloning and nucleotide sequence of a transforming gene detected by transfection of chicken B-cell lymphoma DNA. Nature 302:114-119
4. Diamond A, Cooper GM, Ritz J, Lane MA (1983) Identification and molecular cloning of the human Blym transforming gene activated in Burkitt's lymphomas. Nature 305:112-116
5. Lane MA, Sainten A, Doherty KM, Cooper GM (1984) Isolation and characterization of a stage specific transforming gene, Tlym-I, from T- cell lymphomas. Proc Natl Acad Sci USA 81:2227-2231
6. Brickell PM, Latchman DS, Murphy D, Willison K, Rigby PWJ (1983) Activation of a Qa/TLa class I major histocompatibility antigen gene is a general feature of oncogenesis in the mouse. Nature 306:756-760.
7. Evans GA, Margulies DH, Camerini-Otero RD, Ozato K, Seidman JG (1982) Structure and expression of a mouse major histocompatibility antigen gene H-2Lα . Proc Natl Acad Sci USA 79:1994-1998
8. Steinmetz M, Winoto A, Minard K, Hood L (1981) Clusters of genes encoding mouse transplantation antigens. Cell 28:489-498
9. Flaherty L: TLA-region antigens. In: The role of the major histocompatibility complex in immunology. Garland STPM Press, New York, p 33

12

ONCOGENES INVOLVED IN CHRONIC MYELOCYTIC LEUKEMIA

NORA HEISTERKAMP, JOHN R. STEPHENSON, GERARD GROSVELD[+], ANNELIES DE KLEIN[+] AND JOHN GROFFEN; Oncogene Science Inc., 222 Station Plaza North, Mineola, New York 11501, [+]Department of Cell Biology and Genetics, Erasmus University, P.O. Box 1738, 3000 DR Rotterdam, The Netherlands.

1. INTRODUCTION

The Abelson strain of murine leukemia virus (MuLV) represents a recombinant between Moloney-MuLV and a cellular oncogene of mouse origin, c-abl (1). We have molecularly cloned human v-abl homologous sequences (human c-abl) from a human cosmid library and have localized this oncogene on the long (q) arm of chromosome 9(2). This observation was of interest in view of the frequent involvement of chromosome 9 in the translocation with chromosome 22, the t(9;22) characteristic of chronic myelocytic leukemia (CML)(3). By analysis of a series of rodent human somatic cell hybrids containing either the $9q^{+}$ or the $22q^{-}$ (Philadelphia, Ph') chromosome, we have demonstrated the translocation of human c-abl from chromosome 9 to the Ph' chromosome. This finding localized c-abl to the q34-qter region of human chromosome 9 and established that the translocation between chromosome 22 and 9 is reciprocal.

Subsequently, we isolated a chimeric DNA fragment from one CML patient containing sequences from chromosome 9 and 22 and located 14 kb immediately 5' of the human c-abl oncogene. This suggests a role for this oncogene in CML. Similar rearrangements in this specific area were not detected in leukemic cells of either of two other CML patients (4). We used the chromosome 22 specific sequences of the chimeric DNA fragment to isolate an extended region on chromosome 22 from non-CML human DNA. The presence of Ph' breakpoints in this area was also investigated in a number of other Ph'-positive CML patients; they all exhibited abnormal restriction enzyme patterns indicating that in Ph'-positive CML a breakpoint occurs within a breakpoint cluster region (bcr) of 4.2 - 5.8 kb on chromosome 22. More recently we have isolated cDNAs with homology to bcr, establishing that this region encodes a protein. By nucleic acid hybridization experiments, the 5' end of this protein-encoding region on chromosome 22 was oriented toward the centromere of the chromosome. The availability of the *bcr* homologous cDNA clones will allow a comparative nucleotide sequence analysis and a determination of whether in Ph'-positive CML cells, aberrant mRNAs are produced which are possibly chimerics of human c-*abl* and *bcr*.

2. RESULTS

2.1. Isolation of v-abl Homologous Sequences from a Cosmid Library of Human Cellular DNA

For use as a molecular probe, a 4.5 kb BamHl restriction fragment encompassing all but a short region of the Abelson MuLV proviral DNA, was excised from -AM-1, kindly provided by E.P. Reddy and S.A. Aaronson and subcloned into pHEP (5). A v-*abl* DNA probe was prepared from pHEP-Ab by digestion with BstEII and BamHI. For identification of v-*abl* homologous human sequences, high molecular weight mouse and human cellular DNAs were digested with EcoRI, electrophoresed, transferred to nitrocellulose filters and hybridized to the v-*abl* BamHI/BstEII probe. V-*abl* homologous human DNA restriction fragments of 11 kb, 7.2 kb, 5 kb, 4.1 kb, 4.0 kb, 3.4 kb, 2.9 kb and 2.5 kb were resolved. The demonstration of numerous human DNA EcoRI restriction fragments hybridizing to v-*abl*, which itself encompasses a region of only 3.0 kb provided an initial indication that the human v-*abl* homologue must contain extensive intervening sequences. It was also apparent that although the strength of homology of human and mouse cellular DNAs with v-*abl* were comparable, the restriction patterns were quite distinct, a finding consistent with previous reports (1, 6).

To facilitate further characterization of v-*abl* homologous human DNA sequences, a previously described (7) cosmid library of human carcinoma DNA was utilized. Upon screening with the v-*abl* BamHI/BstEII probe, nine positive cosmid clones were identified.

Restriction maps of v-*abl* homologous sequences within three of these cosmids, cos 8, 15 and 18, were generated using various combinations of EcoRI, KpnI, BamHI, HindIII and BglII. As summarized in Figure 1A, the three cosmid clones contain overlapping cellular sequences corresponding to a single contiguous region of human cellular DNA of around 64 kb. Based upon hybridization with four individual subgenomic v-*abl* probes, seven distinct regions of v-*abl* homology (region I to VII; Fig.1A), interspersed by six nonhomologous regions representing probable intervening sequences (introns)

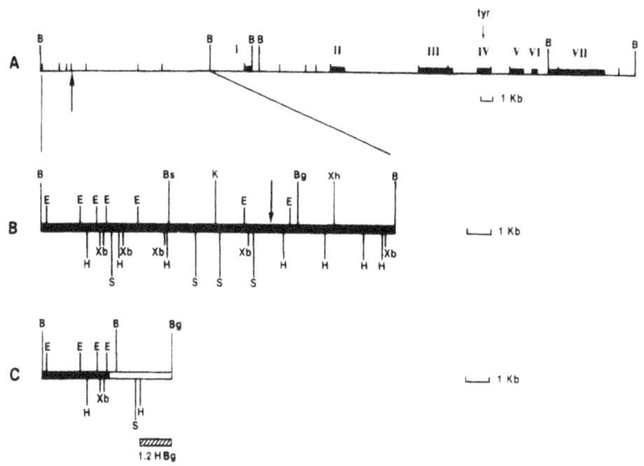

FIGURE 1. Restriction map of the human c-abl oncogene and pBglII 9q+.A. Regions of homology to the v-abl specific probes are represented by solid bars and designated I through VII. EcoRI sites are marked by small vertical lines. The vertical arrow points to the breakpoint in the DNA of CML 0319129. A restriction map of p5'-c-abl is shown in B. The pBglII-9q+ fragment in C is a subclone of a 6.0 kb BglII fragment isolated from CML patient 0319129. The solid bar indicates sequences from chromosome 9 while the open bar represents sequences for chromosome 22. Restriction enzymes include: BamHI (B); BglII (Bg); BstEII (Bs); HindIII (H); SstI (S); XbaI (Xb); XhoI (Xh): EcoRI (E); and KpnI (K).

were identified. In addition, colinearity of sequences within the human v-abl homologue and the viral v-abl gene was established.

We have identified sequences encoding the tyrosine phosphorylation acceptor sites of v-abl and human c-abl (region IV, Fig. 1A) and have determined the nucleic acid sequence of these regions (8). Extensive homology between this region of c-abl and acceptor domains of the v-src, v-yes and v-fps/fes family of viral oncogenes was found, as well as more distant relatedness to the catalytic chain of the mammalian cyclic AMP-dependent protein kinase. These findings suggest that all the homologues of retroviral oncogenes with tyrosine specific protein kinase activity examined to date were probably derived from a common progenitor and may represent members of a diverse family of cellular protein kinases.

2.2 Translocation of c-abl to Chromosome 22 (Ph' Chromosome) in CML

In experiments not described here, we have localized c-abl to the long arm of chromosome 9 (2). These findings are of interest because of the involvement of the long arm of chromosome 22 (22q11-qter) in a specific translocation with the long arm of chromosome 9 (band 9q34), the Philadelphia translocation (Ph'), occurring in CML. The abnormal chromosomes are designated $9q^+$ and $22q^-$; of these, the $22q^-$ (Ph') chromosome is observed in 96% of CML cases.(Fig. 2)

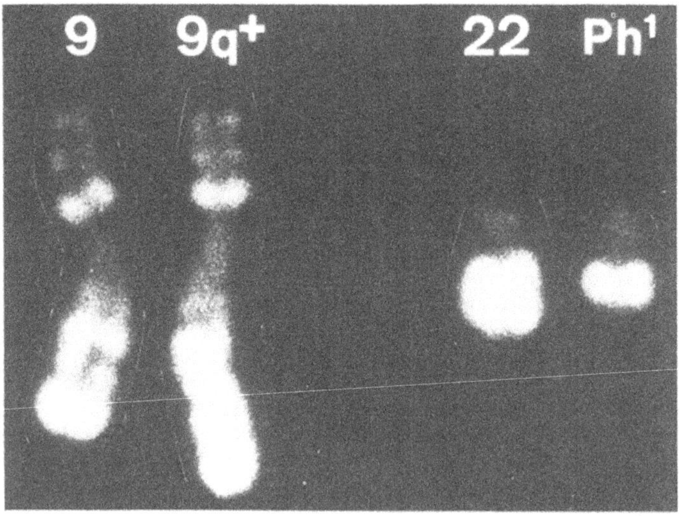

FIGURE 2. Chromosomes involved in the Philadelphia translocation.

We investigated the chromosomal location of the human c-abl gene in cases of CML where the Philadelphia translocation is present. Southern blot analyses with c-abl and v-abl probes were performed on EcoRI digested DNAs from somatic cell hybrids segregating the $9q^+$ and $22q^-$ chromosomes (9).

The cell hybrids used each contain a full complement of mouse or Chinese hamster chromosomes and a limited number of human chromosomes. The hybrid cell lines were obtained by fusion of cells from mouse or Chinese hamster origin with leukocytes from different CML patients and from a normal donor. To maximize specificity for c-abl detection, two restriction fragments corresponding with the most 5' and 3' v-abl homologous EcoRI fragments of human c-abl were isolated. Using these probes, EcoRI restricted DNAs of hybrid cell lines containing chromosomes 22, 9, $9q^+$ or $22q^-$ were analyzed for human c-abl sequences. As controls, DNAs from human placenta and from the mouse and Chinese hamster fusion partners were analyzed. Human c-abl specific restriction fragments detected in human placenta DNA, were present in DNA from the hybrid cell lines 10CB-23B (chromosome 9), 1CB-17a NU and WESP-2A (both containing chromosome $22q^-$). These bands were not detected in DNA from PgMe-25Nu (chromosome 22), 14CB-21A (chromosome $9q^+$), Pg19 and WEHI-3B (mouse controls) or E36 and a3 (Chinese hamster controls). Because all other c-abl EcoRI fragments which hybridize to v-abl sequences are flanked by the 2.9 kb and 5.0 kb EcoRI fragments, it seems highly probable that these fragments are also included in the translocation to the Philadelphia chromosome. To test this possibility directly, hybridization was performed using a v-abl $P_{1.7}$ probe. This probe detects human v-abl homologous fragments of 11, 7.2, 4.0, 3.4, 2.9 and 2.5 kb. Of these fragments, the 11 kb band has been shown to map outside the main human c-abl locus and will not be considered here. The human 2.9, 3.4, 4.0 and 7.2 kb c-abl fragments were readily detected in WESP-2A DNA. The 2.5 kb EcoRI human c-abl fragment comigrates with a mouse fragment of similar size and thus could not be identified in this analysis.

The hybrid cell lines containing the $9q^+$ and $22q^-$ chromosomes examined in the present study were obtained from fusion experiments with CML cells from three different individuals. Therefore, we conclude that in the Philadelphia translocation the transposed fragment includes the human c-abl sequences (Fig. 3). This finding establishes that the translocation is reciprocal, a general assumption which is demonstrated unequivocally by these results. Moreover, the data raise the possibility of involvement of the human c-abl gene in the generation of CML.

In addition, we investigated if c-abl is translocated in variant forms of CML. Employing in situ hybridization techniques (10), no translocation of human c-abl to chromosome 22 was found in two Ph'-negative CML patients; however, in two patients with complex Philadelphia translocations, a t(9;11;22) and a t(1;9;22), the c-abl oncogene was moved to the Ph' chromosome. The latter data suggest that in patients with complex Ph' translocations, c-abl moves consistently to chromosome 22. Moreover, recent in situ hybridization data suggest that yet in another variant form of CML, in which chromosome 22 was previously not thought to be involved, human c-abl is translocated to chromosome 22 (A. Hagemijer, unpublished observation.)

2.3 Search For a t(9;22) Chimeric Fragment

To investigate the possibility that the chromosome 9 breakpoint in the t(9;22) may be localized either within or in close proximity to the human c-abl oncogene, high molecular weight DNA was isolated from biopsy samples of the spleens of three CML patients and from an erythroleukemic cell line, K562, (11) established from a CML patient in blast crisis. Each DNA was digested with BamHI and subjected to Southern blot analysis. The restriction enzyme patterns of each of the four CML DNAs were indistinguishable from those of control DNA, when hybridized either to the above described v-abl probe, v-abl $P_{1.7}$, or probes isolated from different regions of the human c-abl locus (data not shown.)

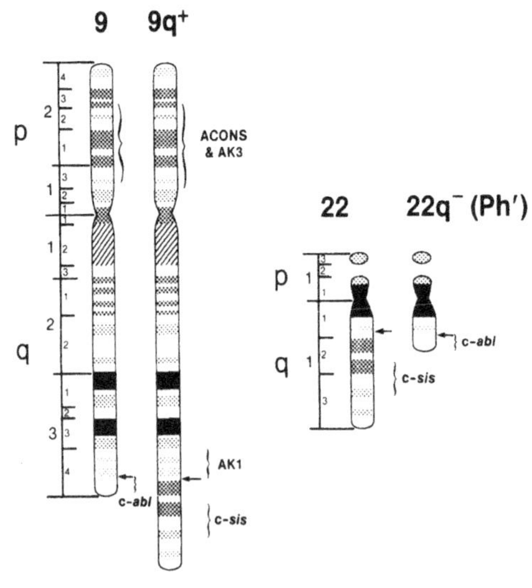

FIGURE 3. Diagramatic representation of the involvement of c-abl and c-sis in the Ph' translocation. Map positions of ACONS, AK3 and AK1 are as previously reported (23). Localization of c-abl within the terminal portion of chromosome 9(q34), is as described in the text. Sublocalization of c-sis to the region of chromosome 22 q12.3 to q13.1 is as previously described (13, 14).

As no rearrangements could be detected in the v-abl homologous cellular DNA region encompassed by the cosmid clones, a probe was prepared corresponding to an 0.4 kb HindIII/EcoRI fragment (0.4 HE) mapping within the 5' domain of the human c-abl locus. Upon analysis of total human DNA, a BamHI fragment of approximately 14.5 kb was found to hybridize to the 0.4 HE probe. To further characterize this restriction fragment, a library of size fractionated BamHI digested human DNA was constructed in Charon 30. The insert of one positive clone was subcloned into pBR328 (p5'-c-abl) and subjected to detailed restriction enzyme analysis as shown in Figure 1B. No sequences in the 14.5 kb fragment hybridized to v-abl specific probes.

An 0.2 kb probe was prepared from the most 5' terminus of p5'-c-abl by digestion with BamHI and EcoRI. As expected, a fragment of 14.5 kb was detected upon hybridization of normal human BamHI digested DNA; however, in DNA of one CML patient, 0319129, an additional BamHI fragment of 3.1 kb was detected. Moreover, additional abnormal fragments were detected in the DNA of patient 0319129 with other restriction enzymes using the same probe.

2.4 Molecular Cloning of a Chromosomal Junction Fragment

Since human c-abl is translocated to the Philadelphia chromosome ($22q^-$) in CML, we reasoned that if the 3.1 kb BamHI fragment of CML patient 0319129 contained a chromosomal breakpoint, the translocated sequences in the DNA of this patient 0319129 should include most of the 14.5 kb BamHI fragment; the 5' sequences of this fragment would presumably remain on chromosome 9, linked to sequences from chromosome 22, thus accounting for the 3.1 kb BamHI fragment.

To test this model, DNA from CML patient 0319129 was digested with BglII. We chose this enzyme because it detects an abnormal, additional 6.0 kb fragment in the DNA of patient 0319129 with the 0.2 kb BE probe; this 6.0 kb BglII fragment should encompass the 3.1 kb BamHI fragment. Upon size fractioning in the 6-7 kb range a library was constructed in BamHI digested Charon 30 phage arms. Three positive clones were identified upon screening with the 0.2 kb BE probe.

As shown in the restriction enzyme map of this fragment (Fig. 1C), the EcoRI site 3' of a 0.52 kb EcoRI fragment is still present. In contrast, an SstI site immediately 3' of it and all other restriction enzyme sites to the 3' are either missing or different from those found in the same region in p5'-c-abl.

To determine the origin of the 6.0 kb BglII fragment, a 1.2 kb HindIII/BglII probe (1.2 HBg, Fig 1C) was prepared. Using stringent washing conditions, this probe hybridized to a 5.0 kb BglII fragment in DNA of the human cell lines A204, but not to sequences in mouse DNA or in rodenthuman somatic cell hybrids containing human chromosome 9. In an independent hybrid (PgMe-25Nu) containing chromosome 22 as its only human component, a 5.0 kb fragment was detected. Moreover, using the same probe both 5.0 kb and 6.0 kb BglII fragments were identified in the DNA of patient 0319129. The 1.2 HBg probe did not hybridize to sequences in the human-mouse somatic cell hybrid WESP-2A, which contains the Ph' chromosome in the absence of 9,9q+ or 22. Thus, the 6.0 kb BglII fragment cloned from patient 0319129 DNA must contain, in addition to sequences from chromosome 9, sequences originating from the translocated region of chromosome 22.

2.5 Molecular Cloning of Ph' Breakpoint Region of Normal Chromosome 22

To define the region in the 6.0 kb BglII fragment which originated from chromosome 22, it was necessary to isolate 1.2 kb HBg-homologous sequences on chromosome 22 from non-CML DNA. For this purpose, a previously described (7) human lung carcinoma cosmid library was screened with the 1.2 kb HBg probe. Three cosmid clones were isolated, which contained overlapping portions of the same region.

As shown in Fig. 4A, a region of approximately 46 kb was molecularly cloned; the 1.2 kb HBg probe hybridized to a BglII fragment of 5.0 kb, located centrally in the cloned region. No homology is apparent between the restriction map of this region and that of human c-*sis* (12), an oncogene situated on chromosome 22 but translocated to chromosome 9 in the Ph' translocation (13). This confirms earlier reports which indicated that c-*sis* is not located in the immediate proximity of the Ph' breakpoint (14). The immunoglobulin light chain constant region (C) and the Ph' chromosomal breakpoint have been localized to chromosome 22 band q11 (3,15,16); this suggests that analogous to the translocation of c-*myc* in Burkitt lymphoma, c-*abl* could be translocated into C in CML. However, a probe isolated from the lambda constant region showed no cross-homology with the above described chromosome 22 sequences. Additionally, no hybridization to a murine-lambda

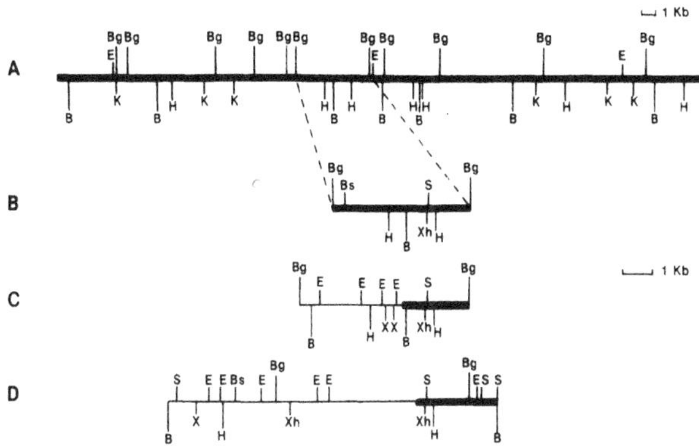

FIGURE 4. Comparative restriction enzyme analysis of the breakpoint region on chromosome 22 with two 9q+ breakpoint regions. A previously described (7) human cosmid library was screened with a 1.2 kb HBg probe according to published methods (26). Three positive cosmid clones were isolated and mapped independently. A restriction enzyme map of the cloned region of chromosome 22 is shown in A; a subclone containing the 5.0 kb BglII fragment in B is compared with the 6.0 kb BglII and 11.3 kb BamHI restriction enzyme fragments of the 9q+ chromosomes in C and D; heavy lines indicate sequences from chromosome 22, whereas light lines indicate sequences originating from chromosome 9. B=BamHI; Bg=BglII; Bs=BstEII, E=EcoRI; H=HindIII; K=KpnI; S=SstI; Xh=XhoI.

variable region probe (17) was observed (results not shown).

Upon hybridization of the DNA of another CML patient (02120185) with the 1.2 kb HBg probe, an abnormal 11.3 kb BamHI fragment was observed in addition to the normal 3.3 kb BamHI fragment. This abnormal fragment was molecularly cloned and could subsequently be shown to represent another 9q+ chimeric DNA fragment (27). In the 11.3 kb BamHI fragment (Fig. 4D) approximately 2.5 kb of DNA, including the 3' BamHI site and extending to the 3' XhoI site, originates from chromosome 22.

2.6 Clustering of Ph' Breakpoints on Chromosome 22 in CML patients

Since in each of the above two CML DNAs the breakpoint in the t (9;22) on chromosome 22 was localized within a common region, we decided to investigate this area in other CML DNAs. As the 1.2 HBg probe had detected abnormal ($9q^{+}$) BglII restriction fragments in DNAs 0319129 and 02120185, we subjected 17 additional independent CML DNAs to similar analysis; 6 of these were from spleen tissue, 9 were from patient blood, and 2 were from bone marrow. All Ph^{+} CML DNAs contained additional BglII fragments hybridizing to the 1.2 HBg probe. The DNAs of the four patients did not exhibit abnormal BglII fragments; two of these showed deviant restriction enzyme patterns with other restriction enzymes (this will be discussed below).

No extra BglII fragments were found in DNA isolated from cultured fibroblasts of a Ph'-positive CML patient H80-251 although DNA isolated from the leukemic cells of this patient clearly contained an extra BglII fragment. Moreover, DNA isolated from the fibroblast cell line, AG 1732, established from a Ph'-positive CML patient, also lacked abnormalities in this region. Finally, in DNA isolated from leukemic cells of a Ph'-negative CML patient and of a 2-year-old child with juvenile Ph'-negative CML, no visible rearrangements were found confirming our results of previous experiments (10) in which no translocations concerning c-*abl* or c-*sis* were found in Ph'-negative CML.

2.7 Sublocalization of Ph' Breakpoints within bcr

As is apparent from the detailed restriction enzyme analysis of the breakpoint fragments of the DNAs of patients 0319129 and 02120185 (Fig. 4C and D), the exact breakpoints are not localized at identical sites on chromosome 22 but rather within a breakpoint cluster region (bcr); in 0319129, the break was between a HindIII and a BamHI site (region 1, Fig. 6), whereas in 02120185 the breakpoint fell in an adjacent BamHI/HindIII fragment (region 2). In DNA 0311068, the BamHI site between region 1 and 2 (Fig. 6) seems to be present on the $9q^{+}$ chromosome, as only one (normal) BamHI fragment is seen upon BamHI digestion and hybridization to the 1.2 kb HBg probe (Fig. 5 lane 1). If, however, BglII digested DNA is hybridized to an 0.6 kb HindIII/BamHI probe, two abnormal fragments become apparent, presumably a $22q^{-}$ and a $9q^{+}$ fragment (Fig. 5 lane 2). Therefore, the breakpoint in DNA 0311068 seems to occur in region 1. In DNA of patient 7701C an abnormal BamHI fragment but no abnormal HindIII fragment is visible

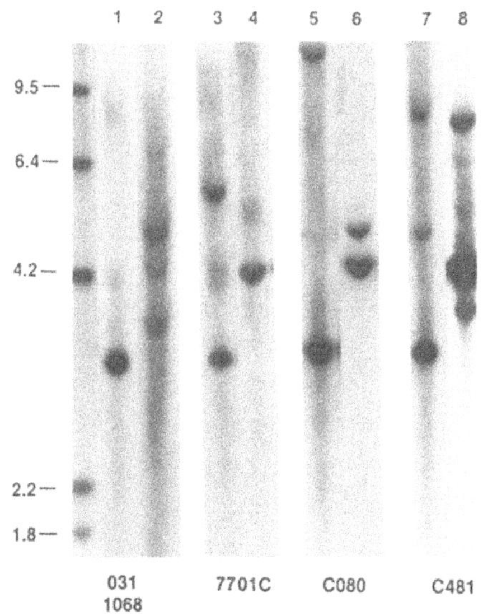

FIGURE 5. Analysis of Ph' translocation breakpoints on chromosome 22. DNA of patients was digested with BamHI (lane 1,3,5,7), BglII (lane 2) or HindIII (lane 4,6,8). Hybridization was with the 1.2 kb HBg probe; lane 2 is hybridized with a 0.6 kb HB probe (Region 1, Fig.6). High molecular weight DNA isolation (24), gel electrophoreses and blotting (25) were as described. Hybridization was with a previously described (4) 1.2 kb HBg probe; filters were washed to 0.3xSSC at 65°. Molecular weights of marker fragments in kb are indicated in the left of the figure.

after hybridization to 1.2 HBg (Fig. 5 lanes 3 and 4), placing the breakpoint in region 2. Patients C481 apparently has a breakpoint in region 3, as two abnormal fragments are visible after digestion with BamHI and HindIII (Fig. 5 lanes 7 and 8) and hybridization to the 1.2 HBg probe. The situation in patient C080 is less clear; although no extra BglII fragments were visible, both after HindIII and BamHI digestion, extra restriction enzyme fragments are found (Fig. 5 lanes 5 and 6), with the 1.2 HBg probe. We have therefore tentatively placed the breakpoint in this DNA in region 4 (Fig. 6). Using different restriction enzymes and probes from the 5.0 kb BglII fragment, we

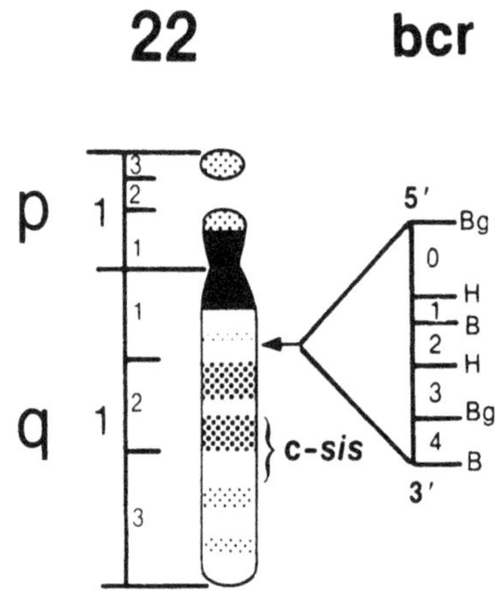

FIGURE 6. Diagrammatic representation of the Ph' translocation. The horizontal arrow indicates the chromosomal breakpoint on chromosome 22. Mapping of c-sis to the region of chromosome 22 (q12.3 to q13.1) translocated to chromosome 9 is a previously described (13, 14). The size of bcr from the 5'BglII to the 3'BamHI site is 5.8kb.

have analyzed the location of the breakpoint in a number of Ph^+ CML DNAs. These data suggest that the breakpoints are dispersed over the region 1,2 and 3 of bcr (Fig. 6, 27) in a random fashion. The region that encompasses the Ph' breakpoints, bcr, is probably encoding a protein as we recently have been able to isolate cDNA clones containing sequences homologous to this region. (J. Groffen, unpublished results). Because the orientation of the cDNA in the plasmid is known we have determined that the 5' region of the bcr gene remains on chromosome 22 in the Ph' translocation: The 5' region of this gene is oriented towards the centromere. (Fig.6). We and others (28) have recently shown that in the cell line K562 and in the leukemic cells of CML patients an additional c-abl RNA transcript of approximately 8 kb can be found. These data strengthen the previous findings which strongly implicate a role for human c-abl in CML; they also enable us to postulate a theory that explains the existence of this 8 kb c-ablmRNA. (see Fig.7): In the Ph' translocation a break occurs in the bcr gene, the tip of chromosome 9 containing the human c-abl is translocated to this truncated gene. In our theory, this construct would give rise to a chimeric 8 kb c-abl in mRNA that contains in its 5' end bcr encoding sequences while its 3' end is formed by human c-abl RNA sequences.

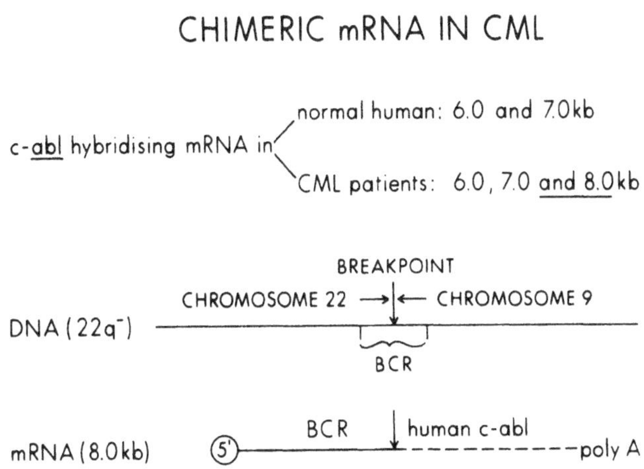

FIGURE 7: Chimeric mRNA in CML

2.8 Amplification of c-abl in K562 DNA

Although the K562 cell line has been shown to lack a cytogenetically indentifiable Ph' chromosome (Bartram, et al., unpublished observation), it was reported to contain a small ring chromosome, probably derived from a Ph' chromosome (18). As shown in Figure 8D, using the 1.2 HBg probe, a nonamplified 5.0 kb BglII fragment was detected in K562 DNA. In contrast,

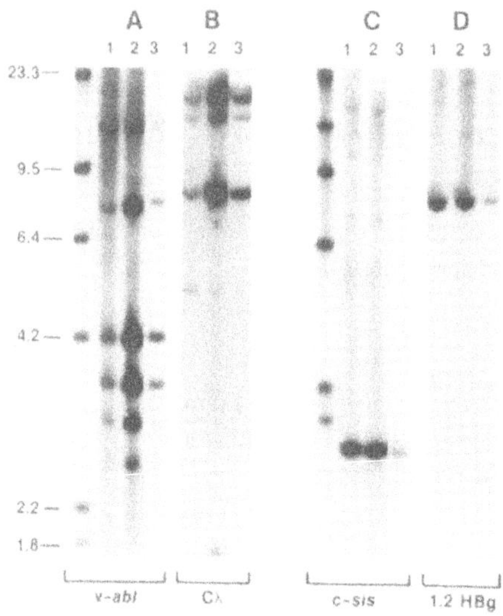

FIGURE 8. Amplification of c-abl in the erythroleukemic cell line K562. Control human DNA (10 ug, lanes 1 in each panel) was run next to 10 ug (lanes 2) and 2.5 ug (lanes 3) K562 DNA. ^{32}P-labelled HindIII digested DNA is included as a molecular weight standard for panels A+B (0.6% agarose gels) and for panels C+D (0.75% agarose gels). Panel A: DNAs were digested with EcoRI, and hybridized to v-abl $P_{1.7}$. Panel B: EcoRI digested DNAs were hybridized to a BglII/HindIII probe, isolated from a human C clone, Hu 5 (19). Panel C: BamHI digested DNA hybridized to a previously described (13) 1.7 kb BamHI probe prepared from a human c-sis cosmid clone. Panel D: BglII digested DNAs hybridized to the 1.2 HBg probe described in Figure 1C.

human c-abl sequences were found to be amplified at least fourfold in K562 DNA, as were sequences up to 17 kb upstream of the most 5' v-abl homologous EcoRI fragment (Fig. 8A). The 11.0 kb EcoRI fragment (Fig. 8A) that hybridizes to the v-abl $P_{1.7}$ probe but has not linkage with the main human c-abl locus is nonamplified and thus served as an internal control (Fig.8A). The immunoglobulin lambda light chain constant region (C), (19) is also amplified at least fourfold (Fig. 8B). This latter observation is consistent with the localization of human c-abl and C sequences on the same amplification unit, presumably a part of the Ph' chromosome. In concordance with this conclusion is the finding that C remains on the Ph' chromosome in the t(9;22) (Bartram et al, unpublished observation). In contrast, c-sis which is located on chromosome 22 and transferred to chromosome 9 in the Ph'translocation (13, 14), is nonamplified (Fig. 8C). Finally, the fact that the 5.0 kb BglII fragment normally localized on chromosome 22, is nonamplified in K562, supports the assumption that it is translocated to chromosome 9 in this cell line.

3. CONCLUSIONS

The present findings localize c-abl to human chromosome 9 and demonstrate its translocation to chromosome $22q^-$ (the Ph' chromosome) in CML. In one of three CML patient DNAs examined, the Ph' chromosomal breakpoint has been localized 14 kb from the most 5' v-abl homologous region. The possibility that the t(9;22) breakpoint may even map within the 5' coding region of the human c-abl locus cannot be excluded, since at present the position of the most 5' exon in human c-abl has not been determined. Although, as yet, we have not localized the breakpoints on chromosome 9 in the DNAs of the two other CML patients or in DNA of the cell line WESP-2A, containing the $22q^-$ chromosome, the results of cytogenetic analysis suggest that variability in Ph' translocation breakpoints must be very minor. Our findings establish that the site of the Ph' translocation breakpoint on chromosome 9 is not identical in each patient and suggests that breakpoints of other CML DNAs may be located 5' of the approximately 80 kb of cloned DNA encompassing the human c-abl locus. Similarly, the t(8;14) translocation breakpoint in Burkitt lymphoma, involving the human c-myc oncogene, has been shown to be variable in position (20, 21, 22) However, the possible involvement of c-*abl* in CML is further indicated by its translocation to the Ph' chromosome in the t(9;11;22) and the t(1;9;22) complex translocations associated with CML and the specific amplification of c-*abl* and C sequences in the K562 cell line. Moreover in cell line K562 and in the leukemic cells of Ph' positive CML patients a novel 8 kb c-*abl* mRNA is found. Finally, we identified a region on chromosome 22 that is specifically involved in the Ph' translocation; the DNAs of all Ph'-positive CML patients examined have a breakpoint within a breakpoint cluster region (bcr) of 4.2-5.8 kb on chromosome 22. Therefore, although our data strongly implicate human c-*abl* in CML, we believe that the chromosome 22 breakpoint region may also contribute to the tumorigenicity of Ph'-positive cells in CML.

ACKNOWLEDGEMENT

We thank Anne Hagemeijer and Ton van Agthoven for supplying patient material and for cytogenetical analysis; P. Leder and U. Storb for the generous gifts of Hu 5 and pV 1; Pamela Hansen and Gail Blennerhasset for technical assistance; Freyda Sussman for typing of the manuscript. This work was supported by the Netherlands Cancer Society (Koningin Wilhelmina Fonds) and under NCI PHS contract NOI-CP-75380.

REFERENCES

1. Goff, S.P., Gilboa, O.N. Witte, D. Baltimore. Structure of the Abelson murine leukemia virus genome and the homologous cellular gene: studies with cloned viral DNA. Cell 22:777. 1980
2. Heisterkamp, N., J. Groffen, J.R. Stephenson, N.K. Spurr, P.N. Goodfellow, B. Solomon, B. Garritt, W.F. Bodmer. Chromosomal localization of human cellular homologues of two viral oncogenes. Nature 299:747. 1982
3. Rowley, J.D. A new consistent chromosomal abnormality in chronic myelogenous leukemia identified by quinacrine fluorescence and Giemsa staining. Nature 243, 290-293. 1983
4. Heisterkamp, N., Stephenson, J.R., Groffen, J., Hansen, P.F., de Klein, A., Bartram, C.R., and Grosveld, G. Localization of the c-*abl* oncogene adjacent to a translocation breakpoint in chronic myelocytic leukemia. Nature, 306:239. 1983
5. Heisterkamp, N., J. Groffen, J.R. Stephenson. The human v-*abl* cellular homologue. J. Mole. Appl. Genet. 2:57. 1983
6. Srinivasan, A., E.P. Reddy, S.A. Aaronson. Abelson murine leukemia virus: Molecular cloning of infectious integrated proviral DNA. Proc. Natl Acad. Sci. USA 78: 2077. 1981
7. Groffen, J., N. Heisterkamp, G. Grosveld, W. Van de Ven, J.R. Stephenson. Isolation of human oncogene sequences (v-*fes* homolog) from a cosmid library. Science 216:1136. 1982

8. Groffen, J., N. Heisterkamp, F. Reynolds, Jr., J.R. Stephenson. Human c-abl phosphotyrosine acceptor site. Nature 304:57. 1983
9. de Klein, A., A. Geurts van Kessel, G. Grosveld, C.R. Bartram, A. Hagemeijer, D. Bootsma, N.K. Spurr, N. Heisterkamp, J. Groffen, J.R. Stephenson. A cellular oncogene is translocated to the Philadelphia chromosome in chronic myelocytic leukemia. Nature 300:765. 1982
10. Bartram, C.R., A. de Klein, A. Hagemeijer, T. van Agthoven, A. Geurts van Kessel, D. Bootsma, G. Grosveld, M. Ferguson-Smith, T. Davis, M. Stone, N. Heisterkamp, J.R. Stephenson, J. Groffen. Translocation of the human c-abl oncogene occurs in variant Ph'-positive but not Ph'negative chronic myelocytic leukemia. Nature 306:277. 1983
11. Lozzio, C.B., Lozzio, B.B. Human chronic myelogenous leukemia cell line with positive Philadelphia chromosome. Blood 45:321. 1975
12. Dalla-Favera, R., Gelman, E.P., Gallo, R.C. and Wong-Staal, F. A human oncogene homologous to the transforming gene (v-sis) of simian sarcoma virus. Nature 292:31. 1981
13. Groffen, J., N. Heisterkamp, J.R. Stephenson, A. van Kessel, A. de Klein, G. Grosveld, D. Bootsma. c-sis is translocated from chromosome 22 to chromosome 9 in chronic myelocytic leukemia. J. Exp. Med. 158:9. 1983
14. Bartram, C.R., A. de Klein, A. Hagemeijer, G. Grosveld, N. Heisterkamp, J. Groffen. Localization of the human c-sis oncogene in Ph'-positive and Ph'-negative chronic myelocytic leukemia by *in situ* hybridization. Blood, 63:223,1984
15. McBride, O.W., Hieter, P.A., Hollis, G.F., Swan, D., Otey, M.C., and Leder, P. (1982). Chromosomal location of human kappa and lambda immunoglobulin light chain constant region genes. J. Exp. Med. 155:1480.
16. Yunis, J.J. The chromosomal basis of human neoplasia. Science 221:227. 1983
17. Miller, J., Bothwell, A., and Storb, U. Physical linkage of the constant region genes for immunoglobulins I and III. Proc. Natl. Acad. Sci. USA 78:3829. 1982
18. Klein, E., H. Ben-Bassat, H. Neumann, P. Ralph, J. Zeuthen, A. Polliack and F. Vånky. Properties of the K562 cell line derived from a patient with chronic myeloid leukemia. Int. J. Cancer 18:421. 1976
19. Hieter, P.A., G.F. Hollis, S.J. Korsmeyer, T.A. Waldmann, P. Leder. Clustered arrangement of immunoglobulin lambda constant region genes in man. Nature 294:536. 1981
20. Taub, R., I. Kirsch, C. Morton, G. Lenoir. Translocation of the c-myc gene into the immunoglobulin heavy chain locus in human Burkitt lymphoma and in murine plasmacytoma cells. Proc. Natl. Acad. Sci. 79:7837. 1982
21. Adams, J.M., S. Gerondakis, E. Webb, L.M. Corcoran, S. Gary. 1983 Cellular myc is altered by chromosome translocation to an immunoglobulin locus in murine plasmacytomas and is rearranged similarly in human Burkitt lymphomas. Proc. Natl. Acad. Sci. USA 80:1982.
22. Dalla-Favera, S. Martinotti, R. Gallo. Translocation and rearrangement of the c-myc oncogene locus in human undifferentiated B-cell lymphomas. Science 219:963. 1983
23. Carritt, B., S. Povey. Regional assignments of the loci AK3, ACONS and AK1 on human chromosome 9. Cytogenet. Cell Genet. 23:171.1979

24. Jeffreys, A.J., and Flavell, R.A. A physical map of the DNA regions flanking the rabbit B-globin gene. Cell 12, 429. 1977
25. Southern, E.M. Detection of specific sequences among DNA fragments separated by gel electrophoreses. J. Mole. Biol. 98:503. 1975
26. Grosveld, F.G, HHM Dahl, E. deBoer, R. Flavell. Isolation of B-globin-related genes from a human cosmid library. Gene 13:227.1981
27. Groffen J, J.R. Stephenson, N. Heisterkamp, A. de Klein, C.R. Bartram, G.Grosveld. Philadelphia chromosomal breakpoints are clustered within a limited region, bcr, on chromosome 22. Cell 36:93.1984
28. E. Canaani, R.P. Gale, D. Steiner-Saltz, A. Berrebi, E. Aghai, E. Januszewicz. Altered transcription of an oncogene in chronic myeloid leukaemia. The Lancet 1:593.1984

13

MONOCLONAL ANTIBODIES GENERATED TO A SYNTHETIC PEPTIDE DEFINE RAS GENE EXPRESSION AT THE SINGLE CELL LEVEL IN HUMAN COLON AND MAMMARY CARCINOMAS

A. Thor, P. Horan Hand, D. Wunderlich, M. Weeks, A. Caruso, R. Muraro, and J. Schlom

National Cancer Institute, Bethesda, Maryland

1. INTRODUCTION

Ras oncogenes were first recognized as the transforming genes of two rat-derived viruses, the Harvey (Ha) and Kirsten (Ki) strains of murine sarcoma virus (MuSV) (1). Molecular cloning studies have identified Ha-*ras*, Ki-*ras*, and subsequently, N-*ras*, as members of a gene family present in a wide range of species including humans (2). At least two mechanisms have been identified by which *ras* activation can mediate transformation of NIH 3T3 cells: (a) a point mutation in the *ras* gene resulting in an alteration of a single amino acid in the 21,000 dalton (p21) *ras* gene product (3), or (b) increased expression of the normal cellular p21 *ras* gene product (1,4,5).

Ras activation has been detected in certain human tumor cell lines and selected biopsy materials from a variety of cancers by the demonstration of the transforming potential of DNA from those specimens for NIH 3T3 cells; only a small percentage (usually less than 10% to 20%) of specimens tested from any given human tumor system, however, have proven positive for activated *ras* in this system (6, S. Aaronson, personal communication). One possible explanation for this is that the mechanism of *ras* activation in these tumors may involve the increased expression of a normal cellular *ras* gene and gene product (e.g., via hormone activation of a *ras* inducing promoter sequence (7), or via gene amplification (5)).

An alternative approach to determining whether correlations exist between enhanced *ras* gene expression (activation) and a particular neoplastic state would be the use of immunologic assays directed against the p21 *ras* gene product. Radioimmunoassays (RIAs) would provide a quantitative determination of *ras* gene expression, while immunohistochemical studies would define *ras* gene expression in circumstances in which other methods are not suitable, i.e., the determination of *ras* gene expression at the single cell level in normal epithelium, hyperplastic lesions, and adjacent malignant tissues from the same patient. In light of the provocative findings on *ras* gene activation in selected colon carcinoma cell lines (6) and a human breast carcinosarcoma cell line (8), and the recent finding of *ras* gene activation in carcinogen induced rat mammary tumor models (9,10), we undertook the development of monoclonal antibodies (MAbs) to a human *ras* gene product. Since the DNA sequence of the entire human Ha-*ras* gene has been defined (3), and the studies of Lerner (11) have demonstrated an extremely efficient utilization of polyclonal antibodies prepared against synthetic peptides, the approach of preparing MAbs to a predefined set of *ras* amino acid sequences was undertaken.

2. PROCEDURE

The following peptides (positions 10-17 of the Hu-*ras* gene product) were synthesized as predicted from the *ras* DNA sequence: (Hu-ras^{T24}): Gly-Ala-Val-Gly-Val-Gly-Lys-Ser, and (Hu-ras^{Ha}): Gly-Ala-Gly-Gly-Val-Gly-Lys-Ser. Tyrosine was added to the amino terminus of each peptide for ease of iodination and lysine was added to the carboxy terminus to facilitate solubilization of the peptides. Peptide Hu-ras^{T24} was coupled to thyroglobulin and used as immunogen. All resulting hybridoma cell lines were cloned twice. MAbs B1.1 (directed against carcinoembryonic antigen (12)), UPC-10 (a purified mouse myeloma protein of the IgG_{2a} isotype (13)) and YA6 259 (a rat anti-rat *ras*, supplied by Dr. M. Furth (14)) have been described elsewhere. Purified immunoglobulins were prepared as described (15). The avidin-biotin-complex (ABC) immunoperoxidase assay was performed on 5 micron sections from formalin fixed paraffin embedded tissues as described (16,17). In all cases an isotype identical primary antibody (UPC-10) was used as a negative control.

3. RESULTS

3.1. Generation of MAbs

Hybridoma cultures were assayed via solid phase RIA for synthesis of Ig demonstrating differential reactivity with the Hu-ras^{T24} peptide or the Hu-ras^{Ha} peptide, and no reactivity with thyroglobulin. Five doubly cloned hybridoma cultures, representing the widest spectrum of differential reactivities to the Hu-*ras*^{T24} peptide vs. the Hu-*ras*^{Ha} peptide were chosen and designated RAP-1 through RAP-5 (RA:*ras*; P:peptide). Each was determined to be of the IgG_{2a} isotype. Figure 1 shows the binding of purified Ig of MAb RAP-5 to the Hu-*ras*^{T24} vs. the Hu-*ras*^{Ha} peptide. As little as 250 pg of purified RAP-5 Ig can detect 10 ng of the Hu-*ras*^{T24} peptide, while no reactivity has been observed to as much as 120 ng thyroglobulin using 32 times more RAP-5 MAb. Similarly, MAb UPC-10 showed no binding to either peptide (Fig. 1). In solid phase RIAs employing a constant MAb amount (1:100 dilution of cell culture supernatant) vs. dilutions of peptides, MAb RAP-5 could detect as little as 400 pg of Hu-*ras*^{T24} peptide vs. 2000 pg of Hu-*ras*^{Ha} peptide. Since these RIAs utilize a solid phase substrate, one must view with caution the differential reactivity observed to equal quantities of Hu-*ras*^{T24} vs. Hu-*ras*^{Ha} (See Discussion).

Initial attempts to immunoprecipitate native p21 from extracts of transformed cells proved unsuccessful. This was not unexpected as the determinants detected by the RAP MAbs have been predicted to be internally located in the native p21 molecule (19,20). Western blotting experiments in which extracts were treated with SDS-mercaptoethanol were thus used to demonstrate binding to p21.

3.2. RIAs for ras p21

Several RAP MAbs showed weak binding in solid phase RIAs (18) to undenatured cell extracts (18) of T24 human bladder carcinoma cells and T24 DNA-transfected NIH 3T3 cells (3); no binding to NIH 3T3 cells was detected. As discussed above, one would not predict efficient binding of these MAbs to native *ras* p21; therefore, extracts were treated with 10% buffered formalin in an attempt to alter the configuration of p21 and thus expose the determinants detected by the RAP MAbs. As shown in Fig. 2, formalin treatment of extracts of either the T24 line or the MCF-7 human mammary carcinoma cell line appreciably enhanced detection of *ras* p21 by MAb RAP-1. It is interesting to note that formalin had no effect on the binding of either MAb UPC-10 to T24 cell extracts (Fig. 2A, insert) or MAb B1.1 to extracts of MCF-7 cells (Fig. 2B, insert). Formalin did eliminate, however, the binding of MAb YA6 259 to T24 cells. Preliminary studies using extracts of biopsy material or cell lines indicate that fixation of extracts with 2%

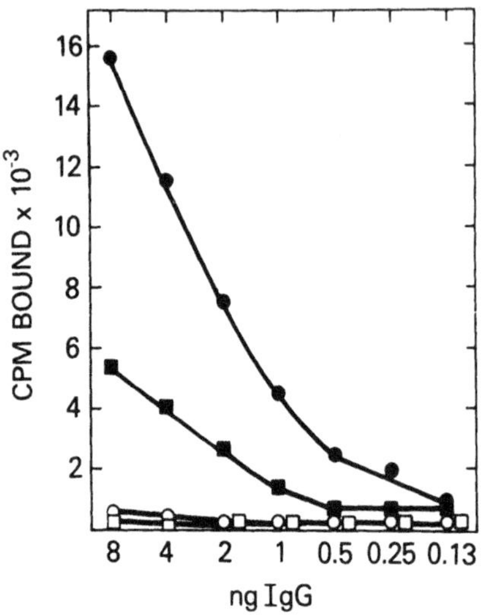

FIGURE 1. Reactivity of MAb RAP-5 with Hu-<u>ras</u>^{T24} and Hu-<u>ras</u>^{Ha} peptides. Using a solid-phase RIA (18), increasing amounts of purified IgG of MAb RAP-5 were assayed for binding to 10 ng Hu-<u>ras</u>^{T24} (●), 10 ng Hu-<u>ras</u>^{Ha} (■), and 120 ng thyroglobulin (□). Purified IgG of MAb UPC-10 was also assayed for binding to <u>ras</u> peptides (○).

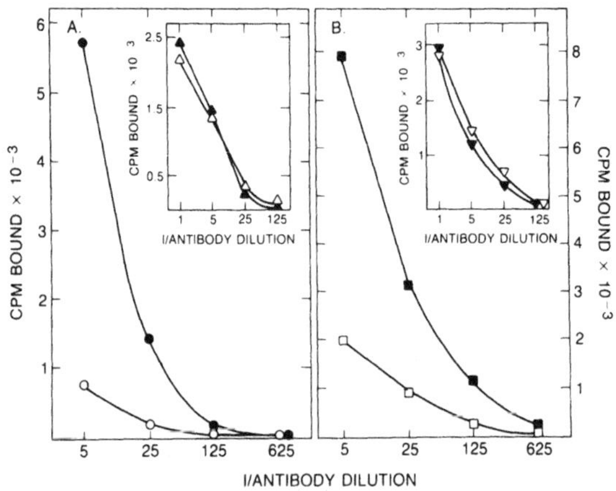

FIGURE 2.Reactivity of MAb RAP-1 to Cell Extracts. Using a solid-phase RIA, MAb RAP-1 was used to detect <u>ras</u> p21. Panel A: undenatured T24 cell extract (○), and formalin-fixed (10% buffered formalin for 1 hr at 25°C) T24 cell extract (●); Panel B: undenatured MCF-7 cell extract (□), formalin fixed MCF-7 cell extract (■). Panel A Insert: MAb UPC-10 reactivity to unfixed (△) and formalin-fixed (▲) T24 cell extract. Panel B Insert: MAb B1.1 reactivity to unfixed (▽) and formalin-fixed (▼) MCF-7 cell extract.

glutaraldehyde is even more efficient than formalin in detection of ras p21 by the RAP MAbs.

3.3. Analysis of Human Mammary Carcinomas

Thirty formalin fixed infiltrating ductal carcinomas (IDCs) from 30 patients were examined for ras gene activation with each of several RAP MAbs (RAP 1, 2, and 5), all with similar results. Twenty-seven of 30 (90%) of the IDCs scored positive (see Fig. 3A). RAP MAb dilution experiments demonstrate that most "positive" mammary carcinomas contain cells that score positive for ras expression at MAb endpoint dilutions 32-fold to 320-fold higher than cells in the vast majority of benign lesions (Table 1). As seen in Fig. 4, however, a natural separation of this group of carcinomas is seen with those tumors scoring ⩽ 5% of carcinoma cells positive (11/30) vs. those with ⩾ 20% of carcinoma cells scoring positive (19/30). Using this criteria, i.e. ⩾ 20% of tumor cells scoring positive, only 2 of the 21 benign breast lesions (0/11 fibrocystic disease and 2/10 fibroadenomas) scored positive (Fig. 4). It is interesting to note that the two fibroadenomas positive for ras gene expression (Fig. 4B, denoted a and b) were from two patients with multiple fibroadenomas (See Discussion).
The one of eleven fibrocystic disease lesions examined (Fig. 4B, patient c) with 10% of cells scoring positive for ras expression, was

Table 1. Titration of MAb RAP-5 with malignant and benign breast lesions

MAb RAP-5 μg/200 μl	Percent ras positive tumor cells: Malignant IDC-1	IDC-2	IDC-3	Benign FA1	FA2	FD1
16	85	95	70	<1	<1	<5
8	100	45	90	0	0	0
4	70	65	90	0	0	0
2	90	1	70	0	0	0
1	30	1	70	0	0	0
0.5	30	1	60	0	0	0
0.1	0	0	5	0	0	0
0.05	0	0	<1	0	0	0

Sequential tissue sections were assayed via the immunoperoxidase method. IDC is infiltrating ductal carcinoma; FA is fibroadenoma; FD is fibrocystic disease (percent positive cells based on the percent of epithelial cells scoring positive).

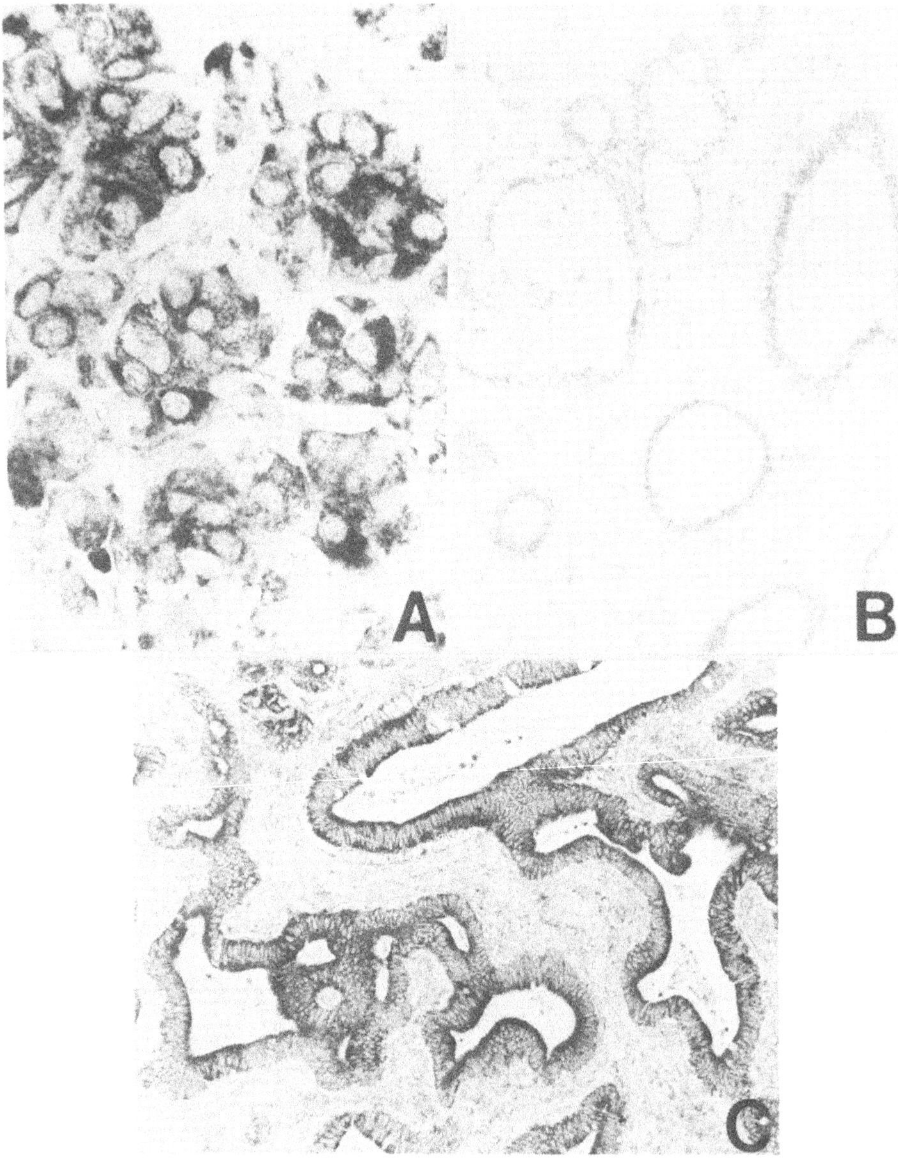

FIGURE 3. Reactivity of MAb RAP-5 (1:8 dilution of tissue culture fluid) with paraffin embedded, formalin fixed surgical specimens using the ABC immunoperoxidase method. A. Positive reaction with infiltrating ductal carcinoma of the breast, 540X, B. Negative reaction with a fibrocystic disease of the breast, 220X, C. positive reaction with a infiltrating adenocarcinoma of the colon, 130X.

from a patient with a clinical history of severe chronic mastitis and a histologic diagnosis of fibrocystic disease and focal chronic inflammation (See Discussion). MAb dilution experiments demonstrated that the cells positive for ras expression in the lesions of patients a, b, and c (Fig. 4B) were as strong as those found in most carcinomas. However, the vast majority of all abnormal ducts and lobules from fibroadenoma patients and fibrocystic disease patients (Fig. 3B) were negative. Normal lobules and ducts from breasts of fibroadenoma patients and fibrocystic disease were also routinely negative for ras gene expression.

In most primary mammary carcinomas, a heterogeneity in the number of tumor cells expressing ras was observed. Several mammary tumor metastases from five patients with ras positive primary mammary tumors were reacted with MAb RAP-1 and also showed some degree of heterogeneity of ras gene expression within individual metastatic masses. The possible reasons for this will be discussed below. However, all five regional lymph node metastases assayed, as well as all four distal metastases, (skin, chest wall, rib, adrenal) demonstrated ras gene expression.

3.4. Assay of Colon Carcinomas

Extracts of six human colon carcinoma biopsies were denatured with 2% glutaraldehyde and assayed in solid phase RIA for ras p21 using MAb RAP-5. As seen in Fig. 5, the six colon carcinomas varied over at least a 30-fold range in their content of ras p21 per mg of protein extract. While one could arbitrarily assign nanogram values of ras p21 per cell for each tumor biopsy, these numbers would be extremely artificial since each biopsy mass will vary greatly in actual percent tumor cells out of total cells present (ranging from less than 1% to over 90%). Immunohistochemical examination of individual surgical specimens would thus be better suited to define which cell type(s) are actually expressing ras p21.

Five micron sections of formalin fixed colon carcinomas were assayed for Hu-ras p21 content using purified immunoglobulin preparations of MAb RAP-5 and the ABC immunoperoxidase method. Using a 40-fold range of purified MAb and serial sections of tumors, 4 of the 6 colon carcinomas were clearly positive for ras p21 expression

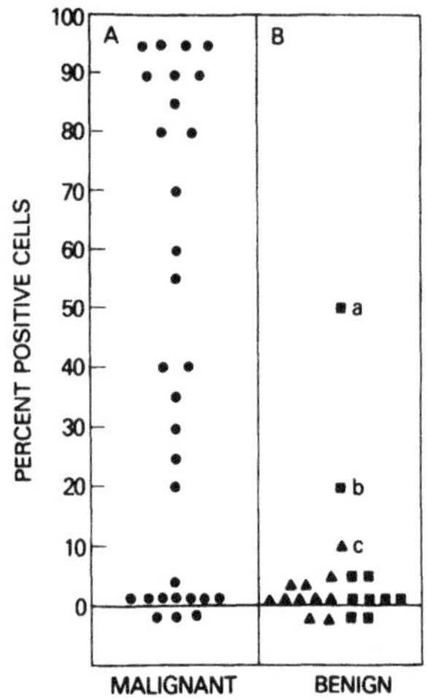

FIGURE 4. MAb RAP-1 (at a 1:8 dilution of supernatant fluid) was reacted with mammary carcinomas (●) and benign lesions: (■) fibroadenoma, (▲) fibrocystic disease. Each symbol represents a paraffin embedded formalin fixed tumor or lesion from a different patient. The percent cells positive denote: (A) for carcinomas and fibroadenomas: the number of tumor cells scoring ras positive divided by the total number of tumor cells X 100; (B) for fibrocystic disease lesions: the number of epithelial cells scoring ras positive divided by the total number of epithelial cells X 100. Tumors a and b are from patients with multiple fibroadenomas; lesion c is from a patient with severe chronic mastitis.

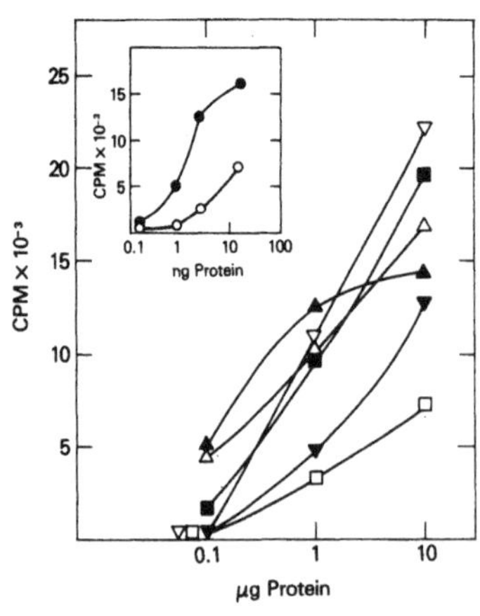

FIGURE 5. Reactivity of MAb RAP-5 with ras synthetic peptides and extracts of colon carcinoma biopsies in solid phase RIA (18) [Insert: Reactivity of MAb RAP-5 (1:100 dilution of tissue culture supernatant fluid) with various amounts of Hu-ras^{T24} (closed circles) and Hu-ras^{Ha} (open circles) synthetic peptides.] Reactivity of MAb RAP-5 (1:50 dilution of culture fluid) with various amounts of 2% glutaraldehyde treated extracts of 6 colon carcinoma biopsies from patients A through F in solid phase RIA.

(Fig. 6). The cell type expressing *ras* in these sections was the carcinoma cells (Fig. 3C), with percent carcinoma cells positive ranging from 20% to greater than 90% (Fig. 6); the percent reactive cells could be reduced in a linear fashion by decreasing the concentration of the RAP MAb used. Colonic stroma and smooth muscle were negative for *ras* p21. Two of the six colon carcinomas showed only a few (< 1%) of carcinoma cells reacting with MAb RAP-5 at any of the concentrations employed. In all assays of this study, equal concentrations of an isotype identical (IgG_{2a}) control MAb UPC-10 were used in place of the RAP MAbs, always with negative results. Normal colonic mucosa from carcinoma patients (when seen within the same section containing carcinoma cells) was either negative for reactivity with MAb RAP-5 at all immunoglobulin (Ig) concentrations used or demonstrated less than 1% of normal epithelial cells expressing *ras* p21 (Fig. 6). Normal colonic epithelium from a non-cancer patient also contained less than 1% positive cells at all MAb RAP-5 concentrations (Fig. 6, open circles).

Four benign colon tumors (2 tubular adenomas and 2 tubulovillous adenomas) were also assayed for *ras* p21 expression using identical MAb RAP-5 concentrations and assay conditions described above. Both types of lesions have been implicated as potentially premalignant (21,22) with a higher incidence of carcinoma arising from tubulovillous adenomas (23-25).The tumor cells from all four lesions assayed were either negative for MAb RAP-5 binding or contained only a few cells positive over the 40-fold range of MAb concentrations used (Fig. 6, open squares and triangles).

To further define if biologic correlations exist in *ras* p21 expression, 32 colon carcinomas, 22 benign colon tumors, inflammatory lesions, or hyperplastic colon lesions, and 9 specimens of normal colon from non-cancer patients were examined for reactivity with MAb RAP-1 using the ABC immunoperoxidase method. Thirty-one of the 32 colon carcinomas contained some *ras* positive carcinoma cells; however, a distinction could be observed (Fig. 7A) with 16/32 (50%) of the tumors from individual cancer patients containing greater than 20% of tumor cells expressing *ras* p21 at the MAb concentration used. In contrast, 2 of the 9 normal colon samples from non-cancer patients contained $\leq$1% of positive cells with the remainder scoring negative (Fig. 7C). Several

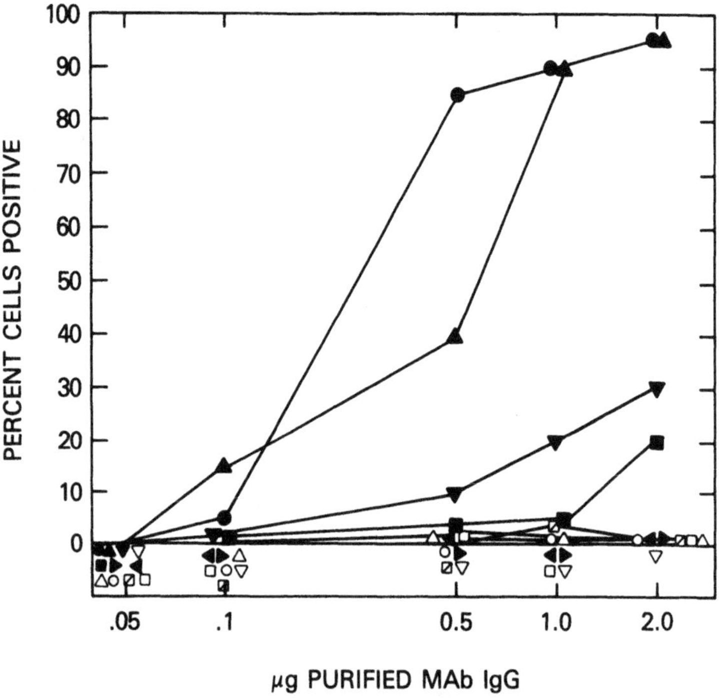

FIGURE 6. Titration of purified MAb RAP-5 (in ug purified IgG/200 ul) with paraffin embedded formalin fixed colonic tissues. Serial sections of adenocarcinomas of the colon (Patients G-L, solid figures), tubulo-villous adenomas (open and slashed squares), tubular adenomas (open triangles) and normal colonic epithelium (open circles) were assayed for ras p21 using the ABC immunoperoxidase technique and purified IgG of MAb RAP-5. The percent positive cells is a semiquantitative value (evaluated two times independently) for tumor cells scoring ras positive divided by the total tumor cells x 100 (for carcinomas, and adenomas), and the percent of normal colonic epithelial cells scoring ras positive divided by the total number of normal colonic epithelial cells. For all tissues an IgG_{2a} isotype identical primary antibody (UPC-10) was used at the same Ig concentrations as negative control, and no positivity was demonstrated.

types of benign, hyperplastic, or inflammatory colon lesions were also assayed. These included eleven tubular adenomas, 8 tubulovillous adenomas, 2 diverticulitis and one ulcerative colitis specimen. As seen in Fig. 7B, 21 of the 22 lesions were either negative for *ras* p21 expression or contained less than 5% of tumor or epithelial cells scoring positive; one severe diverticulitis lesion demonstrated 10% of cells expressing *ras* p21 (Fig. 7B, patient "a"). It thus appears that, at the RAP MAb concentration and conditions used for these assays, enhanced *ras* p21 expression can be observed (using > 20% cells positive as an arbitrary criterion - see Fig. 7) in 16 of 32 colon carcinomas as opposed to none of 31 benign colon tumors, hyperplastic lesions (with possibly one exception, i.e., patient "a"), or normal colon specimens from 31 different patients.

A great deal of antigenic heterogeneity has been observed within most human carcinomas using MAbs directed against several distinct tumor associated antigens (26). As seen here, virtually all colon and breast carcinoma specimens also varied in the percent of tumor cells within a given tumor mass expressing *ras* p21. MAb RAP-5 was used to examine five metastatic lesions from two colon carcinoma patients whose primary tumors were positive for *ras* p21 expression (40% and 80% of tumor cells, respectively). All five metastatic lesions (to ovary, liver, omentum, and 2 lymph nodes) also displayed antigenic heterogeneity with levels ranging from 5% to over 90% of cells scoring positive for *ras* p21 expression.

4. DISCUSSION

Several possible explanations exist for the heterogeneity in *ras* expression observed within carcinoma masses: (a) the assays employed are not sensitive enough to detect low levels of *ras* expression in some cells; (b) cell cycle influences p21 expression, as has been observed for other tumor associated antigens (27) and recently for *ras* (28); (c) the milieu of individual tumor cells or tumor cell clusters including apocrine, paracrine, and/or endocrine factors influences *ras* expression; (d) *ras* is not involved in the etiology of colon cancer, and its expression is an effect of the neoplastic process in some cells or lesions; and/or (e) *ras* may be involved in the initial transformation event, but other mechanisms of conferring immortality may come into play in

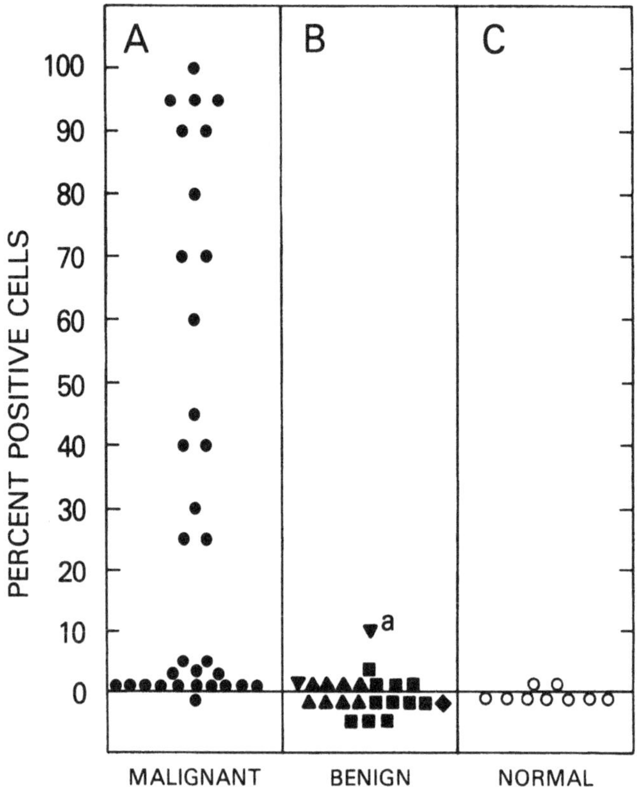

FIGURE 7. Reactivity of MAb RAP-1 with various colonic disease states. MAb RAP-1 (at a 1:8 dilution of supernatant fluid) was reacted with formalin fixed five micron sections of colonic adenocarcinomas (Panel A, closed circles), diverticulitis (Panel B, inverted triangles), tubular adenomas (Panel B, squares), tubulovillous adenomas (Panel B, triangles), ulcerative colitis (Panel B, diamond) and normal colon (Panel C, open circles), using the ABC immunoperoxidase method. Each symbol represents a tumor or tissue from a different patient. The percent positive cells denotes: for carcinomas and benign tumors (Panels A and B) the number of tumor cells scoring ras p21 positive divided by the total number of tumor cells x 100; for diverticulitis (B) and normal colon (C) the percent cells positive is the number of epithelial cells scoring ras p21 positive divided by the total number of epithelial cells x 100. Benign lesion "a" (Panel B) is from a patient with severe diverticulitis and acute perforation.

the approximately 10 to 30 years that have been theorized to elapse between the initial cell transformation and the detection and removal of a carcinoma mass (29,30).

Whether ras gene activation is actually involved in the etiology of human breast or colon cancer remains to be proven. The immunologic studies reported here do provide, however, data that ras p21 is differentially expressed in many breast and colon carcinomas versus tumors, hyperplastic or inflammatory lesions of these tissues. Furthermore, preliminary studies indicate that enhanced ras expression (a) appears to correlate with the depth of invasion (presumed degree of malignancy) in at least some colon carcinoma lesions, and (b) appears to be a late event, at least within some lesions, in the multistep process of colon carcinogenesis.

The percent of human colon carcinomas in which activated ras was detected with the RAP MAbs was much higher than that reported with DNA transfection experiments. The finding of activated ras gene expression in a majority of human mammary carcinomas was even more unexpected in light of the fact that DNA transfection experiments looking for activated ras expression in human breast cancers have been thus far unsuccessful. Two possible explanations for these observations could be that (a) the NIH 3T3 foci indicator system is not efficient for this particular ras gene, or (b) the mechanism of ras activation in many colon and mammary carcinomas involves the enhanced expression of a normal c-ras gene, perhaps at times, via a hormonally controlled promoter sequence; DNA transfection experiments would not score positive for this type of mechanism. It is interesting to note that the only two benign breast lesions that scored with similar percentages of tumor cells positive as the mammary carcinomas were from patients (Fig. 4B, patients "a" and "b") with multiple fibroadenomas (a total of 7 tumors removed from the two patients prior to 24 years of age). Hormonal factors have been implicated in the development of these lesions and for severe chronic mastitis (Fig. 4B, patient c (31)).

The studies reported here demonstrate that MAbs prepared against a set of predefined amino acid sequences, believed to be internally located in a molecule and thus not efficiently exposed for antibody binding in the native conformation, can be rendered available by simply altering the tertiary structure of the molecule with a substance such as formalin or glutaraldehyde (Fig. 2).Fortunately, formalin fixed tissue sections have several advantages over frozen sections: finer histologic detail, ease of processing, and availability. Conversely, we have been unable to detect ras p21 with the YA6 259 antibody (prepared against native p21) in formalin fixed tissues.

The detection of ras p21 in solid phase RIAs by the RAP MAbs provides, to our knowledge, the first quantitative radioimmunoassay for any onc gene product. The purified Ig dilution experiments shown in Table 1 also provide semi-quantitative evaluation of the relative amounts of p21 in individual cells in tissue section, since we have determined linear binding to purified peptides within the range of Ig concentrations employed (data not shown).

The RAP MAbs generated thus far do not discriminate among the Hu-ras genes being detected, i.e., the human Ha-, Ki-, and N-ras genes. Thus, the immunoassays employed here should be termed "group specific" in that they recognize translational products from members of a group of related genes within a given species. Clearly "type specific" immunoassays, employing antibodies directed against peptides reflecting variable regions of the ras gene, will eventually be utilized to determine which of the Hu-ras genes is being expressed in a given cell.

The quantitative ras p21 RIAs developed, as well as the use of formalin fixed tissue specimens for identification of particular cell types expressing ras p21, now make possible the direct evaluation (both retrospective as well as prospective) of clinical material in an attempt to define the precise role, if any, of ras gene translational products in the processes of carcinoma initiation, promotion, and progression.

REFERENCES

1. Ellis, RW, DeFeo, D, Shih, TY, Gonda, MA, Young, HA, Tsuchida, N Lowy, DR, Scolnick, EM: The p21 src genes of Harvey and Kirsten sarcoma viruses originate from divergent members of a family of normal vertebrate genes. Nature (292): 596-511, 1981.

2. Shimizu, K, Goldfarb, M, Suard, Y, Perucho, M, Kamata, T, Feramisco, J., Stavnezer, E, Fogh, J, Wigler, M: Three transforming genes are related to the viral ras oncogenes. Proc. Natl. Acad. Sci., USA (80): 2112-2116, 1983.

3. Reddy, EP, Reynolds, RK, Santos, E, Barbacid, M: A point mutation is responsible for the aquisition of transforming properties by the T24 human bladder carcinoma oncogene. Nature (300): 149-152, 1982.

4. Tabin, CJ, Bradley, SM, Bargmann, CI, Weinberg, RA, Papageorge, AG, Scolnick, EM, Dhar, R, Lowy, DR, Chang, EH: Mechanism of activation of a human oncogene. Nature (300): 142-148, 1982.

5. Schwab, M, Alitalo, K, Varmus, HE, Bishop, JM: A cellular oncogene (c-Ki-ras) is amplified, overexpressed, and located within karyotypic abnormalities in mouse adrenocortical tumour cells. Nature (303): 497-501, 1983.

6. Pulciani, S, Santos, E, Lauver, AV, Long, LK, Aaronson, A, Barbacid, M: Oncogenes in human solid tumors. Nature (300): 539-542, 1982.

7. Huang, AL, Ostrowski, MC, Berard, D, Hager GL: Glucocorticoid regulation of Ha-MuSV p21 gene conferred by sequences from mouse mammary tumor virus. Cell (27): 245-255, 1981.

8. S. Aaronson: A position 12-activated H-ras oncogene in all HS57T mammary carcinosarcoma cells but not normal cells of the same patient. RNA Tumor Viruses (Abstracts of Meeting May 22-27, 1984). Cold Spring Harbor Laboratories, Cold Spring Harbor, New York, 1984. p. 126.

9. Sukumar, S, Notario, V, Martin-Zanca, D, Barbacid, M: Induction of mammary carcinomas in rats by nitroso-methylurea involves malignant activation of H-ras 1 locus by single point mutations. Nature (306): 658-661, 1983.

10. Cho-Chung, YS and Huang, FL: (Abstract) Enhanced expression and suppression of c-ras^{H} oncogene during growth and regression of hormone dependent mammary tumors. In Proceedings of the 16th Miami Winter Symposium. ICSU Press, Miami. pp. 142-143.

11. Lerner, RA: Tapping the immunological repertorire to produce antibodies of predetermined specificity. Nature (299): 592-596, 1982.

12. Colcher, D, Horan Hand, P, Nuti, M, Schlom, J: Differential binding to human mammary and non-mammary tumors of monoclonal antibodies reactive with carcinoembryonic antigen. Cancer Invest. (1): 127-138, 1983.

13. Potter, M: Immunoglobulin-producing tumors and myeloma proteins of mice. Physiol. Rev. 52, 631-719.

14. Furth, ME, Davis, LJ, Fleurdelys, B, Scolnick, EM: Monoclonal antibodies to the p21 gene products of the transforming gene of the Harvey murine sarcoma virus and of a cellular ras gene family. J. Virol.(43): 294-304, 1982.

15. Colcher, D, Zalutsky, M, Kaplan, W, Kufe, D, Austin, F, Schlom, J: Radiolocalization of human mammary tumors in athymic mice by a monoclonal antibody. Cancer Res. (43): 736-742, 1983.

16. Nuti, M, Teramoto, YA, Mariani-Constantini, R, Horan Hand, P, Colcher, D, Schlom, J: A monoclonal antibody (B72.3) defines patterns of distribution of a novel tumor assoicated antigen in human mammary carcinoma cell populations. Int. J. Cancer (29): 539-545, 1982.

17. Hsu, SM, Raine, L, Fanger, HJ: Use of avidin-biotin-complex (ABC) in immunoperoxidase technique: a comparison between ABC and unlabed antibody (PA) procedures. Histochem. Cyto.(29): 577-580, 1981.

18. Colcher, D, Horan Hand, P, Teramoto, YA, Wunderlich, D, Schlom, J: Monoclonal antibodies define divewrsity of mammary tumor viral gene products in virions and mammary tumors of the genus Mus. J. Cancer Res. (41): 1451-1459, 1981.

19. Wierenga, RK, Hol, WGJ: Predicted nucleotide-binding properties of the p21 protein and its cancer associated variant. Nature (302): 842-844, 1983.

20. Pincus, MR, van Renswoude, J, Harford, JB, Chang, EH, Carty, RP, Klaussner, RD:Prediction of the three-dimensional structure of the transforming region of EJ/T24 human baldder oncogene product and its normal cellular homologue. Proc. Natl. Acad. Sci USA (80): 5253-5257, 1983.

21. Muto, T, Bussey, HRJ, Morson, BC: The evolution of cancer of the colon and rectum. Cancer (36): 2251-2270, 1975.

22. DeVita, VT, Hellman, S, Rosenberg, SA (eds) Cancer principles and practice of oncology. J.B. Lippincott, Philadelphia, 1982, pp. 647-650.

23. Spratt, JS, Ackerman, LV, Moyer, CA: Relationship of polyps of the colon to colonic cancer. Ann. Surg. (148): 682-698, 1958 .

24. Castleman, B, Krickstein, HI: Do adenomatous polypsof the colon become malignant? New Eng. J. Med. (267):469-475, 1962.

25. Fung, CHK, Goldman, H: Incidence and significance of villous change in adenomatous polyps. Am. J. Clin. Path. (53): 21-25, 1970.

26. Horan Hand, P, Nuti, M, Colcher, D, Schlom, J: Definition of antigenic heterogeneity and modulation among human mammary carcinoma

cell populations using monoclonal antibodies to tumor associated antigens. Cancer Res. (43): 728-735, 1983.

27. Kufe, DW, Nadler, L, Sargent, L, Shapiro, H, Horan Hand, P, Austin, F, Colcher, D, Schlom, J: Cell surface-binding properties of monoclonal antibodies reactive with human mammary carcinoma cells. Cancer Res. (43): 851-857, 1983.

28. Campisi, J, Gray, HE, Pardee, AB, Dean, M, Sonenshein, GE: Cell cycle control of c-myc but not c-ras expression lost following chemical transformation. Cell (36): 241-247, 1984.

29. Spratt, JS, Ackerman, LV: The growth of a colonic adenocarcinoma. Am. Surg. (27): 23-28, 1961.

30. Welin, S, Youker, J, Spratt, JS: Rates and patterns of growth of 375 tumors of the large intestine and rectum observed serially by double contrast enema study (Malmo Technique). Am. J. Roentgenol., Radium Therapy and Nuclear Med. (90): 673-687, 1963.

31. Slamon, DJ, deKernion, JB, Verma, IM, Cline, MJ: Expression of cellular oncogenes in human malignancies. Science (224):256-262, 1984.

32. Robbins, SL, Cotran, SR: Pathologic Basis of Disease, 2nd Ed. WB Saunders Co., Philadelphia, 1979, pp. 1317-1318.

14

WHICH CANCERS ARE CAUSED BY ACTIVATED PROTO-ONC GENES?*

PETER H. DUESBERG,[1] MICHAEL NUNN,[2] NANCY KAN,[3] DENNIS WATSON,[3] PETER H. SEEBURG,[4] TAKIS PAPAS[3]

1 Department of Molecular Biology and Virus Laboratory, University of California, Berkeley, California 94720
2 The Salk Institute, P.O. Box 85800, San Diego, California 92138-9216
3 Laboratory of Molecular Oncology, National Cancer Institute, Frederick Cancer Research Facility, Frederick, MD 21701
4 Genentech, Inc., 460 Point San Bruno Boulevard, South San Francisco, California 90007

Proto-onc genes are conserved cellular genes defined by their sequence homology with the transforming (onc) genes of retroviruses. Proto-onc genes differ significantly from viral onc genes both structurally and functionally (1). About twenty different proto-onc genes corresponding to 20 different retroviral onc genes are known (1). At this time the normal function of proto-onc genes has not yet been determined. One of them is structurally related to a growth factor, another to a growth factor receptor (2) and a third one is related to a yeast cell cycle gene (3). It is now widely believed that proto-onc genes can upon transcriptional or mutational activation function like viral onc genes. Activation in oncogene research refers to the conversion of a non-oncogenic proto-onc gene into a carcinogenic variant. Indeed mutationally or transcriptionally altered proto-onc genes have been found in certain tumors. However, the known mutationally or transcriptionally altered proto-onc genes are structurally different from viral onc genes and have not been shown to be the causes of tumors. There is as yet no adequate functional assay for oncogenicity and no consistent correlation between any proto-onc alteration and a certain tumor. As yet viral onc genes are the only proven examples of "activated" proto-onc genes. The proto-onc genes are only a subset of a larger group of cellular genes thought to play a role in cancer (4).

---

*This paper was also presented at the sixth meeting on "Modern trends in human leukemia" at Wilsede, Germany, June 17-21 (1984).

1. RETROVIRAL ONC GENES AND PROTO-ONC GENES

Retroviral onc genes are the fastest acting, obligatory carcinogens known to date. They are the only genes known that initiate and maintain cancers per se. This has been proven genetically with temperature-sensitive (ts) mutants of Rous (RSV) (5), Kirsten (KiSV) (6), and Fujinami sarcoma viruses (7, 8), with avian erythroblastosis virus (9), and with deletion mutants of these and other retroviruses (10-15). It is likely that all retroviral onc genes are sufficient to intiate and maintain neoplastic transformation, because all susceptible cells infected by retroviruses with onc genes become transformed as soon as they are infected. This high transformation efficiency virtually excludes selection of preneoplastic cells initiated by another gene.

The structural characteristic of retroviral onc genes is a specific sequence that is unrelated to the three essential virion genes gag, pol and env. Typically the onc-specific sequence replaces essential virion genes and thus renders the virus replication-defective, or it is added to the essential genes as in the case of RSV and is readily deleted (1, 10, 11, 16). Thus, onc sequences are parasitic and have no survival value for the virus (1, 16). It is this onc-specific sequence that is related to one or several proto-onc genes. However, despite this relationship, viral onc genes and proto-onc genes are not isogenic (1). About 17 of the 20 known viral onc genes are hybrids of specific subsets of proto-onc genes linked to elements of essential retroviral genes (1, 16-24).

In our laboratories we are studying the structural and functional relationships between viral onc genes and corresponding proto-onc genes with particular emphasis on the onc genes of avian carcinoma, sarcoma and leukemia viruses. The onc gene of avian carcinoma virus MC29 was the first among viral onc genes to be diagnosed as a hybrid gene (17) (Fig. 1). About one-half of its information (1.5 kb) is derived from the gag gene of retroviruses; the other half (1.6 kb), termed myc, is derived from the proto-myc gene. The gene is defined by a 110,000 dalton Δgag-myc protein, termed p110 (1). The proto-myc gene of the chicken has at least 3 exons. The 5' end of the gene is as yet undefined (23, 24). The myc region of MC29 derives from the 3' end of the first exon and includes the second and third proto-myc exons (Fig. 1).

Three other avian carcinoma viruses MH2, OK10 and CMII also have onc genes with myc sequences (18). The myc-related gene of MH2 is derived from the second and third proto-myc exon and includes the splice acceptor of the first proto-myc intron (Fig. 1) (21-23). It also appears to be a hybrid consisting of six gag codons up to the splice donor of the gag gene. It is expressed via a subgenomic

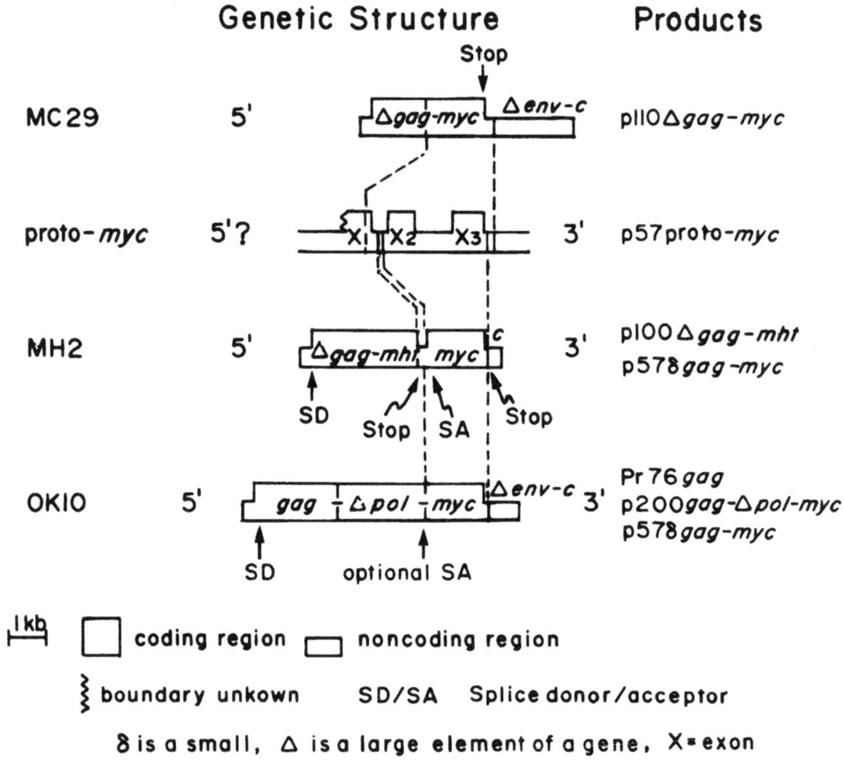

FIGURE 1. Comparison of the genetic structures and gene products of the myc-related genes of MC29, MH2, OK10 and chicken proto-myc.

mRNA as a p57 myc-related protein product (Fig. 1) (23). In addition, MH2 contains a second potential transforming gene, Δgag-mht. The mht sequence is very closely related to the onc gene of murine sarcoma virus MSV3611 (21, 22). We are currently preparing mht and myc deletion mutants of MH2 to determine whether both onc genes are necessary for MH2 transforming function or whether each gene may function on its own. We are also analyzing the myc related genes in OK10 virus (Fig. 1). As in MH2, the myc sequence of OK10 is derived from the second and third proto-myc exons and includes the splice acceptor of the first proto-myc intron (Fig. 1) (P. Seeburg, T. Papas and P. Duesberg unpublished). It is expressed via a subgenomic mRNA as a p57 protein (Fig. 1) (25). At the same time, the myc sequence of OK10 is also part of a large hybrid onc gene, gag-Δpol-myc, similar to the hybrid myc gene of MC29. This gene is defined by a 200,000 dalton protein termed p200 (Fig. 1) (18). Again, it remains to be determined whether both of these two onc gene products are necessary for transforming function.

Similar comparisons are being carried out between the Δgag-fps genes of Fujinami, PRCII and PRCIIp sarcoma viruses and cellular proto-fps (Fig. 2) (20, 26, 27). In these cases, the sarcoma viruses share with proto-fps a two to three kb fps domain including probably the 3' translation stop codon. However, the viral genes each initiate with retroviral gag regions, whereas proto-fps initiates with a proto-fps-specific exon(s) (Fig. 2) (20).

Analysis of the onc genes of the leukemia viruses avian myeloblastosis (AMV) and erythroblastosis virus (E26), and of proto-myb, the common cellular proto-type of the myb sequence shared by these viruses, are schematically summarized in Figure 2. Unlike the myc and fps containing onc genes, the onc genes of each of these viruses share an internal domain with the cellular proto-type (19, 28-30). In E26, the myb region is flanked by a gag-related region at its 5' and by a newly discovered onc-specific domain, termed ets, at its 3' end to form a tripartite onc gene (19, 30). In AMV the myb region includes a proto-myb splice acceptor that is presumably served in the virus by the splice donor of Δgag. The myb region of AMV is flanked at its 3' end by an element derived from the env gene of retroviruses.

It is concluded that the onc-specific sequences of each of these carcinoma, sarcoma and leukemia viruses are subsets of proto-onc genes linked to elements of essential retrovirus genes. Since proto-onc genes are not related and not linked to essential genes of retroviruses, all viral hybrid onc genes are by definition structurally different from proto-onc genes. A few viral onc genes, like the src gene of RSV and probably the onc genes of Harvey, Kirsten and Moloney sarcoma viruses (termed Ha- and Ki-ras and mos, respectively) are derived entirely from proto-onc sequences. Nevertheless, even these onc genes differ from proto-onc genes in extensive deletions and point mutations (see Fig. 4). For example, the src gene of RSV is a hybrid of genetic elements derived from at least three proto-src regions (1, 31).

Two arguments indicate that these qualitative differences between onc and proto-onc genes are essential for transforming function of the viral genes. First, there is the overwhelming evidence that many proto-onc genes are regularly expressed in normal cells without altering the normal phenotype (1, 32). Second, there is more indirect evidence that proto-onc sequences cloned in retroviral or

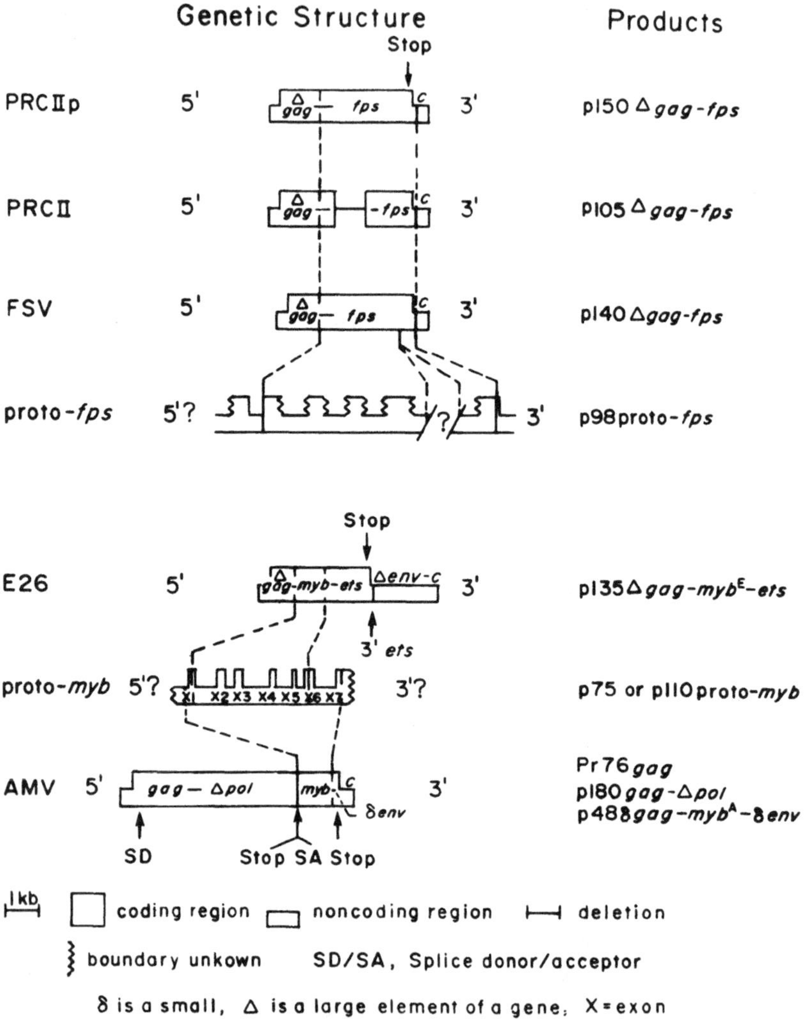

FIGURE 2. Comparison of the genetic structures and gene products the fps-related genes of avian Fujinami, PRCIIp and PRCII sarcoma viruses and the chicken proto-fps gene (top) and of the myb-related genes of avian leukemia viruses E26 and AMV and the chicken proto-myb gene (bottom).

plasmid vectors do not transform normal, diploid cells. For example, phage or plasmid vectors carrying the viral src-related region (but not a complete complement of the major proto-src gene) (33, 34; T. Parsons and D. Shalloway, personal communication), or proto-fos, the precursor of the transforming gene of

FBJ murine osteosarcoma virus (35), or proto-myc, the precursor of avian MC29 virus (T. Robins, P. Duesberg and G. Vande Woude, unpublished), do not transform cells in culture. The src-related region of the major proto-src gene also fails to transform in a RSV vector (36). Further, proto-src and proto-Ha-ras fail to transform in a reticuloendotheliosis virus vector while the corresponding viral onc genes have transforming function (W. Tarpley and H. Temin, personal communication).

Apparent exceptions are proto-mos and proto-ras which, after ligation to retroviral promoters, transform the preneoplastic NIH 3T3 cell line (37, 38). The proto-mos and ras regions used in these constructions are essentially the same as those found in Moloney and Harvey sarcoma viruses but are not complete proto-onc genes (see Fig. 4). Conceivably, the proto-onc regions that were not included in these constructions and are not in the viruses, might in the cell suppress transforming potential of the complete proto-onc genes (1). Moreover, it will be detailed below that transforming function in 3T3 cells is not a reliable measure of transforming function in diploid embryo cells or in the animal. Neither the proto-ras nor the proto-mos construction were found to transform diploid embryo cells (39, 40; G. Vande Woude, personal communication). Thus, normal proto-onc genes and viral onc genes are related, but are structurally and functionally different. The question is now whether there are conditions under which proto-onc genes can cause cancer.

2. THE SEARCH FOR ACTIVATION OF PROTO-ONC GENES TO CANCER GENES

The only clear, although indirect proof for activation of proto-onc genes to cancer genes is based on the rare cases in which proto-onc genes functioned as accidental parents of retroviral onc genes. It has been deduced from structural analyses of retroviral genes and proto-onc genes that viral onc genes were generated by transduction of specific domains from proto-onc genes (1, 16). Because no significant sequence homology exists between retroviruses and proto-onc genes, such transductions must procede via two rare, nonhomologous recombinations (1, 23). It is probably for this reason, that only 50 to 100 sporadic cancers from which retroviruses with onc genes were isolated have been reported and that no reproducible system of transduction has been described (41-43). Thus, such transductions or "activations" are extremely rare, even though all cells contain proto-onc genes and many animal species contain retroviruses without onc genes.

Their role as accidental progenitors of viral onc genes has made proto-onc genes the focus of the search for cellular cancer genes. Their possible function in cancer is currently being tested in many laboratories in view of a "one gene-one cancer" and a "multigene-one cancer" hypothesis. The one gene-one cancer hypothesis, essentially the oncogene hypothesis of Huebner and Todaro, postulates that activation of inactive cellular oncogenes is sufficient to cause cancer (44). Some investigators have postulated that activation is the result of increased dosage of a given proto-onc gene product. This view, termed the quantitative model, received support from early experiments which suggested that the src gene of RSV and proto-src and their products were equivalent (45-49). In the meantime, significant structural and functional differences between these genes have been found (1, 31, 33, 34, 36, see above). Others have suggested that proto-onc genes are activated by mutations or rearrangements in the primary DNA sequence (50, 51). This view is termed the qualitative model (1).

The multigene-one cancer hypothesis postulates that an activated proto-onc gene is necessary, but unlike the corresponding viral gene, not sufficient to cause cancer. A quantitatively or qualitatively activated proto-onc gene is postulated to function either as initiation or as maintenance gene together with another proto-onc gene, in a multistep process (39, 40, 52-58). This hypothesis fits the view of how virus-negative tumors are thought to arise in general and provides identifiable candidates to test the hypothesis. However, since retroviral onc genes have yet to be dissociated into initiation and maintenance functions, this hypothesis is without viral precedent.

Two kinds of assays have been performed to test these hypotheses. One assay correlates transcriptional activation and mutation of proto-onc genes with cancer; the other directly measures transforming function of proto-onc genes upon transfection into certain recipient cells, typically the mouse 3T3 cell line. Such experiments have most frequently linked cancers with alterations of proto-myc and proto-ras.

Is proto-myc activation the cause of B-cell lymphomas? Based on the observation that transcription of the cellular proto-myc is enhanced in retroviral lymphomas of chicken, it has been suggested that transcriptional activation of proto-myc is the cause of B-cell lymphoma (49, 59). Chicken B-cell lymphoma is a clonal cancer that is caused in a small fraction of animals infected by one of the avian leukosis viruses (which have no onc genes) after latent periods of over six months (43). The hypothesis, termed downstream promotion, postulates that the gene is activated by the promoter of a retrovirus integrated upstream (Fig. 3) and

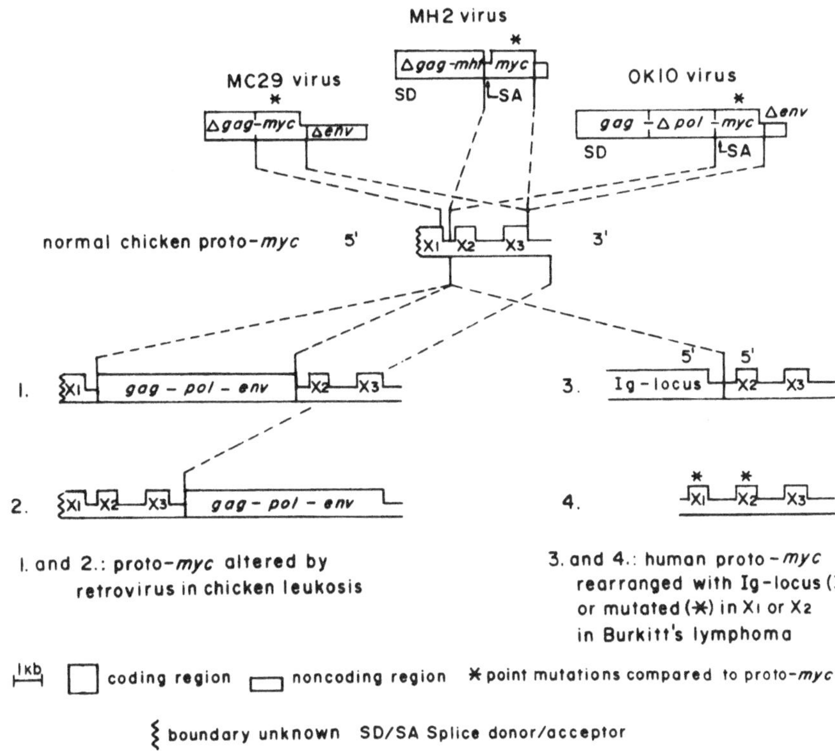

FIGURE 3. Myc-related genes in avian carcinoma viruses and in normal and lymphoma cells. The common and specific myc domains of avian carcinoma viruses MC29 (23, 52), MH2 (21, 22) and OK10 (18 and unpublished), of normal proto-myc (23, 56), and of the proto-myc genes of avian leukosis (41, 51) and human Burkitt's lymphoma (47, 49, 54) are graphically compared. Proto-myc has three exons (X1, X2, X3) the first of which is thought to be noncoding (23, 56). Gag, pol, env are the three essential virion genes of retroviruses and Δ marks incomplete complements of these genes.

that activated proto-myc functions like the transforming gene of MC29 (49). Subsequently, samples were found in which the retrovirus is integrated 3' of proto-myc. In these cases, the virus is thought to function as an enhancer of proto-myc (Fig. 3) (59).

However, proto-myc differs from the 3-kb Δgag-myc gene of MC29: (a) in a 5' noncoding, probable regulatory exon that is not shared with MC29 (except for the last 4 codons); (b) in the absence of Δgag (1.5 kb); and (c) in several bases within the common myc domain (Fig. 3) (23, 24). Further, it has been argued previously (1) that the hypothesis fails to explain the origin of about 20% of viral lymphomas in which proto-myc is not activated (49); the discrepancies between the phenotype of the disease and the cancers caused by MC29; and the clonality of the tumors, defined by a single integration site of the retrovirus with regard to proto-myc as well as the long latent period of the disease. Given about 10^6 kb of chicken DNA and activation of proto-myc by retrovirus integration within about 5 kb of proto-myc (59), one in 2 X 10^5 infections should generate the first tumor cell. Since the chicken probably has over 10^7 uncommited B-cells and many more virus particles, the critical carcinogenic integration event should occur after a short latent period. The tumor should also not be clonal, since integration by retroviruses is not site-specific and there could be numerous infections during the latent period of about six months. Further, the model has not been confirmed in viral leukemia of other animal species (1).

Recently, it was suggested that mutation may have activated proto-myc because mutations have been observed in viral lymphoma (60). However, the proto-myc mutations have not been shown to be the cause of the viral lymphoma.

Activation of proto-myc has also been postulated to cause the retrovirus-negative, human Burkitt's lymphomas, and mouse plasmacytomas. In these cases, chromosome translocation has been proposed as a mechanism of activating proto-myc function (55, 56, 61, 62). The human proto-myc is related to that of the chicken from which carcinoma viruses have been derived (Fig. 3). The two genes have unique first exons, similar second exons with unique regions and colinear third exons (23). In man, proto-myc is located on chromosome 8 and an element of this chromosome is reciprocally translocated in many Burkitt's lymphoma lines to immunoglobulin (Ig) loci of chromosome 14 and less frequently of chromosome 2 or 22. Since the crossover points of chromosome 8 are near proto-myc, translocation was initially suspected to activate proto-myc transcriptionally by rearranging proto-myc (Fig. 3) or by altering its immediate environment and thus bringing it under the influence of new promoters or enhancers (61). However, in many lymphomas rearranged proto-myc is not linked to a new promoter, instead the first presumably noncoding exon is replaced by the Ig locus, linked to it 5'-5' in the opposite transcriptional orientation (Fig. 3) (50, 61). Despite these inconsistencies the altered proto-myc is thought to function as a cellular oncogene in these tumors. Further this model cannot explain how proto-myc would be activated when the complete proto-myc gene, including its known promoters and flanking regions, is translocated (55, 57, 63), or recent observations that in a significant minority of Burkitt's lymphomas proto-myc remains in its original chromosomal location while a region 3' of proto-myc is translocated (64-68).

Moreover, there is no consensus at this time whether proto-myc expression is enhanced in Burkitt's lymphoma cells, as compared to normal control cells. Some investigators report elevated expression compared to normal B-lymphoblasts or lines (69), while others report essentially normal levels of proto-myc mRNA (55, 63, 67, 68, 70-73). Further, enhanced proto-myc transcription is not specific for B-cell lymphomas, since high levels of proto-myc expression are seen in non-Burkitt's lymphomas (72), in other tumors (58), and in chemically transformed fibroblast cell lines in which proto-myc is not translocated or rearranged (32). The view that enhanced expression of proto-myc may be sufficient to cause Burkitt's lymphoma is also challenged by the observations that proto-myc transcription reaches cell cycle-dependent peak levels in normal cells similar to those in tumor cells (32, 74).

The possibility that mutations of proto-myc may correlate with Burkitt's lymphoma has also been investigated. In some Burkitt's cell lines mutations have been observed in translocated, but un-rearranged, proto-myc (Fig. 3) (73, 75). Initially it was proposed that these mutations may activate proto-myc by altering the gene product (75), but in at least one Burkitt's lymphoma line the coding sequence corresponding to proto-myc exons 2 and 3 was identical to that of the normal gene (Fig. 3) (63). Recently it has been proposed that mutations in the first noncoding exon may activate the gene (Fig. 3) (73, 76). However, there is no functional evidence for this view and an activating mutation that is characteristic of Burkitt's lymphomas has not been identified. A sequence comparison between translocated proto-myc of a mouse plasmacytoma with the germline proto-myc found the two genes to be identical except for one nucleotide difference in the first exon. It was concluded that proto-myc mutations are not required for oncogenesis (77).

Therefore, no translocation, rearrangement, elevated expression, or characteristic mutation of proto-myc is common to all Burkitt's lymphomas investigated. This casts doubt on the concept that any of the known proto-myc alterations are necessary for Burkitt's lymphoma.

The question of whether proto-myc has transforming function has been tested directly using the 3T3 cell transformation assay with DNA from chicken or human B-cell lymphomas. However, no myc-related DNA was detected even though its presumed functional equivalent, the Δgag-myc gene of MC29, is capable of transforming 3T3 cells (78, 79) and other rodent cells (80). Instead, another DNA sequence, termed Blym, was identified by the assay (53, 81). Based on these results the role of proto-myc in lymphomas has been interpreted in terms of a two-gene hypothesis. It has been suggested that activated proto-myc is necessary but not sufficient to cause the lymphoma (53, 55). It is postulated to have a transient early function that generates a lymphoma maintenance gene, Blym. This gene appears to be the DNA that transforms 3T3 cells and is thought to maintain the B-cell tumor. There is no proof for this postulated role of proto-myc as a lymphoma initiation gene, because the 3T3 cell transformation assay does not measure proto-myc initiation function, and because there is no evidence that the two genes jointly (or alone) transform B-cells. Furthermore, the hypothesis does not address the question why proto-myc should have any transforming function at all, if it is not like MC29. (MC29 does not require a second gene to transform a cell.) It is also not known whether Blym is altered in primary Burkitt's lymphomas, since all of the transfection experiments were done with DNA from cell lines.

It is conceivable that translocation between the proto-myc chromosome 8 and chromosomes carring immunoglobulin genes and that proto-myc mutations may be specific consequences, rather than the cause of the lymphoma (82). Human B-cell lymphomas with translocations that do not involve chromosome 8 have indeed been described (83-84). In the case of clonal myeloid leukemias with consistent translocations, like the Philadelphia chromosome, it has been convincingly argued that translocation is preceded by clonal proliferation of certain stem cells with the same isoenzyme markers as leukemic cells but without chromosomal or clinical abnormalities (85).

Perhaps primary Burkitt's lymphomas should be analysed now and more emphasis should be given to the question whether proto-myc alteration contributes to Burkitt's lymphoma, rather than to speculation about possible mechanisms.

Proto-ras mutations, the cause of human and rodent carcinomas? Use of the 3T3 cell assay to measure transforming function of DNA from a human bladder carcinoma cell line has identified DNA homologous to the ras gene of Harvey sarcoma virus (Fig. 4) (51, 86). Based on the viral model, the proto-Ha-ras gene is thought to be a potential cancer gene because it encodes a 21,000-dalton protein, p21, which is colinear with an onc gene product p21 of Ha-MuSV (Fig. 4) (87). The proto-Ha-ras gene from the bladder carcinoma cell line differs from normal proto-Ha-ras in a point mutation which alters the codon 12 in exon 1 from normal gly to val (51, 88). This mutation does not cause overproduction of the ras gene product (p21) in the 3T3 cell line (51) and does not change known biochemical properties of p21 (89). The single base change is thought to activate the gene to a functional equivalent of Ha-MuSV and to be the cause of the carcinoma because it is the apparent cause for 3T3 cell transforming function (51, 90). However, this

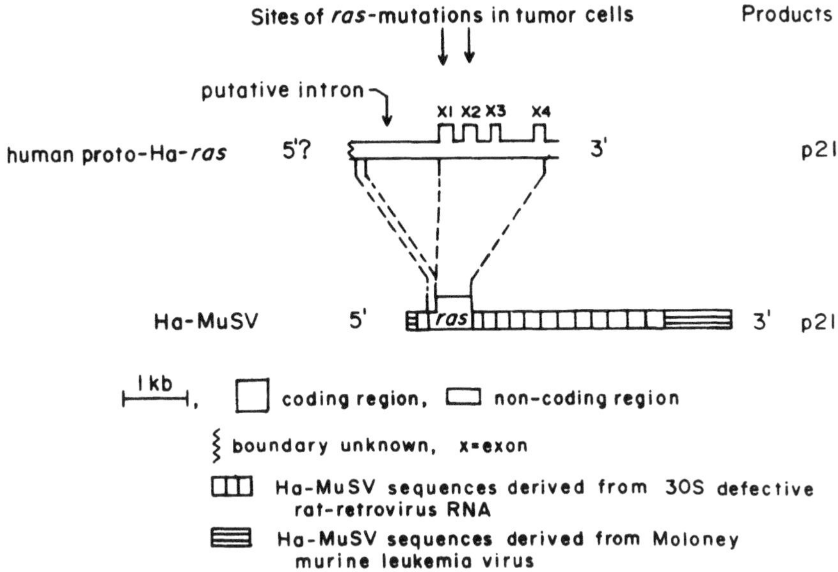

FIGURE 4. Comparison of the genetic functions and gene products of the human proto-Ha-ras gene (88,89) and the 5.5 kb RNA genome of Harvey sarcoma virus (Ha-MuSV). Ha-MuSV is a genetic hybrid of the rat proto-ras gene, a 30S defective retrovirus RNA from rat cells and of Moloney leukemia virus (88, 108).

mutation has not been found in over 60 primary human carcinomas, including 10 bladder, 9 colon and 10 lung carcinomas (91), in 8 other lung carcinomas (92), and 14 additional bladder and 9 kidney carcinomas (R. Muschel and G. Khoury, personal communication). Further, the mutated human proto-Ha-ras, which transforms 3T3 cells, does not transform primary rat embryo cells (39, 54) and, more significantly, does not transform human embryo cells (93). Transformation of primary cells would be expected from a gene that causes tumors in animals. Thus the mutated proto-ras gene does not correspond to the viral model which transforms primary mouse, rat (94-95) and human cells (96-100). In addition, the 12th amino acyl residue (val) of 3T3 cell-transforming proto-ras is different from the arg of the viral counterpart (88).

Other mutations have since been found to confer 3T3 cell-transforming function to proto-Ha-ras DNA. Proto-Ha-ras with a mutation in codon 61 was isolated from a human tumor cell line (101) 3T3 cell-transforming proto-Ha-ras DNAs were also isolated from 2 out of 23 primary urinary tract tumors analyzed. One of these contained a mutation in codon 61, the other was not identified (102). The mutations were not found in the normal tissue of the respective patients. Nevertheless, this does not prove that these mutations were necessary for tumor formation since each was associated with only 1 out of 23 histologically indistinguishable tumors.

A 3T3 cell-transforming mouse proto-Ha-*ras* DNA was also found in some (not all) chemically induced benign papillomas and malignant carcinomas of mice (103). Since only a small (5-7%) portion of the benign tumors progressed to carcinomas, it would appear that the mutation was not sufficient to cause the carcinomas, and since not all carcinomas contained the mutation, it would appear that it was not necessary either. A high proportion, i.e. 14 out of 17 methylnitrosourea-induced mammary carcinomas of rats, were found to contain 3T3 cell-transforming proto-Ha-*ras* DNA (M. Barbacid, personal communication). This suggests that the mutation may be important, although not necessary for the tumor. The original study reported 9 out of 9 positives (104). However, the hormone-dependence and high tissue specificity of the carcinogen in this study suggests that other genes must be involved, because mutated proto-*ras* has been found in association with other tumors and transforms 3T3 cells without hormones. It is plausible that other genes, which may be involved in tumorigenesis but which do not register in the 3T3 assay, were also altered by the carcinogen.

In an effort to explain why mutated proto-Ha-*ras* transforms 3T3 cells, but not rat or human embryo cells and is only infrequently associated with cancers, it has recently been proposed that mutated proto-Ha-*ras* is only one of at least two activated genes that are necessary to induce cancer (39, 40, 54). This two gene-hypothesis has been tested by transfecting primary rat cells with a mixture of the mutated human proto-Ha-*ras* and either MC29 provirus or activated proto-*myc* from mouse plasmacytoma (39) or the EIA gene of adenovirus (54) as helper genes. None of these genes were able to transform rat embryo cells by themselves, but some cells were transformed by the artificial mixed doubles. The study that used the adenovirus helper gene showed that proto-*ras* expression varied from high to normal levels in transformed cells and that normal proto-*ras* was inactive in the assay (54). The study that used *myc*-related helper genes did not show that the transformants expressed the added DNAs. It also did not test whether unaltered forms of proto-*myc* or proto-*ras* were sufficient for a mixture of these genes to register in this assay. This appears to be a particularly relevant question since a proto-*myc* clone from a mouse plasmacytoma with an SV40 enhancer at its 3' end but without its natural promoter (56) was reported to be active (39) although such a construction is not expected to activate proto-*myc*.

The *myc*-related genes were proposed to convert rat embryo cells to cells that are capable of dividing indefinitely, like 3T3 cells, a function termed immortalization (39, 40). The supposed immortalization function of MC29 or of activated proto-myc was not demonstrated independently. The proposal did not explain why an immortalization gene was necessary. Since embryo cells are capable of sufficient rounds of mitoses (up to 50) in cell culture, immortalization is not necessary for focus formation and probably not for tumor formation (105). In the avian system, MC29 transforms primary cells and causes tumors in chicken independently without the benefit of secondary oncogenes, and most MC29 tumor cells are not immortal if tested in cell culture. There is also no precedent for a function of proto-ras in a multistep transformation mechanism, because the transforming genes of Harvey or Kirsten sarcoma viruses transform rat and mouse embryo cells (94, 95) or human embryo cells (96-100) with single hit kinetics and without helper genes. Likewise, there is no precedent for the artifical mixtures of the two activated proto-onc genes in any natural tumors.

Other 3T3 cell-transforming proto-ras genes, namely proto-Ki-ras (which is more closely related to the ras gene of Kirsten sarcoma virus than to Harvey virus) and N-ras (which is related to both viruses) (106), have also been found in tumors or cell lines. Proto-Ki-ras encodes a p21 protein that is related to the p21 protein encoded by proto-Ha-ras (88, 106, 107). One group has found transforming proto-Ki-ras DNA in three primary human tumors and five tumor cell lines out of 96 samples tested (92, 108) and in one out of eight lung carcinomas tested (92). The DNA from the latter tumor, but not that from normal tissue of the same patient, had a mutation in codon 12. As pointed out above, the infrequent occurrence of proto-Ki-ras among these tumors raises the question of whether the mutations were necessary for tumorigenesis.

In a study of human melanomas, only one of five different metastases from the same human melanoma patient was found to contain 3T3 cell-transforming proto-Ki-ras DNA (109). A 3T3 cell-transforming Ki-ras DNA was also detected in a metastatic variant but not in a primary methylcholanthrene-induced T-cell lymphoma of mice (110). An example of a spontaneous proto-ras mutation appearing in tumor cells cultured in vitro has been described recently (111). This suggests that these proto-ras mutations were consequences rather than the causes of these tumors.

Since 3T3 cell-transforming or mutated proto-ras genes are only rarely associated with human and murine tumors, and since mutated proto-Ha-ras does not transform human or rat embryo cells (39, 54, 94; proto-Ki-ras was not tested), there is as yet no proof that mutated proto-ras is sufficient or even necessary for any of the above tumors.

The failure of the mutated proto-Ha or Ki-ras to behave like the viral model suggests that structural differences between the cellular and viral genes are responsible (Fig. 4). Proto-Ha-ras differs from the genome of Harvey sarcoma virus (112) in a cell-specific 1-kb DNA region 5' of exon 1 that is preceded by a virus-related region (89) (Fig. 4), and in the sizes (1.2 and 5 kb) of the proto-ras transcripts compared to the genomic viral 5.5 kb mRNA (43, 113, 114). The cell-specific proto-Ha-ras region is thought to be an intron, but it may have another function. Proto-Ha-ras with 3T3 cell-transforming function further differs from normal proto-Ha-ras, as well as from the viral ras in point mutations in exons 1 or 2 (Fig. 4) (51, 88). The 5' end of proto-Ha-ras is not as yet defined (88). Moreover, only about 10% of the genomes of Harvey and Kirsten sarcoma viruses are ras-related. Each viral RNA contains about 3 kb of genetic information, derived from a rat 30S defective retrovirus RNA (115) which may contribute to the oncogenicity of these viruses (Fig. 4). Finally, Ha- and Ki-MuSV are not obvious models for proto-ras genes with hypothetical carcinoma function, since these viruses cause predominantly sarcomas.

Does the 3T3 assay detect cancer genes? Since the proto-ras mutations found by the 3T3 assay do not transform primary cells, it is possible that they are not relevant for tumor formation. Available data suggest that these are coincidential or consequential rather than causative mutations occuring in tumor cells, because the mutations are not consistently correlated with specific tumors and because in some cases they precede tumor formation and in others they evolve during tumor progression. The preponderance of 3T3 cell transformation-negatives among the above described tumors further suggests that either no genes have caused the negative tumors or that the assay failed to detect them. It would follow that the test is insufficient to detect genes that cause tumors in animals.

That only ras-related proto-onc genes have been detected in human tumors signals another limitation of the assay. However, other 3T3 cell-transforming (and possibly carcinogenic) DNAs which are not related to viral onc genes have been detected by the assay in certain tumors (4).

3. CONCLUSIONS

There is as yet not a single proven case that an activated proto-onc gene has caused cancer. The only "activations" that have clearly converted proto-onc genes to cancer genes are those that generated retroviral onc genes.

However, proto-onc genes are sometimes mutationally or transcriptionally altered in tumor cells. The alterations that have been found are structurally different from those that set apart proto-onc genes from viral onc genes. No altered proto-onc gene has been found that functions like a viral onc gene. Structural analyses have shown that proto-myc is frequently rearranged or mutated in B-cell lymphomas. But in contrast to MC29, altered proto-myc does not transform cells in culture. Mutated proto-ras from certain tumors has transforming function for the 3T3 cell line, but not for murine or human embryo cells like the ras genes of the Harvey and Kirsten sarcoma viruses. Since the known altered proto-onc genes are structurally and functionally different from viral onc genes and are not consistently associated with specific tumors, the one gene-one cancer hypothesis remains unproven. It remains to be shown in appropriate test systems whether altered proto-onc genes can be sufficient causes of cancer.

The observations that altered proto-onc genes do not behave like viral onc genes and that in some tumors more than one proto-onc gene and in others a whole battery are transcriptionally or mutationally altered (58) have been interpreted in terms of a multigene hypothesis. Activated proto-myc has been proposed to cooperate with the Blym gene to cause chicken and human B-cell lymphoma (53), and it has been reported to cooperate in an artificial system with activated proto-ras to transform rat embryo cells in culture (39, 40). These proposals assume that altered proto-onc genes are necessary but not sufficient for tumor formation. The proposals speculate that altered proto-onc genes behave like functional subsets of viral onc genes but do not explain why these genes are assumed to have unique oncogenic functions that are different from those of the viral models. The speculation is without precedent since it is not known whether viral onc genes can be dissociated into complementary or helper gene-dependent genetic subsets. It is based on the structural relationship between altered (and normal) proto-onc genes and viral onc genes and on the assumption that transformation of 3T3 cells by altered proto-ras and transformation of primary rodent cells by proto-ras in combination with other genes are relevant to carcinogenesis. As yet, no multigene complements that include one or two proto-onc genes have been shown to be consistently associated with specific tumors. Hence, the view that these genes are necessary for multigene carcinogenesis is speculative.

It may be argued that the proto-onc gene alterations that are associated with some cancers play a nonspecific, but nonetheless causative, role in carcinogenesis that could be substituted by another gene. To support this view it would be necessary to know which other genes could substitute for the role that altered proto-onc genes are thought to play in the origin of cancer. Further, one would have to know whether proto-onc gene alterations are more typical than alterations of other genes in cancer cells and which other genes undergo alterations. It is likely that unknown events, additional to the known alterations of resident proto-onc genes, are required for the development of cancer (1, 116).

The fact that proto-onc genes share common domains with viral onc genes remains a persuasive argument that proto-onc genes may be changed, under certain conditions, into cancer genes. The evidence that most normal proto-onc genes are expressed in normal cells suggests that certain cell-specific domains of proto-onc genes may suppress potential oncogenic function. Thus, mutation or removal of suppressors could activate a proto-onc gene as has been predicted for Burkitt's lymphoma. In addition, virus specific onc gene elements may also be essential to activate a proto-onc gene. In this case, a retrovirus without an onc gene (leukemia virus) could activate a proto-onc gene by a single illegitimate recombination which would form a hybrid onc gene. Such an event would be more probable than the generation of a retrovirus with an onc gene for which at least two illegitimate recombinations are necessary. The most important challenge now is to develop functional assays for cellular cancer genes.

ACKNOWLEDGMENTS

We thank Mike Botchan, Mike Carey, G. Steven Martin, Will Phares, Cynthia Romerdahl, Harry Rubin for encouragement and many critical comments and Linda Brownstein for typing numerous drafts of this manuscript. The work from my laboratory is supported by NIH grant CA 11426 from the National Cancer Institute and by grant CTR 1547 from The Council for Tobacco Research - U.S.A., Inc.

REFERENCES

1. Duesberg, P. H. (1983). Nature 304, 219-226.

2. Heldin, C-H., and Westermark, B. (1984). Cell 37, 9-20.

3. Peterson, T. A., Yodren, J., Byers, B., Nunn, M. F., Duesberg, P. H., Doolittle, R. F., and Reed, S. I., (1984). Nature 309, 556-558.

4. Cooper, G. M. (1982). Science 218, 801-806.

5. Martin, G. S. (1970). Nature 221, 1021-1023.

6. Shih, T. Y., Weeks, M. O., Young, M. A., and Scolnick, E. M. (1979). J. Virol. 31, 546-556.

7. Pawson, A., Guyden, J., Kung, T-H., Radke, K., Gilmore, T., and Martin, G. S. (1980). Cell 22, 767-775.

8. Lee, W-H., Bister, K., Moscovici, C., and Duesberg, P. H. (1981). J. Virol. 38, 1064-1076.

9. Palmieri, S., Beug, H., and Graf, T. (1982). Virology 123, 296-311.

10. Duesberg, P. H. and Vogt P. K. (1970). Proc. Natl. Acad. Sci. 67, 1673-1680.

11. Martin, G. S., and Duesberg, P. H. (1972). Virology 47, 494-497.

12. Wei, C-M., Lowy, D. R., and Scolnick, E. M. (1980). Proc. Natl. Acad. Sci. USA 77, 4674-4678.

13. Goff, S. P., and Baltimore, D. (1982). In: Advances in Viral Oncology, Vol. 1, G. Klein, ed., (New York, Raven Press), pp. 217-139.

14. Srinivasan, A., Dunn, C. Y., Yuasa, Y., Devare, S. G., Reddy, E. P., and Aaronson, S. A. (1982). Proc. Natl. Acad. Sci. USA 79, 5508-5512.

15. Evans, L. H., and Duesberg, P. H. (1982). J. Virol. 41, 735-743.

16. Duesberg, P. H. (1980). Cold Spring Harbor Symp. Quant. Biol. 44, 13-29.

17. Mellon, P., Pawson, A., Bister, K., Martin, G. S., and Duesberg, P. H. (1978). Proc. Natl. Acad. Sci. USA 75, 5874-5878.

18. Bister, K., and Duesberg, P. H. (1982). In: Advances in Viral Oncology, Vol. 1, G. Klein, ed. (Raven Press, New York), p. 3-42.

19. Nunn, M. F., Seeburg, P. H., Moscovici, C., and Duesberg, P. H. (1983). Nature 306, 391-395.

20. Seeburg, P. H., Lee, W-H., Nunn, M. F., and Duesberg, P. H. (1984). Virology 133, 460-463.

21. Kan, N. C., Flordellis, C. S., Mark, G. E., Duesberg, P. H., and Papas, T. S. (1984). Proc. Natl. Acad. Sci. USA, 81, 3000-3004.

22. Kan, N. C., Flordellis, C. S., Mark, G. E., Duesberg, P. H., and Papas, T. S. (1984). Science 223, 813-816.

23. Papas, T. S., Kan, N. K., Watson, D. K., Flordellis, C. S., Psallidopoulos, M. C., Lautenberger, J., Samuel, K. P., and Duesberg, P. (1984). In: Cancer Cells 2/Oncogenes and Viral Genes, G. F. Vande Woude, A. J. Levine, W. C. Topp, and J. D. Watson, eds., (Cold Spring Harbor Laboratory, Cold Spring Harbor, New York) p. 153-163.

24. Watson, D. K., Reddy, E. P., Duesberg, P. H., and Papas, T. S. (1983). Proc. Natl. Acad. Sci. USA 80, 2146-2150.

25. Chiswell, D.J., Ramsay, G., and Hayman, M.J. (1981). J. Virol. 40, 301-304.

26. Lee, W-H., Phares, W., and Duesberg, P. H. (1983). Virology 129, 79-93.

27. Duesberg, P. H., Phares, W., and Lee, W. H. (1983). Virology 131, 144-158.

28. Klempnauer, K-H., Gonda, T. S., and Bishop, J. M. (1982). Cell 31, 453-463

29. Rushlow, K. E., Lautenberger, J. A., Papas, T. S., Baluda, M. A., Perbal, B., Chirikjian, J. G., and Reddy, E. P. (1982). Science 216, 1421-1423.

30. Nunn, M., Weiher, H., Bullock, P., and Duesberg, P. H. (1984). Virology, in press.

31. Takeya, T., and Hanafusa, H. (1983). Cell 32, 881-890.

32. Campisi, J., Gray, H. E., Pardee, A. B., Dean, M., and Sonenshein, G. E. (1984). Cell 36, 241-247.

33. Takeya, T. and Hanafusa, H. (1982). J. Virol. 44, 12-18.

34. Parker, R. C., Varmus, H. E., and Bishop, J. M. (1984). Cell 37, 131-139.

35. Miller, A. D., Curran, T. and Verma, I. M. (1984). Cell 36, 51-60.

36. Iba H., Takeya, T., Cross, F.R., Hanafusa, T., and Hanafusa, H. (1984). Proc. Nat. Acad. Sci. USA 81, 4424-4428.

37. Blair, D. G., Oskarsson, M., Wood, T. G., McClements, W. C., Fischinger, P. J., and Vande Woude, G. F. (1981). Science 212, 941-943.

38. Chang, E. H., Furth, M. E., Scolnick, E. M., and Lowy, D. R. (1982). Nature 297, 479-483.

39. Land, H., Parada, L. F., and Weinberg, R.A. (1983). Nature 304, 596-602.

40. Land, H., Parada, L. F. and Weinberg, R.A. (1983). Science 222, 771-778.

41. Gross, L. (1970). Oncogenic Viruses. (Pergamon Press, New York).

42. Tooze, J., ed. (1973). The Molecular Biology of Tumour Viruses. (Cold Spring Harbor Laboratory, Cold Spring Harbor, New York).

43. Weiss, R. A., Teich, N. M., Varmus, H., and Coffin, J. M. eds. (1982). Molecular Biology of Tumor Viruses: RNA tumor viruses. (Cold Spring Harbor Laboratory, Cold Spring Harbor, New York).

44. Huebner, R. J., and Todaro, G. J. (1969). Proc. Natl. Acad. Sci. USA 64, 1087-1094.

45. Bishop, J. M., Courtneidge, S. A., Levinson, A. D., Oppermann, H., Quintrell, N., Sheiness, D. K., Weiss, S. R., and Varmus, H. E. (1980). Cold Spring Harbor Symp. Quant. Biol. 44, 919-930.

46. Bishop, J. M. (1981). Cell 23, 5-6.

47. Wang, L. H., Snyder, P., Hanafusa, T., Moscovici, C., and Hanafusa, H., (1980). Cold Spring Harbor Symp. Quant. Biol. 44 755-764.

48. Karess, R. E., Hayward, W. S., and Hanafusa, H. (1980). Cold Spring Harbor Symp. Quant. Biol. 44, 765-771.

49. Hayward, W. S., Neel, B. G., and Astrin, S. M. (1981). Nature 290, 475-480.

50. Klein, G. (1981). Nature 294, 313-318.

51. Tabin, C. J., Bradley, S. M., Bargmann, C. I., Weinberg, R. A., Papageorge, A. G., Scolnick, E. M., Dhar, R., Lowy, D. R., and Chang, E. H. (1982). Nature 300, 143-149.

52. Cooper, G. M., and Neiman, P. E. (1981). Nature 292, 857-858.

53. Diamond, A., Cooper, G. M., Ritz, J., and Lane, M-A. (1983). Nature 305, 112-116.

54. Ruley, H. E. (1983). Nature 304, 602-606.

55. Leder, P., Battey, J., Lenoir, G., Moudling, C., Murphy, W., Potter, H., Stewart, T. and Taub, R. (1983). Science 222, 765-771.

56. Adams, J. M., Gerondakis, S., Webb, E., Carcoran, L. M., and Cory, S. (1983). Proc. Natl. Acad. Sci. USA 80, 1982-1986.

57. Klein, G. and Klein, E. (1984). Carcinogenesis 5, 429-435.

58. Slamon, D. J., deKernion, J. B., Verma, I. M., and Cline, M. J. (1984). Science 224, 256-262.

59. Payne, G. S., Bishop, J. M., and Varmus, H. E. (1982). Nature 295, 209-214.

60. Westaway, D., Payne, G., and Varmus, H. E. (1984). Proc. Natl. Acad. Sci. USA 81, 843-847.

61. Klein, G. (1983). Cell 32, 311-315.

62. Rowley, J.D. (1983). Nature 301, 290-291.

63. Battey, J., Moulding, C., Taub, R., Murphy, W., Stewart, T., Potter, H., Lenoir, G., and Leder, P. (1983). Cell 34, 779-787

64. Gelmann, E., Psallidopoulos, M. C., Papas, T. S., and Dalla-Favera, R. (1983). Nature 306, 799-809.

65. Croce, C. M., Thierfelder, W., Erikson, J., Nishikura, K., Finan, J., Lenoir, G. M., and Nowell, P. C. (1983). Proc. Natl. Acad. Sci. USA 80, 6922-6926.

66. Erikson, J., ar-Rushidi, A., Drwinga, H.L., Nowell, P.C., and Croce, C.M. (1983). Proc. Natl. Acad. Sci. USA 80, 820-824.

67. Hollis, G. F., Mitchell, K. F., Battey, J., Potter, H., Taub, R., Lenoir, G. M., and Leder, P. (1984). Nature 307, 752-755.

68. Davis, M., Malcolm, S., and Rabbitts, T. H. (1984). Nature 308, 286-288.

69. Erikson, J., Nishikura, K., Ar-Rushdi, A., Finan, J., Emanuel, B., Lenoir, G., Nowell, P. C., and Croce, C. M. (1983). Proc. Natl. Acad. Sci. USA 80, 7581-7585.

70. Westin, E. H., Wong-Staal, F., Gelmann, E. P., Dalla Favera, R., Papas, T. S., Lautenberger, J. A., Eva, A., Reddy, E. P., Tronick, S. R., Aaronson, S. A., and Gallo, R. C. (1982). Proc. Natl. Acad. Sci. USA 79, 2490-2494.

71. Maguire, R. T., Robins, T. S., Thorgersson, S. S., and Heilman, C. A. (1983). Proc. Natl. Acad. Sci. USA 80, 1947-1950.

72. Hamlyn, P. H., and Rabbitts, T. H. (1983). Nature 304, 135-139.

73. Taub, R., Moulding, C., Battey, J., Murphy, W., Vasicek, T., Lenoir, G.M., and Leder, P., (1984). Cell 36, 339-348..

74. Kelly, K., Cochran, B. H., Stiles, C. D., and Leder P. (1983). Cell 35, 603-610.

75. Rabbitts, T. H., Hamlyn, P. H., and Baer, R. (1983). Nature 306, 760-765.

76. Rabbitts, T. H., Forster, A., Hamlyn, P. and Baer, R., (1984). Nature 309, 592-597.

77. Stanton, L.W., Fahrlander, P.D.Tesser, P.M. and Marcu, K.B. (1984). Nature 310, 423-425.

78. Copeland, N. G., and Cooper, G. M. (1980). J. Virol. 33, 1199-1202.

79. Lautenberger, J.A., Schulz, R.A., Garon, C.F., Tsichlis, P.H., and Papas, T.S. (1981). Proc. Natl. Acad. Sci. USA 78, 1518-1522.

80. Quade, K. (1979). Virology 98, 461-465.

81. Goubin, G., Goldman, D. S., Luce, J,, Neiman, P. E., and Cooper, G. M. (1983). Nature 302, 114-119.

82. Rubin, H. (1984). Nature, 309, 518.

83. Erikson J., Finan, J., Tsujimoto, Y., Nowell, P.C. and Croce C. (1984) Proc. Not. Acad. Sci. 81, 4144-4148.

84. Yunis, J.J., Oken, M.D., Kaplan, M.E., Ensurd, K.M., Howe, R.R., Theologides, A. New Engl. J. of Med. 307, 1231-1236 (1982).

85. Fialkow, R. J., and Singer, J. W. (1984). In: Proceedings of the Dahlem Workshop on Leukemia. (Berlin, Germany, Springer-Verlag), in press.

86. Der, J. C., Krontiris, T. G., and Cooper, G. M. (1982). Proc. Natl. Acad. Sci. USA 79, 3637-3640.

87. Ellis, R. W., Lowy, D. R., and Scolnick, E. M. (1982). In: Advances in Viral Oncology, Vol. 1, G. Klein, ed., (New York, Raven Press), pp. 107-126.

88. Capon, D. J., Chen, E. Y., Levinson, A. D., Seeburg, P. H., and Goeddel, D. V. (1983). Nature 302, 33-37.

89. Finkel, T., Channing, J. D., and Cooper G. M. (1984) Cell 37, 151-158.

90. Reddy, E. P., Reynolds, R. K., Santos, E., and Barbacid, M. (1982). Nature 300, 149-152.

91. Feinberg, A. P., Vogelstein, B., Droller, M. J., Baylin, S. B., and Nelkin, B. D. (1983). Science 220, 1175-1177.

92. Santos, E., Martin-Zanca, D., Reddy, E. P., Pierotti, M. A., Della Porta, G., and Barbacid, M. (1984). Science 223, 661-664.

93. Sager, R., Tanaka, K., Lau, C. C., Ebina, Y. Anisowicz, A. (1983). Proc. Natl. Acad. Sci. USA 80, 7601-7605.

94. Harvey, J. J., and East, J. (1971). Int. Rev. of Exp. Pathol. 10, 265-360.

95. Levy, J. A. (1973). J. Nat. Cancer Inst. 46, 1001-1007.

96. Aaronson, S.A. & Todaro, G.I. (1970). Nature 225, 458-459.

97. Aaronson, S.A. & Weaver, C.A. (1971). J. Gen. Virol 13, 245-252.

98. Klement, V., Friedman, M., McAllister, R., Nelson-Rees, W., and Huebner, R.J. (1971). J. Nat. Cancer Inst. 47, 65-73.

99. Pfeffer, L.M. & Kopelvich, L. (1977). Cell 10, 313-320.

100. Levy, J. A. (1975). Nature 253, 140-142.

101. Yuasa, Y., Srivastava, S. K., Dunn, C. Y., Rhim, J. S., Reddy, E. P., and Aaronson, S. A. (1983). Nature 303, 775-779.

102. Fujita, J., Yoshida, O., Yuasa, Y., Rhim, J. S., Hatanaka, M., and Aaronson, S. A. (1984). Nature 309, 464-469.

103. Balmain, A., Ramsden, M., Bowden, G.T., and Smith, J. (1984). Nature 307, 658-660.

104. Sukumar, S., Notario, V., Martin-Zanca, D., and Barbacid, M. (1983). Nature 306, 658-661.

105. Holliday, R. (1983). Nature 306, 742.

106. Wigler, M., Fasano, O., Taparowsky, E., Powes, S., Kataoka, T., Brinbaum, D., Shimizu, K. F., Goldfarb, M. (1984). In: Cancer Cells 2/Oncogenes and Viral Genes, G. F. Vande Woude, A. J. Levine, W. C. Topp, and J. D. Watson, eds., (Cold Spring Harbor Laboratory, Cold Spring Harbor, New York) in press.

107. Capon, D. J., Seeburg, P. H., McGrath, J. P., Hayflick, J. S., Edman, U., Levinson, A. D., and Goeddel, D. V. (1983). Nature 304, 507-513.

108. Pulciani, S., Santos, E., Lauver, A. V., Long, L. K., Aaronson, S. A., and Barbacid, M. (1982). Nature 300, 539-542.

109. Albino, A.P., Le Strange, R., Oliff, A.I., Furth, M.E., and Old, L.J. (1984). Nature 308, 69-72.

110. Vousden, K. M., and Marshall, C. J. (1984). EMBO Journal 3, 913-917.

111. Tainsky, M. A., Cooper, C. S., Giovanella, B. C., Vande Woude, G. F. (1984). Science 225 643-645.

112. Maisel, J., Klement, V., Lai, M.M-C., Ostertag, W. and Duesberg, P. H. (1973) Proc. Nat. Acad. Sci. USA 70, 3536-3540.

113. Ellis, R. W., Defeo, D., Furth, M. E., and Scolnick, E. M. (1982). Molec. Cell. Biol. 2, 1339-1345.

114. Parada, L. F., Tabin, C., Shih, C. and Weinberg, R. A. (1982). Nature 297, 474-478.

115. Scolnick, E. M. Vass, W. C., Howk, R. S., and Duesberg, P. H. (1979). J. Virol 29, 964-72.

116. Temin, H. M. (1983). Nature 302, 656.

15

THE FAMILY OF HUMAN T-CELL LEUKEMIA VIRUSES AND THEIR ROLE IN THE CAUSE OF T-CELL LEUKEMIA AND AIDS

R.C. GALLO, G. SHAW, B. HAHN, F. WONG-STAAL, M. POPOVIC, J. SCHUPBACH, M.G. SARNGADHARAN, S. ARYA, S.Z. SALAHUDDIN, and M.S. REITZ, JR.

Laboratory of Tumor Cell Biology, Developmental Therapeutics Program, Division of Cancer Treatment, National Cancer Institute, Bethesda, Maryland 20205.

1. INTRODUCTION

HTLV is the generic name we gave the first human retroviruses. The majority of isolates are very closely related; we call them human T-cell leukemia virus type I (HTLV-I). HTLV-I is endemic (at low rates) in the Caribbean, South and Central America, southeast U.S., southern Japan, and especially Africa. Viruses closely related to HTLV-I, but distinct from it, have been isolated from Old World monkeys. This and other facts led us to propose that the ancestral origin of HTLV is in Africa. Evidence indicates that HTLV-I is the direct cause of an aggressive form of adult T-cell leukemia and lymphoma. The mechanisms involved in the in vitro immortalization and in vivo malignancy are not yet clear but apparently do not involve any visible consistent chromosomal change, consistent virus expression, or known onc genes. Whichever the mechanism for growth induction by HTLV-I, its efficiency in causing malignancy may be because it has dual major effects on infected cells: (1) immortalization of some T cells, and (2) interference with function and cytopathic changes in many others. In collaboration with D. Golde and colleagues, we also discovered a second class of human T-lymphotropic retroviruses (HTLV-II). It shares many features with HTLV-I but has major genomic differences. It has been isolated only from one patient with hairy cell leukemia, and recently we isolated it again from a patient with AIDS. Finally, we have obtained 96 isolates of HTLV-III. This retrovirus shares some antigenic cross-reactivity and genomic homology with HTLV-I and II, is also highly T4 tropic, but has only cytopathic and not immortalizing effects. All isolates of

HTLV-III have come from patients with AIDS or people at high risk for this disease. Sera from over 85% of AIDS and pre-AIDS patients have antibodies specifically against this virus, whereas 1% of healthy heterosexuals are positive. These and some prospective studies indicate that HTLV-III is the cause of AIDS.

2. HTLV-I AND ADULT T-CELL LEUKEMIA

The first human retrovirus isolates, which we now refer to as HTLV-I, were isolated from black patients in the United States with what were diagnosed as unusually aggressive variants of cutaneous T-cell lymphoma/leukemia (Sézary syndrome and mycosis fungoides) (1-3). The virus has typical retroviral morphology (Fig. 1) and contains reverse transcriptase and high molecular weight polyadenylated RNA. HTLV-I is distinct from other animal

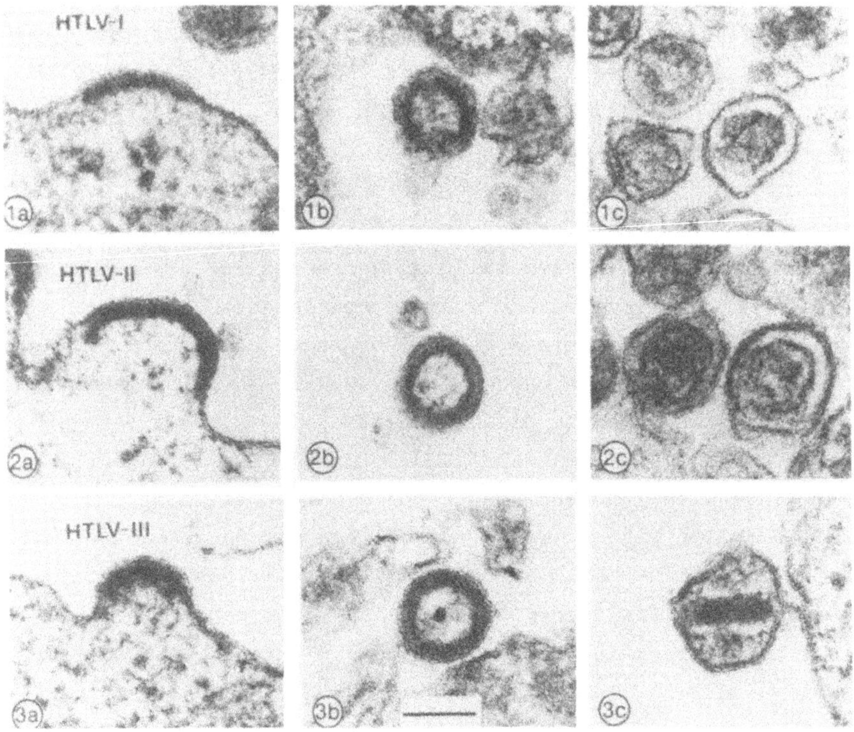

FIGURE 1. Electron microscopy of HTLV-I, II and III. Shown are budding (panels a), immature (panels b) and mature virions of the three types of HTLV. The bar in panel 3b equals 100 nm.

retroviruses by protein serology (4-6) and nucleic acid hybridization (3), and is exogenous to man (3). Transmission of the virus is horizontal and does not seem to occur genetically (7,8).

The availability of HTLV-I proteins and antibodies against viral proteins made it possible to test serum samples for evidence of exposure to this agent. It was apparent that most persons in the United States were negative for HTLV-I, including persons with leukemias and lymphomas. Furthermore, HTLV-I was only sporadically detected in persons from the United States with cutaneous T-cell neoplasms (9), most of whom were blacks in the southeastern United States or of Caribbean origin (10).

Two geographic regions were noted, however, in which diseases were endemic which clinically resembled those from which the first two HTLV isolates originated. These two regions were the Caribbean (11) and southwestern Japan (12). The disease in the Caribbean, then called lymphosarcoma cell leukemia, and that in Japan, called adult T-cell leukemia, were both found to be highly associated with the presence of serum antibodies to HTLV-I (13-15). Both diseases are now considered to be the same and are collectively called adult T-cell leukemia/lymphoma, or ATLL.

These results were confirmed by investigators in Japan, who also isolated a retrovirus from cases of ATLL (8,16). The Japanese isolates are now recognized as examples of HTLV-I (17). Sporadic cases of ATLL as well as sporadic exposure to HTLV-I have also been noted in many other areas of the world (18), and parts of Africa also appear to be endemic for HTLV-I (19).

As is the case for other leukemia viruses, only a small fraction of individuals infected with HTLV-I develop ATLL (20). Other factors such as host immune response, age of exposure, virus dose, and route of infection may be important factors in determining the outcome of infection.

3. IN VITRO TRANSFORMATION AND OTHER BIOLOGICAL EFFECTS OF HTLV-I

HTLV-I was first shown to transform T cells by Miyoshi and colleagues (21), but it was not shown that the target cells were themselves free of virus. Subsequently, transformation was reported for T cells shown to be HTLV-negative (22,23).

HTLV-I selectively infects T cells (particularly those of an $OKT4^+$ phenotype) both in vivo (7) and in vitro (22-24). The cells infected in vitro acquire many of the properties of transformed ATLL cells, including an altered morphology, an increased growth rate, the tendency to grow in clumps, reduced dependence on (or complete independence from) added T-cell growth factor (TCGF), and cell surface expression of high levels of the TCGF receptor and HLA-DR antigens (23-25). Infection with HTLV-I also abrogates the usual crisis period observed with uninfected T cells 4 to 5 weeks after initiation into culture. Transformation in vitro by HTLV-I appears to be much more rapid and efficient than leukemogenesis in vivo.

Infection of functional T cells by HTLV-I causes loss of some of their immune functions. For example, a T-cell line derived from one long-term survivor of ATLL was shown to be cytotoxic for autologous HTLV-I-infected cells (26). These cytotoxic T cells could themselves be infected with HTLV-I, subsequently losing some functions. One clone infected with HTLV-I, called K7, could no longer kill infected cells, but instead stopped dividing and died when presented with the target cells (27). A variety of other changes after infection with HTLV have been observed as well (28,29).

HTLV-I can also infect and transform bone marrow cells (30). The phenotype of these infected cells differs, and can be $OKT4^+T8^-$, $OKT4^-T8^+$, or $OKT4^-T8^-$.

4. HTLV-II

HTLV-II was first isolated from one patient with a hairy cell leukemia (31). Although related to HTLV-I by antigenic determinants on the major gag protein, p24, and on its envelope proteins (31,32), it is quite distinguishable by protein serology (33) and nucleic acid hybridization (34). It shares many biochemical and biological properties with HTLV-I (see Table 1), including its ability to transform T cells and mediate a loss of immune function (29). It has been isolated only rarely, and in spite of its biological properties, it has not at this time been linked epidemiologically to any diseases.

Table 1. Relatedness of HTLV-I, II and III

Property	Subgroup of HTLV		
	I	II	III
1. General infectivity	Lym	Lym	Lym
2. Particular tropism	T4	T4	T4
3. RT size	ω100K	ω100K	ω100K
4. RT divalent cation	Mg^{++}	Mg^{++}	Mg^{++}
5. Major core	p24	p24	p24
6. Common envelope epitope	+	+	+
7. Common p24 epitope	+	+	+
8. Nucleic acid homology to I (stringent)		±	-
9. Nucleic acid homology to I (moderate stringency)		++	+
10. Homology to other retroviruses	0	0	0
11. pX	+	+	+
12. Produces giant multinucleated cells	+	+	+
13. African origin	Likely	?	Likely

5. THE GENOMIC STRUCTURE OF HTLV-I AND HTLV-II

The complete genome of HTLV-I has been sequenced (35). Like other retroviruses, HTLV-I contains two large terminal repeat (LTR) sequences which contain transcriptional promoters for RNA transcription and termination signals, and *gag*, *pol*, and *env* genes. In addition, 3' to the *env* gene is an extensive stretch of DNA which has four open reading frames capable of coding for proteins of 10, 11, 12 and 27 kilodaltons. This region, called the pX region, is presumably not required for viral replication. Although its function is not known, it may play a role in cell transformation (see below). The pX region, like the rest of the HTLV-I genome, has no homology with uninfected human DNA. The structure of the HTLV-I genome is presented in Figure 2.

HTLV-II also has a pX region, and has the same gene order as HTLV-I (36). Under relaxed hybridization conditions, it can be shown that HTLV-I and II are at least distantly related over the length of their genomes. Of all the genes of both viruses, the pX region appears to be the most closely conserved. Recently, this

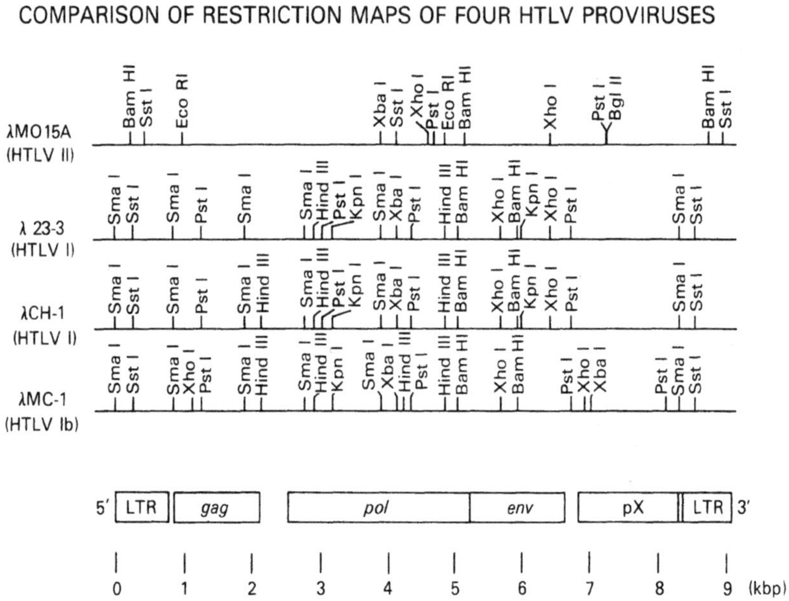

FIGURE 2. Genomes and restriction maps of HTLV-I and II. λMO15A is an example of HTLV-II, λ23-3 and λCH-1 are examples of HTLV-I, and λMC-1 is HTLV-Ib. Genomic regions corresponding to LTR, gag, pol, env, and pX are drawn to scale according to the published nucleotide sequence of an HTLV-I isolate. Two BglII sites in the 5' end of λMO15A are not shown.

region of HTLV-II has been sequenced (37). There is a large open reading frame in the 3' portion of the HTLV-II pX capable of coding for a protein of at least 38 kilodaltons which is highly homologous to a similar region in HTLV-I, suggesting that the product coded for by this region is important for the biological activity of HTLV-I and II.

The env gene of HTLV-II has also recently been sequenced (38). The envelope genes of HTLV-I and II are significantly related (50% overall at the DNA sequence level) except at the extreme carboxy and amino termini of the gene.

The LTRs of I and II show marked differences in their sequences through most of their length (39), but sequences at or near the RNA cap site, the primer binding site, and a 21 base pair sequence repeated four times in the HTLV-II LTR and three times in that of HTLV-I are highly homologous. These could conceivably represent RNA transcriptional enhancers.

6. MOLECULAR MECHANISMS OF TRANSFORMATION BY HTLV-I and II

A central paradox of the biology of HTLV-I (and II) is that transformation of infected T cells appears to be rapid, yet the viral genome does not contain a classically defined (i.e., cell-derived) onc gene. Moreover, leukemogenesis is relatively inefficient, resembling the chronic animal leukemia viruses such as the feline and bovine leukemia viruses.

This paradox is also apparent at the molecular level. The proviral integration site in fresh leukemic blood cells, in cell lines derived from these cells, and in long-term infected cord blood T-cell lines established in vitro is nearly always mono- or oligoclonal (8,27,40',41), suggesting that only a few of the infected cells become transformed. However, there does not appear to be a unique integration site common to different leukemic patients or cell lines (40,41), suggesting that a specific integration event is not required for transformation and that the virus itself therefore contains all the information required for transformation.

How might this paradox be resolved? Recently it has been shown that the RNA polymerase promoter in the HTLV-I and II LTRs are strongly influenced by the type of cell in which they are present (42,43), and are relatively more active in T cells than in other cell types. In fact, the HTLV-I promoter is far more active in cells already infected with HTLV than in uninfected cells, while the HTLV-II promoter appears to have a strong requirement for a factor in HTLV-infected cells. Sodroski et al. (42) interpret these data as indicating the presence of a trans-acting factor (which could be encoded by the pX gene) present in HTLV-infected cells which strongly activates the HTLV promoter. If this were indeed the pX product, and if it were able to also affect the promoters of cellular genes critical for T-cell function and proliferation, it could explain both a rapid transformation of T cells without the requirement for a specific integration site and a cytopathic or dysfunctional effect on infected T cells. This does not, however, explain the rapid monoclonality which occurs after HTLV-I and HTLV-II infection and transformation of T-cells.

7. HTLV-III AND ITS ASSOCIATION WITH AIDS

Acquired immunodeficiency syndrome (AIDS) is a recently recognized, usually fatal disease involving a severe depletion of helper T cells as well as multiple opportunistic infections and/or malignancies among high-risk groups, including promiscuous homosexuals, intravenous drug abusers, Haitians, hemophiliacs, and infants born to members of high-risk groups. Epidemiologic data suggest involvement of a transmissible agent. Because of this as well as the involvement of OKT4^{+} T cells in the disease, it seemed possible that an HTLV-like retrovirus was involved. Indeed, Essex and his colleagues reported the presence of an antibody in a large percentage of AIDS and high-risk populations which reacted against a protein present specifically in HTLV-I-infected cells (44,45).

Recently, we developed a cell system which allowed the reproducible detection of retrovirus from AIDS and pre-AIDS pateints (46). Some of the target cells support the production of high levels of virus, and more than 90 isolates from this group of patients have now been obtained (47 and P. Markham et al., in preparation). Based on electron microscopic examinations, the biochemical properties of the viral reverse transcriptase (46), antigenic determinants of the env and gag proteins (48), and demonstration of distant but significant nucleic acid homology, particularly in the gag-pol region (49,50), this new virus is distantly related to both HTLV-I and II. Its T4 cell tropism, likely African origin, and presence of a pX sequence also indicate that these viruses are of common ancestory. This indicates that it belongs to the HTLV group of viruses, and it has been designated HTLV-III.

This also suggests that the activity detected by Essex and his co-workers reflected a cross-reactivity with antibody to HTLV-III. We have isolated HTLV-III from a majority of pre-AIDS patients and a large fraction of actual AIDS patients (47). Isolation is rare from the normal population. Moreover, the overwhelming majority of such patients have antibodies to HTLV-III (51). A typical Western blot is shown in Figure 3. The major reactivity appears to be

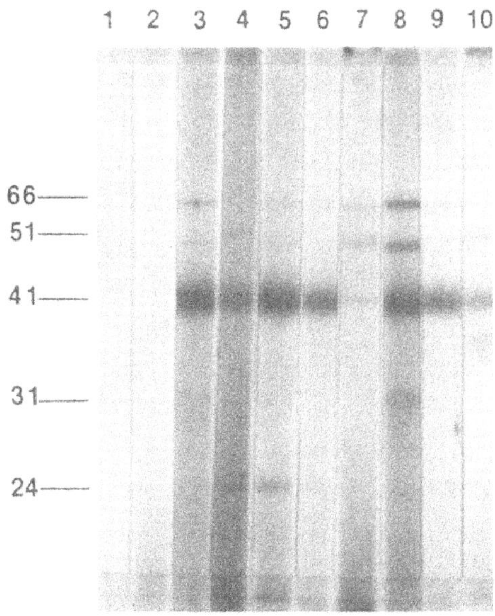

FIGURE 3. Identification of HTLV-III antigens recognized by sera of AIDS patients. HTLV-III was lysed and fractionated by electrophoresis on a 12% polyacrylamide slab gel in the presence of SDS. The protein bands on the gel were electrophoretically transferred to a nitrocellulose sheet and strip solid-phase radioimmunoassays were then performed. The strips were washed, dried, mounted, and exposed to x-ray film. Strip 1, adult T-cell leukemia; strip 2, normal donor; strip 3, mother of a child with AIDS; strips 4 and 6 to 10, AIDS patients; and strip 5, patient with pre-AIDS.

directed against a 41 Kd protein which is the presumed env antigen of HTLV-III. More recent data show that the incidence of such antibodies to HTLV-III in these patients is virtually 100% (52). The striking association of HTLV-III and AIDS suggests that this virus is in fact the etiologic agent of AIDS, and that this family of viruses can cause T-cell depletion as well as the clonal T-cell proliferation seen in ATLL. Recent evidence indicates that the virus called LAV or IDAV detected previously by Sinoussi-Barre et al. is a member of the same HTLV subgroup (53) (see also Montagnier et al. in this book).

8. DISCUSSION

We have used the term HTLV to designate the members of what is at present a family of three highly distinct but related virus groups, HTLV-I, II, and III, which infect and have major effects on OKT4$^+$ T cells. HTLV-I is highly associated with adult T-cell leukemia/lymphoma (ATLL), and its identification in fact helped establish ATLL as a distinct worldwide clinicopathologic entity. Its biology in vitro appears to mimic at least some of its activity in vivo, and provides in many respects a model system for the disease. Infection in vitro results in cell transformation (20-22), loss of immune function (27-29), and in some instances selective T-cell death (27).

HTLV-II, although it brings about many of the same changes in infected T cells as HTLV-I, is at present not associated with any disease and has in fact been isolated only rarely. Its geographic distribution and etiologic role in human disease awaits clarification.

HTLV-III seems highly likely to be the cause of AIDS. Not only is evidence of its presence found in the overwhelming majority of AIDS and pre-AIDS patients, but its cytopathic effect in vitro against OKT4$^+$ cells mimics what occurs in vivo in AIDS.

There are thus a group of related human retroviruses with disparate effects on the same target cell, the OKT4$^+$ T cell. It will be of interest to see if still other members of this virus family remain to be discovered. The identification of the presently recognized members of this group gives us opportunities to study T-cell biology, as well as the potential to intervene in certain now fatal (and, in the case of AIDS, increasingly prevalent) T-cell diseases.

References

1. Poiesz BJ, Ruscetti FW, Gazdar AF, Bunn PA, Minna JD, Gallo RC: Detection and isolation of type C retrovirus particles from fresh and cultured lymphocytes of a patient with cutaneous T-cell lymphoma. Proc Natl Acad Sci USA (77): 7415-7419, 1980.
2. Poiesz BJ, Ruscetti FW, Reitz MS, Kalyanaraman VS, Gallo RC: Isolation of a new type-C retrovirus (HTLV) in primary uncultured cells of a patient with Sezary T-cell leukemia. Nature (294): 268-271, 1981.

3. Reitz MS, Poiesz BJ, Ruscetti FW, Gallo RC: Characterization and distribution of nucleic acid sequences of a novel type C retrovirus isolated from neoplastic human T lymphocytes. Proc Natl Acad Sci USA (78): 1887-1891, 1981.
4. Kalyanaraman VS, Sarngadharan MG, Poiesz BJ, Ruscetti FW, Gallo RC: Immunological properties of a type C retrovirus isolated from cultured human T-lymphoma cells and comparison to other mammalian retroviruses. J Virol (38): 906-915, 1981.
5. Robert-Guroff M, Ruscetti FW, Posner LE, Poiesz BJ, Gallo RC: Detection of the human T-cell lymphoma virus p19 in cells of some patients with cutaneous T-cell lymphoma and leukemia using a monoclonal antibody. J Exp Med (154): 1957-1964, 1981.
6. Rho HM, Poiesz BJ, Ruscetti FW, Gallo RC: Characterization of the reverse transcriptase from a new retrovirus (HTLV) produced by a human cutaneous T-cell lymphoma cell line. Virology (112): 355-360, 1981.
7. Gallo RC, Mann D, Broder S, Ruscetti FW, Maeda M, Kalyanaraman VS, Robert-Guroff M, Reitz MS: Human T-cell leukemia-lymphoma virus (HTLV) is in T- but not B-lymphocytes from a patient with cutaneous T-cell lymphoma. Proc Natl Acad Sci USA (79): 4680-4684, 1982.
8. Yoshida M, Miyoshi I, Hinuma Y: Isolation and characterization of retrovirus from cell lines of human adult T-cell leukemia and its implication in the disease. Proc Natl Acad Sci USA (79): 2031-2034, 1982.
9. Posner LE, Robert-Guroff M, Kalyanaraman VS, Poiesz BJ, Ruscetti FW, Fossieck B, Bunn PA Jr, Minna JD, Gallo RC: Natural antibodies to the human T cell lymphoma virus in patients with cutaneous T cell lymphomas. J Exp Med (154): 333-346, 1981.
10. Blayney DW, Blattner WA, Robert-Guroff M, Jaffe ES, Fisher RI, Bunn PA Jr, Patton MG, Rarick HR, Gallo RC: The human T-cell leukemia-lymphoma virus in the southeastern United States. JAMA (250): 1048-1052, 1983.
11. Catovsky D, Greaves MF, Rose M, Galton DAG, Goolden AWG, McCluskey DR, White JM, Lampert I, Bourikas G, Ireland R, Brownell AI, Bridges JM, Blattner WA, Gallo RC: Adult T-cell lymphoma-leukaemia in blacks from the West Indies. Lancet (i): 639-643, 1982.
12. Takatsuki K, Uchiyama J, Sagawa K, Yodoi J: Adult T-cell leukemia in Japan. In: Seno S, Takaku F, Irino S (eds) Topics in hematology. Excerpta Medica, Amsterdam-Oxford, 1977, pp 73-77.
13. Kalyanaraman VS, Sarngadharan MG, Nakao Y, Ito Y, Aoki T, Gallo RC: Natural antibodies to the structural core protein (p24) of the human T-cell leukemia (lymphoma) retrovirus found in sera of leukemia patients in Japan. Proc Natl Acad Sci USA (79): 1653-1657, 1982.
14. Robert-Guroff M, Nakao Y, Notake K, Ito Y, Sliski A, Gallo RC: Natural antibodies to human retrovirus HTLV in a cluster of Japanese patients with adult T cell leukemia. Science (215): 975-978, 1982.

15. Blattner WA, Kalyanaraman VS, Robert-Guroff M, Lister TA, Galton DAG, Sarin PS, Crawford MH, Catovsky D, Greaves M, Gallo RC: The human type-C retrovirus, HTLV, in Blacks from the Caribbean region, and relationship to adult T-cell leukemia/lymphoma. Int J Cancer (30): 257-264, 1982.
16. Miyoshi I, Kubonishi I, Yoshimoto S, Akagi T, Ohtsuki Y, Shiraishi Y, Nagato K, Hinuma Y: Type C virus particles in a cord T-cell line derived by co-cultivating normal human cord blood leukocytes and human leukemic T-cells. Nature (294): 770-771, 1981.
17. Watanabe T, Seiki M, Yoshida M: HTLV type I (U.S. isolate) and ATLV (Japanese isolate) are the same species of human retrovirus. Virology (133): 238-241, 1984.
18. Gallo RC, Kalyanaraman VS, Sarngadharan MG, Sliski A, Vonderheid EC, Maeda M, Nakao Y, Yamada K, Ito Y, Gutensohn N, Murphy S, Bunn PA Jr, Catovsky D, Greaves MF, Blayney DW, Blattner W, Jarrett WFH, zur Hausen H, Seligmann M, Brouet JC, Haynes BF, Jegasothy BV, Jaffe E, Cossman J, Broder S, Fisher RI, Golde DW, Robert-Guroff M: Association of the human type C retrovirus with a subset of adult T-cell cancers. Cancer Res (43): 3892-3899, 1983.
19. Saxinger WC, Blattner WA, Levine PH, Clark J, Biggar R, Hoh M, Moghissi J, Jacobs P, Wilson L, Jacobson P, Crookes R, Strong M, Ansari AA, Dean AG, Nkrumah FH, Mouvali N, Gallo RC: Human T-cell leukemia virus (HTLV-I) antibodies in Africa. Science (in press).
20. Tajima K, Tominaga S, Suchi T, Kawagoe T, Komoda H, Hinuma Y, Oda T, Fujita K: Epidemiological analysis on distribution of antibody to adult T-cell leukemia-virus-associated antigen (ATLA): possible horizontal transmission of adult T-cell leukemia virus. Gann (in press).
21. Miyoshi T, Yoshimoto S, Kubonishi I, Tagushi H. Shiraishi Y, Ohtsuki Y, Akagi T: Transformation of normal human cord lymphocytes by co-cultivation with a lethally irradiated human T-cell line carrying type C virus particles. Gann (71): 155-156, 1981.
22. Popovic M, Sarin PS, Robert-Guroff M, Kalyanaraman VS, Mann D, Minowada J, Gallo RC: Isolation and transmission of human retrovirus (human T-cell leukemia virus). Science (219): 856-859, 1983.
23. Popovic M, Lange-Wantzin G, Sarin PS, Mann D, Gallo RC: Transformation of human umbilical cord blood T cells by human T-cell leukemia/lymphoma virus. Proc Natl Acad Sci USA (80): 5402-5406, 1983.
24. Mann DL, Popovic M, Murray C, Neuland C, Strong DM, Sarin P, Gallo RC, Blattner WA: Cell surface antigen expression of newborn cord blood lymphocytes infected with HTLV. J Immunol (131): 2021-2024, 1983.
25. Mann DL, Popovic M, Sarin PS, Murray C, Reitz MS, Strong DM, Haynes BF, Gallo RC, Blattner WA: Cell lines producing human T-cell lymphoma virus show altered HLA expression. Nature (305): 58-60, 1983.

26. Mitsuya H, Matis LA, Megson M, Bunn PA, Murray C, Mann DL, Gallo RC, Broder S: Generation of an HLA-restricted cytotoxic T-cell line reactive against cultured tumor cells from a patient infected with human T-cell leukemia/lymphoma virus. J Exp Med (158): 994-999, 1983.
27. Mitsuya H, Guo H-G, Megson M, Trainor CD, Reitz MS, Broder S: Transformation and cytopathic effect in an immune T-cell clone infected by human T-cell leukemia-lymphoma virus (HTLV). Science (223): 1293-1295, 1984.
28. Mitsuya H, Guo H-G, Cossman J, Megson M, Reitz M, Broder S: Functional properties of antigen-specific T-cells infected by human T-cell leukemia/lymphoma virus (HTLV-I). Science (in press).
29. Popovic M, Flomenberg N, Volkman DJ, Mann D, Fauci AS, Dupont B, Gallo RC: Alteration in T-cell functions by infection with HTLV-I or HTLV-II. Science (in press).
30. Markham PD, Salahuddin SZ, Macchi B, Robert-Guroff M, Gallo RC: Transformation of different phenotypic types of human bone marrow T-lymphocytes by HTLV-I. Int J Cancer (33): 13-17, 1984.
31. Kalyanaraman VS, Sarngadharan MG, Robert-Guroff M, Miyoshi I, Blayney D, Golde D, Gallo RC: A new subtype of human T-cell leukemia virus (HTLV-II) associated with a T-cell variant of hairy cell leukemia. Science (218): 571-573, 1982.
32. Lee TH, Coligan JE, McLane MF, Sodroski JG, Popovic M, Wong-Staal F, Gallo RC, Haseltine W, Essex M: Serologic cross-reactivity between envelope gene products of type I and type II human T-cell leukemia virus. Proc Natl Acad Sci USA (in press).
33. Kalyanaraman VS, Jarvis-Morar M, Sarngadharan MG, Gallo RC: Immunological characterization of the low molecular weight gag gene proteins p19 and p15 of human T-cell leukemia-lymphoma virus (HTLV) and demonstration of human natural antibodies to them. Virology (132): 61-70, 1984.
34. Reitz MS Jr, Popovic M, Haynes BF, Clark SC, Gallo RC: Relatedness by nucleic acid hybridization of new isolates of human T-cell leukemia-lymphoma virus (HTLV) and demonstration of provirus in uncultured leukemic blood cells. Virology (126): 688-692, 1983.
35. Seiki M, Hattori S, Hirayama Y, Yoshida M: Human adult T-cell leukemia virus: complete nucleotide sequence of the provirus genome integrated in leukemia cell DNA. Proc Natl Acad Sci USA (80): 3618-3622, 1983.
36. Shaw GM, Gonda MA, Flickinger GH, Hahn BH, Gallo RC, Wong-Staal, F: The genomes of evolutionarily divergent members of the human T-cell leukemia virus family (HTLV-I and HTLV-II) are highly conserved, especially in pX. Proc Natl Acad Sci USA (81): 4544-4548, 1984.
37. Haseltine WA, Sodroski J, Patrarca R, Briggs D, Perkins D, Wong-Staal F: Structure of the 3' terminal region of type II human T-lymphotropic virus: Evidence for a new coding region. Science (225): 419-421, 1984.

38. Sodroski J, Patarca R, Perkins D, Briggs D, Lee TH, Essex M, Coligan J, Wong-Staal F, Gallo RC, Haseltine WA: Sequence of the envelope glycoprotein gene of type II human T lymphotropi virus. Science (225): 421-424, 1984.
39. Sodroski J, Trus M, Perkins D, Patarca R, Wong-Staal F, Gelmann E, Gallo R, Haseltine WA: Repetitive structure in the long terminal repeat element of type II human T cell leukemia virus. Proc Natl Acad Sci USA (in press).
40. Wong-Staal F, Hahn B, Manzari V, Colombini S, Franchini G, Gelmann EP, Gallo RC: A survey of human leukaemias for sequences of a human retrovirus, HTLV. Nature (302): 626-628, 1983.
41. Yoshida M, Seiki M, Yamaguchi K, Takatsuki K: Monoclonal integration of human T-cell leukemia provirus in all primary tumors of adult T-cell leukemia suggests causative role of human T-cell leukemia virus in the disease. Proc Natl Acad Sc USA (81): 2534-2537, 1984.
42. Sodroski JG, Rosen CA, Haseltine WA: Trans-acting transcriptional activation of the long terminal repeat of human T-lymphotropic viruses in infected cells. Science (225): 381-385, 1984.
43. Chen ISY, McLaughlin J, Golde DW: Long terminal repeats of human T-cell leukemia virus II genome determine target cell specificity. Nature (309): 276-280, 1980.
44. Essex M, McLane MF, Lee TH, Falk L, Howe CWS, Mullins JI, Cabradilla C, Francis DP: Antibodies to cell membrane antigen associated with human T-cell leukemia virus in patients with AIDS. Science (220): 859-862, 1983.
45. Essex M, McLane MF, Lee TH, Tachibana N, Mullins JI, Kreiss J Kasper CK, Poon M-C, Landay A, Stein SF, Francis DP, Cabradilla C, Lawrence DN, Evatt BL: Antibodies to human T-cell leukemia virus membrane antigens (HTLV-MA) in hemophiliacs. Science (221): 1061-1063, 1983.
46. Popovic M, Sarngadharan MG, Read E, Gallo RC: Detection, isolation, and continuous production of cytopathic retroviruses (HTLV-III) from patients with AIDS and pre-AIDS. Science (224): 497-500, 1984.
47. Gallo RC, Salahuddin SZ, Popovic M, Shearer GM, Kaplan M, Haynes BF, Palker TJ, Redfield R, Oleske J, Safai B, White G, Foster P, Markham PD: Frequent detection and isolation of cytopathic retroviruses (HTLV-III) from patients with AIDS an at risk for AIDS. Science (224): 500-503, 1984.
48. Schupbach J, Popovic M, Gilden RV, Gonda MA, Sarngadharan MG, Gallo RC: Serological analysis of a subgroup of human T-lymphotropic retroviruses (HTLV-III) associated with AIDS. Science (224): 503-504, 1984.
49. Arya SK, Gallo RC, Hahn BH, Shaw GM, Popovic M, Salahuddin SZ Wong-Staal F: Homology of genome of AIDS associated virus (HTLV-III) with genomes of human T-cell leukemia viruses (HTLV-I and HTLV-II). Science (in press).
50. Hahn BH, Shaw GM, Arya SK, Popovic M, Gallo RC, Wong-Staal F: Molecular cloning and characterization of the virus associate with AIDS (HTLV-III) (Submitted).

51. Sarngadharan MG, Popovic M, Bruch L, Schupbach J, Gallo RC: Antibodies reactive with human T-lymphotropic retroviruses (HTLV-III) in the serum of patients with AIDS. Science (224): 506-508, 1984.
52. Safai B, Sarngadharan MG, Groopman J, Arnett K, Popovic M, Sliski A, Schupbach J, Gallo RC: Seroepidemiological studies of human T-lymphotropic retrovirus type III in acquired immunodeficiency syndrome. Lancet (June 30) 1438-1440, 1984.
53. Barré-Sinoussi F, Chermann JC, Rey F, Nugeyre MT, Chamaret S, Gruest J, Dauguet C, Axler-Blin C, Vézinet-Brun F, Rouzioux C, Rosenbaum W, Montagnier L: Isolation of a T-lymphotropic retrovirus from a patient at risk for acquired immune deficiency syndrome (AIDS). Science (220): 868-870, 1983.

16

A NOVEL HUMAN LYMPHOTROPIC RETROVIRUS (LAV) : NEW DATA ON ITS BIOLOGY AND ROLE IN AIDS

L. MONTAGNIER[1], F. BARRE-SINOUSSI[1], D. KLATZMANN[3], J.C. GLUCKMAN[3], C. ROUZIOUX[2], F. BRUN-VEZINET[2] and J.C. CHERMANN[1]

[1] Department of Virology, Institut Pasteur, Paris, France
[2] Hopital Claude Bernard, Paris, France
[3] U.E.R. Pitié-Salpêtrière, Paris, France.

Retroviruses are known for a long time to be involved in animal diseases : many of the natural retroviruses studied are the causal agents of malignant diseases, involving particularly the lymphoid system. A few others, such as the Visna-Maedi group and the Equine Infectious Anemia Virus (EIAV), are the agents of persistent, occasionally letal infections.

In contrast, the search for similar retroviruses in humans has been unsuccessful until the recent isolation of Human T Leukemia Virus (HTLV-I) or Adult T Cell Leukemia Virus (ATLV) (1) (2) and of HTLV-II(3). In these findings, the earlier discovery of a growth factor allowing sustained culture of T-lymphocytes (T cell growth factor,TCGF or Interleukin 2) (4) was critical, in allowing whole expression of the retrovirus in activated T-lymphocytes, and therefore detection by its reverse transcriptase activity.

A similar approach, combined with the use of antibodies to interferon (5), led our group to discover in 1983 (6) another novel lymphotropic retrovirus, Lymphadenopathy Associated Virus (LAV), and there is now strong evidence suggesting that this virus is indeed the primary agent of the Acquired Immune Deficiency Syndrome (AIDS).

In this presentation, we shall summarize the main characteristics of this new group of retroviruses and the data indicating their involvement in AIDS and related diseases.

1. ISOLATION AND CHARACTERISTICS OF LAV

LAV1 was isolated from a lymph node of a French homosexual with lymphadenopathy syndrome. Cells from the minced lymph node were put in culture in the presence of Phytohemagglutinin (PHA) and anti-interferon α serum. After 3 days, PHA containing medium was removed and replaced by medium containing TCGF and anti-interferon serum. Cells began to release virus-associated reverse transcriptase activity from day 15 until day 25 of the culture. The virus could be propagated in T-lymphocyte cultures from normal donors or from umbilical cord, without co-cultivation.

The viral isolate was shown to be a retrovirus, by all classical criteria (density in sucrose gradient, template requirements of the reverse transcriptase (RT), high molecular weight RNA, morphogenesis by budding).

It has some similarities with HTLV-I and II : Mg^{++} dependence of the RT for optimal reaction, tropism for T-lymphocytes. However, it clearly differs from the latter retroviruses by the following characteristics :

a/ Lack of antigenic cross-reactivity of the major core protein with HTLVI and II p24. The major core protein of LAV migrates in polyacrylamide gels, under denaturing conditions, slightly slower than HTLVI p24. Its apparent molecular weight was deduced to be 25,000. LAV p25 could be immunoprecipitated by serum of the patient from which LAV was isolated, but not by antisera raised against HLTV-I p24 (6). Similarly, in a homologous radioimmunoassay, no competition was found with HTLV-I and HTLV-II p24 (7). Other major proteins include a p18, a small molecular weight protein (p12) and a high molecular weight glycoprotein.

b/ Different ultrastructure. Three types of particles could be seen in ultrathin sections of LAV producing lymphocytes : budding particles on the cell surface with a thin dense crescent separated from the bilayered membrane, free immature particles with also uncondensed core and mature particles with a small dense, eccentric core. The latter resembles mature D-type particles or those of EIAV.

d/ Lack of *in vitro* transforming activity. Whereas HTLVI and II transform T-lymphocytes, giving rise to immortalized T cell lines, such a phenomenon was never observed with LAV. Infection of normal T-lymphocytes with LAV leads to an acute production followed by the decline of cell multiplication and even cell death (see below).

Classification of LAV in the same group as HTLVI and HTLVII is not warranted by such differences and awaits a better knowledge of the whole group of human retroviruses.

We have previously reported (8) some antigenic similarities between LAV p25 and the corresponding core protein of EIAV, a retrovirus whose classification within the three subfamilies of retroviruses remains uncertain.

2. EVIDENCE FOR CAUSAL RELATIONSHIP BETWEEN VIRUSES OF THE LAV TYPE AND AIDS

During the last fifteen months, we have accumulated data which suggest that LAV related retroviruses are not simply opportunistic agents, but are indeed the best candidates for being the AIDS agent (14) (15).

2.1. Frequent isolation of LAV from all groups of patients having AIDS or at risk of AIDS

Using the method previously described for the isolation of LAV1, we have made more than 20 viral isolates from homosexuals, hemophiliacs, Zairians, Haitians, I.V. drug users presenting with AIDS or with lymphadenopathy syndrome. The three following Tables illustrate the origin of the isolates and the high correlation with the presence of antibodies to LAV p25 in the serum of the patients from which the viruses were isolated.

However, one patient (REM) had no detectable antibody against LAV p25, but he was weakly positive in a ELISA using disrupted whole virus and antibodies against the LAV p18 could be detected by the Western Blot technique (unpublished results).

All viral isolates have in common a Mg^{++} dependent reverse transcriptase, an antigenically related p25, the unability to transform T-lymphocytes. Electron microscopy studies, made on some isolates, always revealed the same characteristic morphology.

Isolation was found to be easier from frank AIDS cases than from cases of lymphadenopathy syndrome : only one failure was observed in the case of a Zairian child with AIDS, whereas the virus was readily isolated from blood lymphocytes of his mother, also with AIDS. In LAS, viral isolation was possible from lymphocytes derived from lymph node biopsies, only in 3 cases out of 13. This difference suggests that more lymphocytes express the virus in the cases of frank AIDS than in cases of LAS.

One viral isolate was obtained from an hemophiliac (not yet immunodepressed). The same virus has been isolated from his brother, an hemophiliac with AIDS (9). This result indicates the possible existence of healthy virus carriers, or at least with a long incubation period. It also suggests the likelihood of viral transmission by commercial preparation of antihemophilic factors.

Heterosexual transmission is also suggested by cases N°9-10. By contrast, no virus isolation could be achieved from healthy blood donors or laboratory workers or from patients with malignant diseases.

Table 1. Viral isolates of the LAV type

1.a. from French patients

N°	Patient's initials	Disease	Group	Antibodies to LAV RIPA p25	Antibodies to LAV ELISA	Antibodies to HTLV-I p24
1	RUB	LAS	Homosexual, Caucasian	+	+	-
2	LAI	LAS AIDS(KS)	Homosexual, Caucasian	+	∓	-
3	DL	AIDS(TX)	Hemophiliac B, Caucasian	+	+	-
4	EL	No	Hemophiliac B, brother of patient 3	+	+	-
5	CHA	LAS AIDS(KS)	Homosexual, Caucasian Stay in Haiti in 1980-81	+	+	-
6	ALL	LAS	Caucasian, living in Trinidad	+	+	-
7	REM	LAS AIDS(PC)	Homosexual, Caucasian	-	-	

1.b. from African and Haitian patients

N°	Patient's initials	Disease	Group	Antibodies to LAV RIPA p25	Antibodies to LAV ELISA	Antibodies to HTLV-I p24
8	ELI	AIDS(PC)	Zairian, immigrated to France	+	∓	-
9	NDO	AIDS(CR)	Zairian, immigrated to France	+	+	-
10	MUN	pre-AIDS	Zairian, wife of patient 9	+	+	-
11	EDO	LAS(Tb)	Haitian, living in France since 1973 - LAS since 1970.	+	+	-

1.c. from patients in U.S.A.

N°	Disease	Group	Antibodies to LAV RIPA p25	Antibodies to LAV ELISA	Antibodies to HTLV-I p24
12	AIDS(PC)	IV drug user, NY USA	+	-	-
13	AIDS(PC)	IV drug user, NY USA	+	-	-
14	AIDS(KS)	Homosexual, NY USA	+	+	-
15	AIDS(PC)	Transfusion, LA USA	+	+	-
16	AIDS(PC)	Transfusion, LA USA	+	+	-
17	AIDS(KS)	Homosexual, LA USA	+	+	-

2.2. Viral tropism for T4 (helper) lymphocytes and induction of a cytopathic effect

Immunofluorescence detection of viral antigens in infected lymphocytes indicated that at most 5% of the cells were expressing viral antigens at a time. Therefore, one of our earliest effort was to analyse which fraction of T-lymphocytes was permissive to viral replication.

T4 and T8 lymphocytes of a normal donor were separated by means of affinity chromatography on monoclonal antibodies (16). After PHA stimulation, they were infected with LAV. Only T4 cells did produce the virus.

This result is not an artefact of *in vitro* stimulation. When T4 and T8 lymphocytes of a "healthy" virus carrier were similarly fractionated, only the T4 fraction released virus upon PHA stimulation (14)(16). Only 10% of the T4 population expressed viral antigens at a time. It remains to be determined whether or not this population belongs to a special subset of the T4 fraction.

Inhibition of cell growth was observed at the peak of virus production. Moreover, giant polykaryons, presumably arising by virus-induced cell fusion, were seen at the onset of virus production. At the same time, on the remaining T4 cells, the T3 and T4 cell surface markers decreased. These results indicate that, at least *in vitro*, intensive virus expression was correlated with a cytopathic effect on the target cells. It remains to be determined whether such a cytopathic effect occurs also *in vivo*. Clearly, a selective tropism for T4 cells is what one should expect for the AIDS agent : an almost constant sign of the disease is the decrease of T4 (leu 3) lymphocytes, leading to an inversion of the T4/T8 ratio.

We have not observed direct release of virus by fresh, unstimulated lymphocytes from patients. Only cells first activated by mitogens (lectins) or alloantigens were found to release virus. If we extrapolate from the *in vitro* situation to the *in vivo* situation, this would imply that only activated T4 lymphocytes will express or be infected by the virus. Pictures of virions resembling to LAV were observed in sections of lymph nodes of patients with lymphadenopathy syndrome (T. Warner, personal communication).

Is the virus tropism restricted to T4 lymphocytes ?

Virus production was not observed in short term cultures of macrophages, B-lymphocytes, monocytes from normal donors (upon *in vitro* infection) or from an healthy virus carrier. However, we found recently that the LAV1 strain, after being propagated *in vitro* for several passages, was able to grow on a lymphoblastoid B cell line (FR8), obtained by *in vitro* transformation with Epstein-Barr virus of the B lymphocytes of a healthy donor. Some, but not all, of the lymphoblastoid lines established from others donors or from umbilical cord lymphocytes, were also susceptible to viral infection. The virus produced by the FR8 line was also able to infect a Burkitt lymphoma cell line, BJAB. This line does not contain the EBV genome, but can be supertransformed *in vitro* by EBV. The EBV/BJAB line (BJAB/B95-8) was found to be more susceptible to LAV infection, in having a higher virus yield (10).

All the LAV infected B cell lines could produce the retrovirus in a continuous way, without apparent damage for the cells. A subclone of the BJAB/B95 line, clone 32, was a particularly good virus producer, suitable for mass virus production.

The significance of the tropism of LAV for cells of the B lineage in the pathogeny of AIDS remains to be determined. It is possible that the general B cell activation observed in AIDS patients be a consequence of LAV infection of B cells, or of an interaction with infection by some DNA viruses, such as EBV, CMV or HBV.

2.3. Sero-epidemiological studies

The search for antibodies against LAV antigens has been carried out with the help of two different techniques : RIPA and ELISA. For the radioimmunoprecipitation assay (RIPA), virus (LAV1, isolates 2, 3 or 4) was metabolically labelled with ^{35}S-methionine. Under these conditions, the main viral protein labelled is the p25 ; p18 and p12 are not apparent, presumably because of their low content in methionine.

Complexes of p25 and antibodies are then bound to Protein A-Sepharose beads and after extensive washing analysed in polyacrylamide gel electrophoresis. The test allows clear distinction between unspecific binding of IgG or others serum proteins to cellular proteins accompanying the unpurified virus, and antibody directed to the viral p25.

In the ELISA, plates were coated with gradient-purified whole virus disrupted with detergents and presumably antibodies directed against any viral protein could be detected. In order to take into account unspecific binding by serum proteins, a control adsorption on a cytoplasmic lysate of uninfected lymphocytes was carried out for each serum (11) (14).

Results obtained with both techniques were remarkably similar, suggesting that the main viral antigen was the p25, and not the envelope protein(s). A few sera which were positive in ELISA and negative by RIPA seem to be directed against the p18 core protein.

The main results of these studies, which have been conducted in collaboration with several groups of clinicians in France, Europe and U.S.A. are the following :
Prevalence of antibodies against LAV in all the groups of patients with AIDS or LAS.

Table 2. Antibodies to Lymphadenopathy Associated Virus (LAV) in Zairian patients

	RIPA	ELISA
AIDS	34/36 (94 %)	32/36 (89 %)
CONTROL PATIENTS (infectious and non infectious diseases)	6/26 (23 %)	5/26 (19 %)
CONTROL POPULATION		
1981	ND	5/100 (5 %)
1983	ND	7/100 (7 %)

As Table 2. indicates, this prevalence was very high (94 % by RIPA, 89 % by ELISA) in a group of Zairian patients with AIDS, diagnosed by an international team in Kinshasa, in the fall 1983 (12). It was lower (40-80 % by our ELISA) in French and American patients (11) (13). The lack of antibodies in some advanced cases of AIDS may be secondary to immunological dysfunction of the B cell system. Indeed a progressive drop and even a loss of antibodies was observed in some AIDS patients (9) (11) during progression of the disease.

Alternatively, the tests used may have been not sensitive enough to pick up low titered antibodies, especially those against envelope proteins.

With regard to healthy subjects, belonging to groups at risk of AIDS, a lower, but significant number was also found to be positive : homosexuals with multiple partners, hemophiliacs.

In the latter case, a correlation was found with the way of treatment by antihemophilic factors : the highest percentage of LAV positiveness was found in a group of hemophiliacs intensively treated with commercial preparations of factor VIII , the lowest in a group of Belgian hemophiliacs only treated with local preparations (17). This result clearly suggests a transmission of the virus via preparations of factor VIII made from large pools of donors.

By contrast, the general population was found to be LAV negative : only one case out of 330 French subjects (Blood donors, laboratory workers, prisoneers) was found to be positive by ELISA (it was negative by RIPA).

In Zaire, 5% of sera from healthy mothers taken in 1980 were positive by ELISA, a significantly higher percentage indicating that the virus underwent a broader diffusion in the general population than in Europe.

Preliminary studies indicate a lack of antibodies against LAV in cases of Mediterranean classical Kaposi Sarcoma and in cases of African Kaposi Sarcoma.

Taken all together, all these data are consistent with the involvement of LAV related viruses in AIDS and LAS.

A more direct argument may soon come from inoculation experiments into Primates, made in collaboration with several centers (TNO, Holland ; CDC, Atlanta ; NIH, Bethesda) : LAV can grow *in vitro* in Chimpanzee's activated lymphocytes. Moreover, it could induce an immunodepression syndrome in one chimpanzee (18). The chimpanzee displayed LAV seroconversion, and its blood transmitted into a second chimpanzee induced a similar seroconversion.

The availability of an animal model will allow to study more deeply the immunodepressive action of the virus and the role of co-factors.

We have surmised (14) that many antigenic stimuli could trigger LAV diffusion into the T4 lymphocyte population, since only activated lymphocytes can express the virus and be infected.

Finally, although many questions about the pathogenic role of this new type of retrovirus, its origin, its routes of transmission, remain to be answered, it is gratifying that within one and half year, the viral origin of a new epidemic was elucidated, thanks to an international effort.

Recently the NCI's group of R. Gallo and co-workers has isolated under the name of HTLVIII a group of retroviruses very similar to LAV viruses (19). Studies in progress indicate that the major core protein (p25 of LAV, p24 of HTLVIII) are the same. Possible minor differences due to the propagation of each type of virus in different permanent cell lines may exist, but the biological properties of the viruses and data on their association with AIDS are basically the same.

Others laboratories (D. Francis, this Volume; J. Levy, personal communication) have also isolated viruses similar to LAV in AIDS patients, thus confirming our earlier finding.

References

1. Poiesz BJ, Ruscetti FW, Gazdau AF, Bunn PA, Minna JD, Gallo RC: Detection and isolation of type C retrovirus particles from fresh and cultured lymphocytes of a patient with cutaneous T-cell lymphoma. Proc. Natl. Acad. Sci. USA (77):7415-7419,1980.
2. Yoshida M, Miyoshi I, Hinuma Y: Isolation and characterization of retrovirus (ATLV) from cell lines of human adult T-cell leukemia and its implication in the disease. Proc. Natl. Acad. Sci. USA (79):2031,1982.
3. Kalyanaraman VS, Sarngadharan MG, Robert Guroff M, Blayney D, Golde D, Gallo RC: A new subtype of human T-cell leukemia virus (HTLV-II) associated with a T-cell variant of Hairy cell leukemia. Science (218):571-573,1982.
4. Morgan DA, Ruscetti FW, Gallo RC: Selective *in vitro* growth of T-lymphocytes from normal human bone marrow. Science (193):1007-1008,1976.
5. Barré-Sinoussi F, Montagnier L, Lidereau R, Sisman J, Wood J, Chermann JC: Enhancement of retrovirus production by anti-interferon serum. Ann. Microbiol. (Inst. Pasteur) (130B):349-362,1979.
6. Barré-Sinoussi F, Chermann JC, Rey F, Nugeyre MT, Chamaret S, Gruest J, Dauguet C, Axler-Blin C, Vézinet-Brun F, Rouzioux C, Rozenbaum W, Montagnier L: Isolation of a T-lymphotropic retrovirus from a patient at risk for acquired immune deficiency syndrome (AIDS). Science (220): 868-871,1983.

7. Kalyanaraman VS, Cabradilla CD, Getchell JP, Narayanan R, Braff EH, Chermann JC, Barré-Sinoussi F, Montagnier L, Spira TJ, Kaplan J, Fishbein D, Jaffe HW, Curran, JW, Francis DP: Antibodies to the core protein of Lymphadenopathy Associated Virus (LAV) in patients with AIDS. Science (225):321-323,1984.
8. Montagnier L, Dauguet C, Axler C, Chamaret S, Gruest J, Nugeyre MT, Rey F, Barré-Sinoussi F, Chermann JC: A new type of retrovirus isolated from patients presenting with lymphadenopathy and acquired immune deficiency syndromes : structural and antigenic relatedness with Equine Infectious Anemia Virus. Ann. Virol. (Inst. Pasteur) (135E):119-134, 1984.
9. Vilmer E, Rouzioux C, Brun-Vézinet F, Fischer A, Chermann JC, Barré-Sinoussi F, Gazengel C, Dauguet C, Manigne P, Griscelli C, Montagnier L: Isolation of a new lymphotropic retrovirus from two siblings with haemophilia B, one with AIDS. Lancet i:753-757,1984.
10. Montagnier L, Gruest J, Chamaret S, Dauguet C, Axler C, Guetard D, Nugeyre MT, Barré-Sinoussi F, Chermann JC, Brunet JB, Klatzmann D, Gluckman JC: Adaptation of the Lymphadenopathy Associated Retrovirus (LAV) to replication in EBV-transformed B lymphoblastoid cell lines. Science (225):63-66,1984.
11. Brun-Vézinet F, Barré-Sinoussi F, Saimot AG, Montagnier L, Rouzioux C, Klatzmann D, Rozenbaum W, Chermann JC: Detection of IgG antibodies to Lymphadenopathy Associated Virus (LAV) by ELISA, in patients with acquired immunodeficiency syndrome or lymphadenopathy syndrome. Lancet i:1253-1256, 1984.
12. Brun-Vézinet F, Rouzioux C, Chamaret S, Gruest J, Barré-Sinoussi F, Géroldi D, Chermann JC, Piot P, Taelman H, Bridts C, Stevens W, McCormick JB, Mitchell S, Kapita Bela, Odio Wobin, Mbendi, Mazebo P, Kayembe NN, Desmyter J, Feinsod FM, Quinn TC, Montagnier L: Prevalence of antibodies to lymphadenopathy associated retrovirus in African patients with acquired immune deficiency syndrome. Science, in press.
13. Unpublished results.
14. Montagnier L, Chermann JC, Barré-Sinoussi F, Chamaret S, Gruest J, Nugeyre MT, Rey F, Dauguet C, Axler-Blin C, Vézinet-Brun F, Rouzioux C, Saimot AG, Rozenbaum W, Gluckman JC, Klatzmann D, Vilmer E, Griscelli C, Gazengel C, Brunet JB: A new human T-lymphotropic retrovirus : characterization and possible role in lymphadenopathy and acquired immune deficiency syndromes. *In*: Gallo RC, Essex ME, Gross L (eds) "Human T cell leukemia lymphoma viruses". Cold Spring Harbor Laboratory New York, 1984, pp. 363-379.
15. Montagnier L, Barré-Sinoussi F, Chermann JC: Possible role of a new type of human T lymphotropic virus in the pathogeny of AIDS and related syndromes. Griscelli C, Vossen J (eds) "Proceedings of the Meeting of the European Group for Immunodeficiences, Chateau de Fillerval, France, Elsevier Science Publishers BV., 1984, pp. 367-372.

16. Klatzmann D, Barré-Sinoussi F, Nugeyre MT, Dauguet C, Vilmer E, Griscelli C, Brun-Vézinet F, Rouzioux C, Gluckman JC, Chermann JC, Montagnier L: Selective tropism of Lymphadenopathy Associated Virus (LAV) for Helper-Inducer T-lymphocytes. Science (225):59-63,1984.
17. Rouzioux C, Brun-Vézinet F, Courouce AM, Gazengel C, Vergoz D, Desmyter J, Vermylen J, Klatzmann D, Géroldi D, Barreau C, Barré Sinoussi F, Chermann JC, Christol D, Montagnier L: IgG antibodies to Lymphadenopathy Associated Virus (LAV) in differently treated French and Belgian haemophiliacs. Submitted.
18. Gajdusek DC, Amyx HL, Gibbs Jr. CJ, Asher DM, Yanagihara RT, Rodgers-Johnson P, Brown PW, Sarin PS, Gallo RC, Maluish A, Arthur LO, Gilden RV, Montagnier L, Chermann JC, Barré-Sinoussi F, Mildvan D, Mathur U, Leavitt R. Transmission experiments with human T-lymphotropic retroviruses and human AIDS tissue. Lancet i:1415-1416,1984.
19. Popovic M, Sarngadharan MG, Read E, Gallo RC: Detection, isolation, and continuous production of cytopathic retroviruses (HTLV-III) from patients with AIDS and Pre-AIDS. Science (224):497-500,1984.

19a. Gallo RC, Salahuddin SZ, Popovic M, Shearer GM, Kaplan M, Haynes BF, Palker TJ, Redfield R, Oleske J, Safai B, White G, Foster P, Markham PD: Frequent detection and isolation of cytopathic retroviruses (HTLV-III) from patients with AIDS and at risk for AIDS. Science (224): 500-503,1984.

19b. Schüpbach J, Popovic M, Gilden RV, Gonda MA, Sarngadharan MG, Gallo RC: Serological analysis of a subgroup of human T-lymphotropic retroviruses (HTLV-III) associated with AIDS. Science (224):503-505,1984.

19c. Sarngadharan MG, Popovic M, Bruch L, Schüpbach J, Gallo RC: Antibodies reactive with human T-lymphotropic retroviruses (HTLV-III) in the serum of patients with AIDS. Science (224):506-508,1984.

17

BIOLOGY OF HUMAN T CELL LEUKEMIA VIRUSES IN IMMUNOSUPPRESSION AND AIDS

M. Essex

Department of Microbiology, Harvard School of Public Health, Boston, Massachusetts

1. INTRODUCTION

The concept that retroviruses could induce immunosuppression following natural infections was first appreciated with respect to the feline leukemia viruses (FeLV's). While it was clearly established that FeLV's could cause leukemia or lymphoma following infection by the late 1960's (1), it was in the early to mid 1970's before the same agents were fully appreciated for their potential in causing disease and death due to immunosuppression (2,3). Now, it is generally accepted that the FeLV's cause substantially more deaths in cats by causing immunosuppression than by causing leukemia.

The first hint that FeLV's could be immunosuppressive came when thymic atrophy was observed in cats inoculated with the virus (4). Subsequently, FeLV-inoculated cats were shown to have delayed homograft responses (2). Despite these observations, few if any researchers realized that field strains of FeLV might cause immunosuppression as a frequent outcome of natural infection until about 1975, when studies with clusters of FeLV-infected cats were undertaken (3). It was soon apparent that the major cause of death in households of infected cats was not leukemia, but a variety of bacterial, protozoan, and viral infections ranging from peritonitis to pneumonias and septicemias (5,6). Additionally, animals viremic with FeLV were found to have a relative state of lymphopenia (3), inadequate lymphocyte mitogen stimulation responses (7), abnormal lymphoid cell membrane capping (8), and impaired primary and secondary humoral antibody responses to independent antigens (9).

Very recently, we also observed that colonies of monkeys, where outbreaks of leukemia and lymphoproliferative diseases had been observed, were also infected with a primate retrovirus that was serologically similar to the human T cell leukemia virus (HTLV) (10). The highest rates of infection of macaque monkeys with HTLV appeared in animals with lymphoid diseases, and the lymphoid diseases themselves were associated with outbreaks of AIDS (11). This not only supported the general concept that retroviruses could be associated with outbreaks of immunodeficiency, but also indicated that members of the HTLV family should also be seriously considered as potential immunosuppressants in man. With this background, it became appropriate not only to study members of the HTLV family in relation to the etiology of the newly described disease syndrome, AIDS, but also in relation to situations of infection that occurred apart from AIDS. In the latter category, for example, we could include the cases of various infectious diseases other than AIDS that occurred at elevated rates in HTLV antibody-positive individuals in endemic regions of southwestern Japan as opposed to antibody-negative individuals from the same regions (12).

2. TRANSMISSION AND DISTRIBUTION OF HTLV'S

Although the first isolation of HTLV by Gallo and his colleagues was from a United States citizen with a malignant variant of mycosis fungoides (13), it soon became clear that isolations of this class of agent, subsequently called HTLV-I, were rare in most of North America and Europe. Conversely, the virus could be found in a much greater proportion of individuals with tumors of lymphoid origin that came from such areas as southwestern Japan and the Caribbean basin (14-16). However, the class of leukemia that was associated with the virus, designated adult T cell leukemia in Japan (17) and lymphosarcoma cell leukemia in the Caribbean (18) also occurred at elevated rates where up to 5-25% of the healthy adult population had evidence of prior exposure to the virus.

In a population of about 700 adults we studied in Miyazaki, Japan, for example, 16% of the healthy adults had evidence of infection with HTLV, as did about 42% of the patients with infectious diseases, and 100% of the patients with adult T cell leukemia/lymphoma (12). Other studies indicated that HTLV-I infections occurred in a similar manner in such places as northern South America, various regions of Africa, the southeastern U.S., and Alaska (19). Since only limited studies have been conducted to date in the context of world-wide geographical screening, it seems likely that this virus will be found to be much more widely distributed than was initially envisioned.

A second type of HTLV, designated type II, was isolated from a case of hairy cell leukemia that originated in the western U.S. (20). Since then, several more isolations of HTLV-II have been made, but it is not clear that they have been regularly associated with any particular disease syndrome. Although the HTLV-I and II agents have substantial cross-reactivity by most serological procedures and by nucleic acid hybridization (19), antibodies to the two can be distinguished on the basis of neutralization of HTLV pseudotypes of vesicular stomatitis virus or by blocking of syncitial cell formation (21). The significance and role of HTLV-II in inducing disease has yet to be understood. However, variants that do not appear to completely fit the HTLV-I or II criteria have already been isolated from other types of leukemia in the Gallo laboratory (19), and a new type or class of HTLV has been etiologically linked to AIDS (22-25; see below).

The mechanisms by which HTLV's are transmitted have not yet been established. While it seems almost certain that these agents are transmitted by blood transmission, by sexual intercourse (at least from the male partner), and by mothers to their infant children (26-28), these routes would still seem to be insufficient to account for the unusual geographical limitations, as well as the unusual rise seen late in life. On the Japanese island of Kyushu, for example, from 10 to 30% of the adults in any given city appear to be infected, yet only 1-2% or less of the people are infected in cities only a few miles to the north. Also, the rate of infection continues to increase with age in adulthood, even after the decades of peak sexual activity (12). This suggests that another major mechanism would appear to be involved in virus transmission. Although a blood-sucking arthropod vector might appear to be the most logical missing link, no concrete evidence to support this has yet been produced.

HTLV-I, which has been studied most thoroughly, apparently exists as a persistent latent infection in all individuals that become exposed. Viremia does not occur, and the infection is presumably maintained by the presence of provirus in a limited number of helper T lymphocytes or their precursors. Transmission is inefficient, at least *in vitro*, in the absence of cell-associated virus (29).

3. IMMUNOGENICITY OF HTLV PROTEINS

The genome of HTLV, like other retroviruses, contains *gag*, *pol*, and *env* genes, plus long terminal repeat (LTR) regulatory sequences at both the 5' and 3' ends of the genome (19,30). A major difference from the viruses of lower animals, such as chickens, mice, and cats, is the presence of about 1600 nucleotides between the end of *env* gene and the 3' LTR. Although not fully understood, this "X" region (30) contains a conserved long open reading frame (LOR) on the 3' side (31) that we believe encodes, at least in part, a protein designated p42 that may be involved in the immortalization-transformation process (32).

To attempt to understand the distribution and spread of HTLV's in relation to both leukemia and immunosuppression, including AIDS, we examined the serum of various populations using two general approaches. The first, indirect membrane immunofluorescence, was used as a broad screening approach to determine if group-reactive antibodies were present and directed to any of the major HTLV proteins (12,33). Secondly, to determine which of the virus proteins were the major targets for the antibodies detected, radioimmunoprecipitation (RIP) was conducted using metabolically labelled cells, and subsequently the reactive molecules were analyzed using sodium dodecyl sulfate polyacrylamide gel electrophoresis (SDS-PAGE) and other procedures (12,34,35).

These approaches revealed that essentially all of the ATL cases and 16% of the healthy adults in Miyazaki, Japan had antibodies to membrane antigens of HTLV-infected cells (HTLV-MA) that were not present on uninfected cells. When the anti-HTLV-MA positive serum samples were examined by RIP/SDS-PAGE, varying proportions showed reactivity for the major *gag*-encoded proteins, p24 and p19. Some also had antibodies to a 42 kilodalton (kd) HTLV-specific protein (p42) that was then of unknown coding origin, and essentially all had antibodies to two proteins of 45-50 kd and 61-67 kd, when cells infected with HTLV-I were examined (32-35). In subsequent studies we determined that p42 was also present in cells such as *C81-66-45* that were transformed with HTLV, but lacking other *gag* or *env*-gene encoded proteins. Using radiolabel amino acid sequence analysis of cyanogen bromide fragments we then showed that at least the major portion of p42 was encoded by the *LOR* gene (31) in the "X" region of the viral genome (32).

The major antigens that react with antibodies in people exposed to HTLV, were, however, the 45 kd and 61 kd species, subsequently called gp45 and gp61 because they were found to be glycosylated using a variety of approaches (33). Using lactoperoxidase ^{125}I cell surface labelling, the same gp61 protein was found to be the major HTLV-specific cell surface antigen detected when sera from virus exposed people were tested. This strongly suggests that the gp61 and/or gp45 class of molecules were the species present in HTLV-MA as detected by membrane immunofluorescence (33).

When the gp61 antigen was obtained devoid of the carbohydrate moiety (i.e. by production in the presence of tunicamycin or deglycosylation with endoglycosidase treatment) it still reacted quite efficiently with human antibodies.

This not only established the specificity of the antibodies for the protein rather than the carbohydrate portion of the molecule, it also indicates that the antibodies react with a portion of the molecule that is not dependent on a tertiary structure regulated by the presence of carbohydrates. The gp45 and gp61 were both shown to be encoded by the env gene (33,35). With radiolabelling of selected amino acids combined with a comparison of the predicted amino acid positions based on the primary nucleotide structure, it was established that both gp45 and gp61 had the same amino terminus. Additionally, we showed that gp61 differed from gp45 only in that the former was a polyprotein precursor that contained the transmembrane protein at the carboxy terminus.

Similar studies were also done with analagous proteins of HTLV-II infected MO cells (35). These studies revealed that the env gene products of HTLV-II were a gp67 polyprotein and a gp52 amino terminus protein. Of particular interest, a high degree of cross-reactivity was observed between the HTLV-II env molecules and the comparable HTLV-I proteins. The cross-reactivities were observed regularly with human serum samples from HTLV-infected people, suggesting that the HTLV-MA antigens and/or the env gene proteins were highly immunogenic and particularly appropriate for screening sera from humans that might have been exposed to different strains or types of HTLV's. The latter issue was of particular importance for screening AIDS patients and individuals at risk for developing AIDS, since an HTLV-type agent seemed to be a logical candidate for consideration in the etiology of this disease (36).

4. HTLV AND AIDS

A virus of the HTLV class seemed to be a logical candidate to consider in the etiology of AIDS for several reasons. First, all members of this class have an almost unique tropism for T helper cells; the same cell that is diseased in AIDS patients (29). Second, HTLV's are thought to be transmitted by essentially the same mechanisms that appear to be involved with the AIDS disease: sexual intercourse with preferential transmission from males, transmission by blood, and transmission from the mother to neonates (26-28). Third, those areas where AIDS is believed to have been first observed, such as Haiti and/or Central Africa, are also regions where HTLV agents appear to be endemic (19). This obviously could increase the likelihood that a mutant variant of HTLV that would cause the new syndrome of AIDS might arise in those regions. Fourth, existing strains of HTLV appeared to be involved with an increased sensitivity to selected infectious diseases (12) as well as a reduction in the number of circulating T helper cells (37). Finally, it is clear that another naturally occurring T-lymphotropic retrovirus causes a similar pattern of leukemia development and immunosuppression in cats, and leukemia development and "AIDS" outbreaks in monkeys have also been associated with retroviruses, including at least one retrovirus that is serologically related to HTLV (10).

With such considerations in mind, we used membrane immunofluorescence and radioimmunoprecipitation/SDS PAGE analysis to examine sera from AIDS patients and related "high-risk" groups for evidence of antibodies to HTLV-MA. In our initial analysis, which was limited to cases of AIDS and the AIDS-related complex (ARC) in homosexual men, we found that one-third of the AIDS cases had antibodies to HTLV-MA expressed on Hut-102 cells, which are infected with HTLV-I (38). Such antibodies were only found in 1% of the matched healthy homosexual controls, but were found in much higher proportions of homosexuals that had contact with AIDS patients and in ARC patients (38,39). However, the prevalence rate of HTLV antibodies observed in AIDS patients was distinctly different from that seen for 15-20 other infectious agents tested. For other agents, such as cytomegalovirus or hepatitis B virus, the presence of antibodies was essentially the same in both AIDS cases and matched homosexual controls.

For several reasons, however, it appeared that the HTLV antibodies observed in the AIDS patients were not induced by conventional strains of HTLV-I, but rather by a variant strain of the virus (39). This was predicted primarily because the disease itself was new, whereas the conventional strains of HTLV-I were believed to have been present in such regions as southwestern Japan and the Caribbean basin long before the occurrence of AIDS. Also, the proportion of antibody positive patients ranged from 25-75%, depending on the stage of disease and the number of different samples examined from different patients (38,39). This seemed most logical to explain on the basis of partial cross-reactivity, with the presence of sufficiently high titers of cross-reactive antibodies in only a portion of the patients.

Similar studies with different classes of AIDS patients, including infants, intravenous drug abusers, hemophiliacs, Haitians, blood transfusion-associated cases (TA-AIDS), and European cases, all yielded similar results (39-42). Additionally, pools of blood donors that donated to TA-AIDS cases usually contained one but only one anti-HTLV-MA positive donor: the individual that presumably represented the source of the agent (40).

Very recently, a variant strain of HTLV was isolated by Gallo and colleagues that, although in the HTLV family, was more cytopathic for T helper cells than previously isolated conventional strains (22-25). Although not yet established, many believe that this agent, designated HTLV-III, is the same as the lymphadenopathy-associated virus (LAV) described at the Pasteur Institute (43).

In studies recently conducted in our laboratory using the HTLV-III reference source as viral antigen, we confirmed and extended observations in the Gallo laboratory concerning the prevalence rates of anti-HTLV-III antibodies in AIDS patients and related high risk groups (44,46). Using membrane immunofluorescence and radioimmunoprecipitation we determined that 95-100% of the AIDS patients and about 90% of the ARC patients had antibodies to HTLV-III antigens (44,46). While antibodies were not found in healthy laboratory workers, 30-40% of the healthy male homosexuals had such antibodies.

These results are summarized in Table I.

We also examined serum from asymptomatic hemophiliacs using the same procedures. In those studies, 30 of 47 had antibodies to HTLV-III (45), and there was complete agreement between the presence of antibodies by membrane immunofluorescence and the presence of antibodies to the HTLV glycoproteins. While these results obviously raise concern about the likelihood of widespread exposure of hemophiliacs to HTLV-III via blood products, the possibility that many of the antibody positive hemophiliacs were exposed only to inactivated viral antigens rather than live virus must be considered.

The HTLV-III specific proteins that are most immunogenic in exposed people are the glycoproteins gp42, gp120 and gp160 (44-46). Other HTLV proteins we observed to be reactive with antibodies found in people include non-glycosylated proteins of 55kd, 24kd, and 17kd. The 24kd protein, which has been used most extensively in radioimmunoassay and ELISA procedures, only appears to induce antibodies in about half of the AIDS/ARC patients while the glycoproteins appear to induce antibodies in about 95%. While the glycoproteins appear to be a more important source of antigen for efficient diagnostic tests for blood screening in the future, the concentration and purification of these proteins in usable amounts from virus grown in culture is obviously difficult. While virus that is delicately concentrated and purified is more likely to contain significant amounts of virus glycoproteins, it is also likely to contain non-specific cellular debris. Conversely, highly purified virus is likely to be rich only in p24, the protein that is only immunogenic in about half of the exposed patients. Also procedures such as western blotting and radioimmunoprecipitation are clearly able to detect antibodies to virus glycoproteins without virus purification, these techniques are not easily adaptable for broad-scale testing of large numbers of samples. This suggests that the most efficacious procedures for broad-scale testing in the long run will probably result from <u>env</u> gene proteins produced by recombinant DNA technology.

Table 1. Prevalence of antibodies to HTLV-III.

Category	Membrane Immunofluorescence	Radioimmunoprecipitations/SDS-PAGE p24	gp*
AIDS	51 (98)[+]	33 (42)	33 (97)
ARC	61 (89)	30 (61)	30 (93)
Healthy homosexuals	75 (37)	24 (25)	24 (33)
Laboratory workers	35 (0)	29 (0)	29 (0)

* Virus glycoproteins gp42, gp120, gp160.
\+ Number tested and percent positive.

5. SUMMARY AND CONCLUSIONS

Retroviruses of higher mammals cause both leukemias and immunosuppression. This has been most thoroughly documented for FeLV, which causes more cases of death in cats by immunosuppression than by leukemia induction. The HTLV's represented a logical group of viruses for containing an AIDS-inducing variant because these agents are particularly trophic for T helper cells, they are transmitted by the same general mechanisms that appeared compatible with the epidemiology of AIDS, and they are associated with increased risk for development of various infectious diseases. The most immunogenic proteins of HTLV are those encoded by the <u>env</u> gene, such as gp61 and gp45 for HTLV-I and gp67 and gp52 for HTLV-II. The latter proteins are also highly cross-reactive in that sera from AIDS patients infected with HTLV-III also react with HTLV type I and/or II glycoproteins when present in high titer. A new protein designated p42 is associated with immortalization in the case of HTLV-I and at least partially encoded by the <u>LOR</u> gene in the "X" region of the virus. Antibodies to HTLV-III can be detected in 90-100% of the patients with AIDS and ARC, and in 30-40% of healthy homosexuals. AIDS and ARC patients recognize the virus glycoproteins as the most immunogenic species, while the major core protein, p24, is significantly less immunogenic in people naturally exposed to HTLV-III.

REFERENCES

1. Jarrett WFH: Feline leukemia. Int Rev Exp Pathol (10): 243-263, 1973.
2. Perryman LE, Hoover EA, Yohn DS: Immunological reactivity of the cat: immunosuppression in experimental feline leukemia. J Natl Cancer Inst (49): 1357-1363, 1972.
3. Essex M, Hardy WD Jr, Cotter SM, Jakowski RM, Sliski A: Naturally occurring persistent feline oncornavirus infections in the absence of disease. Infect Immun (11): 470-475, 1975.
4. Anderson LJ, Jarrett WFH, Jarrett O, Laird HM: Feline leukemia virus infection of kittens: Mortality associated with atrophy of the thymus and lymphoid depletion. J Natl Cancer Inst (47): 807-817, 1971.
5. Essex M: Horizontally and vertically transmitted oncornaviruses of cats. Advan Cancer Res (21): 175-248, 1975.
6. Hardy WD Jr, Hess PW, MacEwen EG, McClelland AJ, Zuckerman EE, Essex M, Cotter SM, Jarrett O: Biology of feline leukemia virus in the natural environment. Cancer Res (36): 582-588, 1976.
7. Mathes LE, Olson RG, Hebebrand LC, Hoover EA, Schaller JP: Abrogation of lymphocyte blastogenesis by a feline leukemia virus protein. Nature (274): 687-689, 1978.
8. Dunlap JE, Nichols WS, Hebebrand LC, Mathes LE, Olsen RG: Mobility of lymphocyte surface membrane conconavalin A receptors of normal and feline leukemia virus-infected viremic felines. Cancer Res (39): 956-959, 1979.
9. Trainin Z, Wernicke D, Essex M, Ungar-Waron H: Suppression of the humoral antibody response in natural retrovirus infections. Science (220): 858-859, 1983.
10. Homma T, Kanki PJ, King NW Jr, Hunt RD, O'Connell MJ, Letvin NL, Daniel MD, Desrosiers RC, Yang CS, Essex M: Lymphoma in macaques: association with exposure to virus of human T lymphotropic family. Science (225): 716-718, 1984.
11. Letvin NL, Eaton KA, Aldrich WR, Sehgal PK, Blake BJ, Schlossman SF, King NW, Hunt RD: Acquired immunodeficiency syndrome in a colony of macaque monkeys. Proc Natl Acad Sci (80): 2718-2722, 1983.
12. Essex M, McLane MF, Tachibana N, Francis DP, Lee TH: Seroepidemiology of HTLV in relation to immunosuppression and the acquired immunodeficiency syndrome. In: Gallo RC, Essex M, Gross L (eds) Human T cell leukemia viruses. Cold Spring Harbor Laboratory, New York, 1984, pp 355-362.
13. Poiesz BJ, Ruscetti FW, Gazdar AF, Bunn PA, Minna JD, Gallo RC: Detection and isolation of type C retrovirus particles from fresh and cultured lymphocytes of a patient with cutaneous T cell lymphoma. Proc Natl Acad Sci (77): 7415-7419, 1980.

14. Robert-Guroff M, Nakao Y, Notake K, Ito Y, Sliski A, Gallo RC: Natural antibodies to human retrovirus HTLV in a cluster of Japanese patients with adult T cell leukemia. Science (215): 975-978, 1982.
15. Blattner WA, Kalyanaraman VS, Robert-Guroff M, Lister A, Galton DAG, Sarin PS, Crawford MH, Catovsky D, Greaves M, Gallo RC: The human type C retrovirus, HTLV, in blacks from the Caribbean region, and relationship to adult T cell leukemia/lymphoma. Int J Cancer (30): 257-264, 1982.
16. Hinuma Y, Komoda H, Chosa T, Kondo T, Kohakura M, Takenaka T, Kikuchi M, Ichimaru M, Yunoki K, Sato M, Matsuo R, Takuichi Y, Uchino H, Hanaoka M: Antibodies to adult T cell leukemia virus associated antigen (ATLA) in sera from patients with ATL and controls in Japan: a nation-wide sero-epidemiologic study. Int J Cancer (29): 631-635, 1982.
17. Uchiyama T, Yodoi J, Sagawa K, Takatsuki K, Uchino H: Adult T cell leukemia: clinical and hematological features of 16 cases. Blood (50): 481-491, 1977.
18. Catovsky D, Greaves MF, Rose M, Galton DAG, Goolden AWG, McClusky DR, White JM, Lampert I, Bourikas G, Ireland R, Brownell AI, Bridges JM, Blattner WA, Gallo RC: Adult T cell lyphoma-leukemia in blacks from the West Indies. Lancet (1): 639-643, 1982.
19. Shaw GM, Broder S, Essex M, Gallo RC: Human T cell leukemia virus: its discovery and role in leukemogenesis and immunosuppression. Advan Intern Med (30): in press.
20. Kalyanaraman VS, Sarngadharan MG, Robert-Guroff M, Miyoshi I, Blayney D, Golde D, Gallo RC: A new subtype of human T cell leukemia virus (HTLV-II) associated with a T cell variant of hairy cell leukemia. Science (218): 571-573, 1982.
21. Clapham P, Nagy K, Weiss RA: Pseudotypes of human T cell leukemia virus types 1 and 2: neutralization by patients' sera. Proc Natl Acad Sci (81): 2886-2889.
22. Popovic M, Sarngadharan MG, Read E, Gallo RC: Detection, isolation, and continuous production of cytopathic retroviruses (HTLV-III) from patients with AIDS and pre-AIDS. Science (224): 497-500, 1984.
23. Gallo RC, Salahuddin SZ, Popovic M, Shearer GM, Kaplan M, Haynes BF, Palker TJ, Redfield R, Oleske J, Safai B, White G, Foster P, Markham PD: Frequent detection and isolation of cytopathic retroviruses (HTLV-III) from patients with AIDS and at risk for AIDS. Science (224): 500-503, 1984.
24. Schupbach J, Popovic M, Gilden RV, Gonda MA, Sarngadharan MG, Gallo RC: Serological analysis of a subgroup of human T lymphotropic retroviruses (HTLV-III) associated with AIDS. Science (224): 503-505, 1984.
25. Sarngadharan MG, Popovic M, Bruch L, Schupbach J, Gallo RC: Antibodies reactive with human T lymphotrophic retroviruses (HTLV-III) in the serum of patients with AIDS. Science (224): 506-508, 1984.
26. Miyoshi I, Fujishita M, Taguchi H, Ohtsuki Y, Akagi T, Morinoto YM, Nagasaki A: Caution against blood transfusion from donors seropositive to adult T cell

leukemia associated antigens. Lancet (1): 683, 1982.
27. Saxinger WC, Gallo RC: Possible risk to recipients of blood from donors carrying serum markers of human T cell leukemia virus. Lancet (1): 1074, 1982.
28. Hinuma Y: Association of a retrovirus (ATLV) with adult T-cell leukemia: review of serologic studies. Gann (28): 211-221, 1982.
29. Popovic M, Sarin PS, Robert-Guroff M, Kalyanaraman VS, Mann D, Minowada J, Gallo RC: Isolation and transmission of human retrovirus (human T cell leukemia virus). Science (219): 856-859, 1983.
30. Seiki M, Hattori S, Yoshida M: Human adult T cell leukemia virus: molecular cloning of the provirus DNA and the unique terminal structure. Proc Natl Acad Sci (79): 6899-6902, 1982.
31. Haseltine WA, Sodroski J, Patarca R, Briggs D, Perkins D, Wong-Staal F: Structure of the 3' terminal region of type II human T lymphotropic virus: evidence for new coding region. Science (225): 419-421, 1984.
32. Lee TH, Coligan JE, Sodroski JA, Haseltine WA, Wong-Staal F, Gallo RC, Essex M: Antigens encoded by the 3' terminal region of human T cell leukemia virus: evidence for a functional gene flanked by the _env_ gene and 3' LTR. Submitted for publication.
33. Lee TH, Coligan JE, Homma T, McLane MF, Tachibana N, Essex M: Human T cell leukemia virus associated membrane antigens (HTLV-MA): identity of the major antigens recognized following virus infection. Proc Natl Acad Sci (81): 3856-3860, 1984.
34. Lee TH, Homma T, Schultz KT, McLane MF, Tachibana N, Howe CWS, Essex M: Antigens expressed by human T cell leukemia virus transformed cells. In: Gallo RC, Essex M, Gross L (eds) Human T cell leukemia viruses. Cold Spring Harbor Laboratory, New York, 1984. pp 111-120.
35. Lee TH, Coligan JE, McLane MF, Sodroski JG, Popovic M, Wong-Staal F, Gallo RC, Haseltine W, Essex M: Serological cross-reactivity between envelope gene products of type I and type II human T cell leukemia virus. Proc Natl Acad Sci, in press.
36. Francis DP, Curran JW, Essex M: Epidemic acquired immune deficiency syndrome: epidemiological evidence for a transmissable agent. J Natl Cancer Inst (71): 1-4, 1983.
37. Evatt BL, Stein SF, Lawrence DN, McLane MF, McDougal JS, Lee TH, Spira TJ, Cabradilla C, Mullins JI, Francis DP, Essex M: Antibodies to human T cell leukemia virus associated membrane antigens (HTLV-MA) in hemophiliacs: evidence for infection prior to 1980. Lancet (2): 698-701, 1983.
38. Essex M, McLane MF, Lee TH, Falk L, Howe CWS, Mullins JI, Cabradilla C, Francis DP: Antibodies to cell membrane antigens associated with human T cell leukemia virus in patients with AIDS. Science (220): 859-862, 1983.
39. Essex M, McLane MF, Lee TH: Prevalence of antibodies to human T cell leukemia virus cell membrane antigens (HTLV-MA) in patients with AIDS. In: Gottlieb MS, Groopman JE (eds) Acquired immune deficiency syndrome,

UCLA Symp Molec Cell Biol (16): in press.

40. Jaffe HW, Francis DP, McLane MF, Cabradilla C, Curran JW, Kilbourne BW, Lawrence DN, Haverkos HW, Spira TJ, Dodd RY, Gold J, Armstrong D, Ley A, Groopman J, Mullins JI, Lee TH, Essex M: Transfusion-associated acquired immunodeficiency syndrome: serologic evidence of human T cell leukemia virus infection of donors. Science (223): 1309-1312, 1984.
41. Essex M, McLane MF, Lee TH, Tachibana N, Mullins JI, Kreiss J, Kasper CK, Poon MC, Landay A, Stein SF, Francis DP, Cabradilla C, Lawrence DN, Evatt BL: Antibodies to human T cell leukemia virus membrane antigens (HTLV-MA) in hemophiliacs. Science (221): 1061-1064, 1983.
42. Mathez D, Leibowitch J, Catalan P, Essex M, Zaguri D: HTLV and AIDS in France. Lancet (1): 799, 1984.
43. Barré-Sinoussi F, Chermann JC, Rey F, Nugeyre MT, Chamaret S, Gruest J, Dauguet C, Axler-Blin C, Vezinet-Brun F, Rouzioux C, Rozenbaum W, Montagnier L: Isolation of a T lymphotropic retrovirus from a patient at risk for acquired immune deficiency syndrome. Science (220): 868-871, 1983.
44. McLane MF, Hirsch M, Schooley R, Ho D, Barin F, Essex M: Prevalence of antibodies to HTLV-MA of type III HTLV in AIDS patients. Submitted for publication.
45. Kitchen L, Barin F, McLane MF, Sullivan JL, Brettler DB, Levine PH, Essex M: Antibodies to human T cell leukemia virus (type III) in asymptomatic hemophiliacs and hemophiliac AIDS cases. Submitted for publication.
46. Barin F, Lee TH, McLane MF, Groopman J, Essex M: Antigens of human T cell leukemia virus (type III) detected by antibodies in patients with AIDS. Submitted for publication.

18

Human Retrovirus in Acquired Immunodeficiency Syndrome (AIDS)

Donald P. Francis, Cirilo D. Cabradilla, Paul M. Feorino, and V.S. Kalyanaraman

Division of Viral Diseases, Center for Infectious Disease, Centers for Disease Control, Atlanta, Georgia 30333

In terms of suffering, acquired immunodeficiency syndrome (AIDS) ranks high among diseases which have spread misery around the world. With its slow but inexorable progression towards death, AIDS recruits various opportunistic organisms to produce some remarkably uncomfortable disease states. Whether from the air hunger of pneumocystis carinii or cytomegalovirus pneumonia, or from the cutaneous or oral discomfort of herpesvirus or candida albicans infection, or from the local or the generalized discomfort of cryptococcal meningitis or toxoplasma gondii meningoencephalitis, or from the lassitude resulting from the wasting and emaciation, patients with AIDS suffer. Unfortunately, the numbers of cases of AIDS continues to rise. Although, recently many have tried to find optimism in the "plateauing" of the AIDS epidemic, the reality is that, although the rate of increase is slightly less, the slope of the epidemic curve is still upward (Figure 1). Over 5000 cases of AIDS have been reported as of July 1, 1984 - unfortunately, half of these have been reported in the last 6 months.

A good sign, at least for the long run, is that progress has been made in identifying the causative agent. Historically this progress has followed a rather logical course, moving from one lead to the next. Fundamental in initiating this progress was the epidemiologic information which suggested that a transmissible agent was ultimately responsible. This information allowed some researchers to recognize the similarity between AIDS and other infectious agents. Most noteable among these was the epidemiologic similarity of AIDS and hepatitis B and the pathogenic similarity of AIDS and diseases caused by feline leukemia virus (1). The latter encouraged the pursuit of retroviruses as a cause

Figure 1

CASES OF ACQUIRED IMMUNODEFICIENCY SYNDROME (AIDS) BY QUARTER OF REPORT, SECOND QUARTER 1981 THROUGH JUNE 4, 1984, UNITED STATES

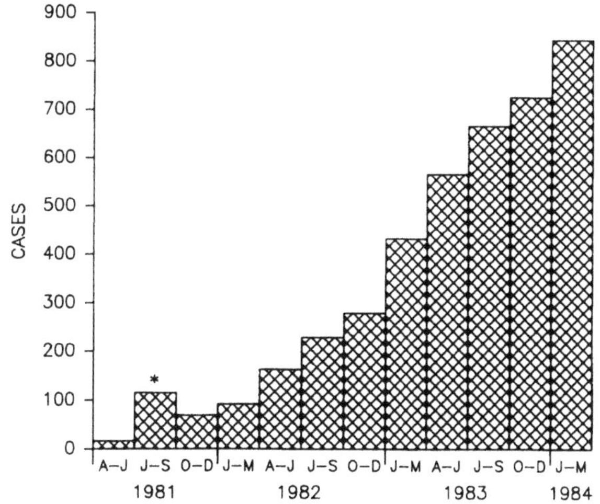

*Includes backlog of cases identified at beginning of CDC surveillance

of AIDS. Early in this pursuit, the application by Essex et al (2) of techniques used in feline leukemia research identified antibodies in AIDS patients which reacted to the cell membrane antigens of human T-cell leukemia virus-infected cells (HTLV-MA). The importance of finding markers of a retrovirus infection relatively early in the etiologic search should be stressed as it allowed limited resources to be applied to a specific etiologic area instead of to broad searches for multiple agents. Although antibodies to HTLV-MA were only found in about 30% of AIDS patients, they were almost never present in any groups not at risk of AIDS (2). Initially the significance of these antibodies was unknown, but their presence in blood donors suspected as being the source of infection in the transfusion AIDS setting (3) gave special credence to their importance. And later, their specificity as a marker of retrovirus infection was documented (4).

With the suspicion of possible retrovirus involvement, attempts were made to isolate the actual agent. Several laboratories set out to isolate retroviruses by applying techniques previously found useful for culture of HTLV, type 1 and HTLV, type 2 (5). However, the infrequent isolation of these viruses from AIDS patients and the lack of other serologic markers of infection, especially antibodies to the major core proteins of HTLV-1 (6), led to the conclusion that a variant of HTLV-1 may be involved. In this regard, a variant retrovirus, called lymphadenopathy-associated virus (LAV), isolated by Barre-Sinoussi and her colleagues at the Institut Pasteur in Paris (7) received increasing attention. The information on this virus, together with the recent important contributions of Gallo and his colleagues at the National Cancer Institute in Bethesda (8-11) who described additional isolates of a variant retrovirus called human T-cell lymphotropic virus, type-3 (HTLV-3), have led the way to the agent which is the presumed cause of AIDS. The comparison of the prototype viruses which have been isolated, LAV and HTLV-3, have not been completed, but preliminary experiments indicate that they are closely related, if not identical.

Assuming that LAV and HTLV-3 are the same virus, what is the evidence that this virus is the cause of AIDS? To answer this several different criteria required to establish the etiologic link between an agent and a disease needs to be addressed (12). These are: 1) Markers of infection should be found in all or almost all AIDS patients while such markers should be rare in control patients; 2) The prevalence and incidence of infection should be high in groups exposed to the infection and low in those not exposed; 3) Infection should occur before the onset of disease; 4) Experimental or natural infection should reproduce disease; and 5) The whole thing should make biologic sense. Portions of each of these criteria have already been met for LAV/HTLV-3:

Infection in AIDS patients. In other contributions to this volume, Dr. Gallo and Dr. Montagnier described their data showing a high proportion of AIDS patients with markers (both antibody and virus) of infection. We have developed antibody tests using prototype LAV (kindly provided by Dr. J-C Chermann) as the target antigen. Two tests have been developed. One an ELISA test using whole disrupted virus and the other a radioimmunoprecipitation test using purified p25, the major core protein. The ELISA test detects antibody in a high proportion of AIDS (78%) and lymphadenopathy syndrome (95%) patients while control blood donors are rarely (1.4%) positive. As we have observed a high rate of false positivity of AIDS serum against several antigens in ELISA testing (presumably because of the high concentrations of immune complexes in AIDS serum), we have begun dissecting the virion antigens for use in subunit-specific assays which, at least in our hands, have not been interfered with by AIDS serum. Our first subunit test developed uses the 24-25,000 MW core protein as the precipitation antigen in a radioimmunoprecipitation assay. Some AIDS patients apparently have decreasing titers of antibody to this antigen as their disease progresses (see below). Possibly as a result, a lower proportion of patients with frank AIDS have antibody (41%) than do patients with lymphadenopathy (88%) (13). No serum from over 300 control patients has reacted in this test.

Regarding the similarity of virus isolated from American AIDS patients to the prototype LAV isolated from a Frenchman, we have examined three isolates in some detail. Two of these were from homosexual men (one from the west coast and the other from the east coast) and one from a woman with transfusion-associated AIDS. By competitive radioimmunoassays, these three isolates were indistinguishable from the prototype LAV (Figure 2). HTLV-3 was not used in these experiments because it was not available at the time.

Prevalence of antibody in groups at risk of AIDS. All testing has not been completed, but from preliminary data it is clear that groups at risk for AIDS are going to have high prevalences of antibodies to LAV/HTLV-3. From our initial data it appears that the majority of Georgia hemophiliacs and New York intravenous drug users have antibody. In addition, we have examined the changing prevalence of antibody in homosexual men over time and have observed a remarkable increase. In collaboration with the San Francisco City/County Health Department we have collected serum from homosexual or bisexual men who have been attending the San Francisco City Clinic. In 1978 1 of 100 (1%) men were

HOMOLOGOUS COMPETITIVE RADIOIMMUNOASSAY COMPARING VARIOUS RETROVIRUS ISOLATES FROM AIDS PATIENTS WITH LAV, HTLV-I, AND HTLV-II

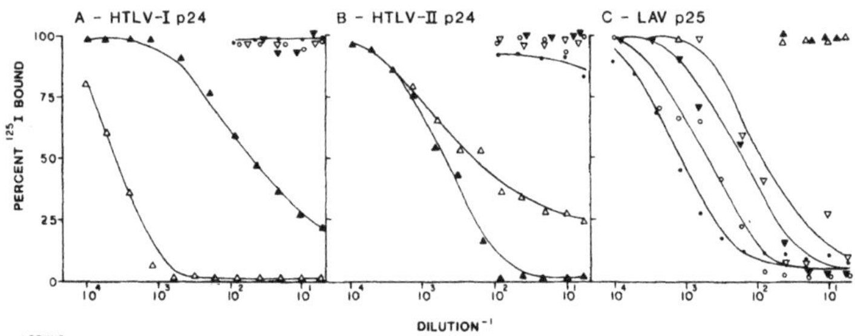

LEGEND:

•-• LAV; △-△ HTLV-I; ▲-▲ HTLV-II,
○-○ HOMOSEXUAL MAN (EAST COAST) WITH AIDS;
▼-▼ HOMOSEXUAL MAN (WEST COAST) WITH AIDS;
▽-▽ TRANSFUSION-ASSOCIATED AIDS CASE;

Figure 2

positive for antibody to LAV p25. This increased to 12 of 48 (25%) in 1980 and 140 of 215 (65%) in 1984.

Infection before onset of AIDS. Because of ongoing studies of hepatitis B in San Francisco, we have prospectively obtained serum specimens from homosexual men. Three AIDS patients whose serum was available were tested for antibody. Each of these three patients seroconverted from antibody negative to antibody positive prior to the onset of AIDS. Interestingly, all three showed different patterns of seroconversion (Figure 3). One patient had a transient positivity and then reverted to antibody negative, only to seroconvert again and remain positive after onset. Another patient seroconverted but over time steadily lost antibody titer until at the time of onset was negative by RIP. The third patient seroconverted prior to onset and remained positive (Figure 3).

Experimental infection. Several primate and non-primate animal species have been inoculated with AIDS patient material and, to date, none has been infected or developed disease. In the absence of an animal model, we have turned to natural transmission settings to

Figure 3

ANTIBODIES TO LAV p25 IN RELATION TO ONSET OF DISEASE, SAN FRANCISCO COHORT, 1978–MARCH 1984

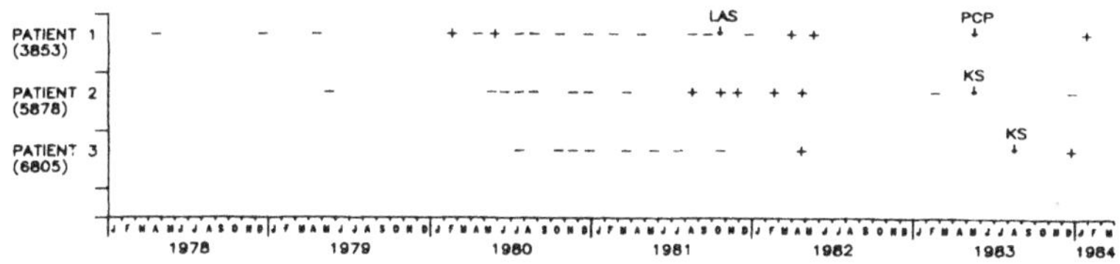

LEGEND:
KS=KAPOSI'S SARCOMA
LAS=LYMPHADENOPATHY SYNDROME
PCP=*PNEUMOCYSTIS CARINII* PNEUMONIA

determine if LAV/HTLV-3 could be isolated from epidemiologically-linked AIDS patients. We studied a blood donor/recipient pair both of whom developed AIDS. The donor was a homosexual man who developed AIDS a month after donating blood to a woman who required transfusions for uterine bleeding. She developed AIDS 13 months after receiving the transfusion. A retrovirus, immunologically indistinguishable from the prototype LAV, was isolated from peripheral lymphocytes of both the donor and the recipient (14).

Biologic sense. The etiologic association between LAV/HTLV-3 does make biologic sense. The major pathologic finding in AIDS is the dramatic decrease and dysfunction of the helper-inducer subset of T-cells. Similar to other human retroviruses, LAV/HTLV-3 is tropic for T- lymphocytes. Specifically, it preferentially replicates in the helper-inducer subset of T-cells (T4 cells). In contrast, however, to other human retroviruses which induce persistent infection in lymphocytes resulting in transformation, this virus is cytopathic for human T4 cells (9,15). Thus, this agent is attractive as the cause of AIDS, not only because of the epidemiologic evidence, but also because of its biologic properties.

In summary, the probable etiologic agent for AIDS has been found. The evidence for the etiologic link is strong, but considerable questions remain. First is the question of the similarity of LAV and

HTLV-3. From multiple aspects, they appear to be the same virus, but complete comparisons will be necessary to solidify the relationship. Next, further studies are necessary to fill in the gaps in our knowledge to complete the etiologic association. Also, a great deal needs to be uncovered regarding the natural history of this infection to determine why some patients develop severe disease and why some may not. Finally, the question of source of this virus remains to be determined. With the descriptions of AIDS in central Africa, one wonders if that is indeed the birth place of the virus. In addition, one wonders whether this is a new virus of humans or one that has existed for a long time.

References

1. Francis DP, Curran JW, Essex M: Epidemic acquired immune deficiency syndrome: epidemiologic evidence for a transmissible agent. J. Natl Cancer Inst (71):1-4, 1983.

2. Essex M, McLane MF, Lee TH, Falk L, Howe LWS, Mullins JI, Cabradilla C, Francis DP: Antibodies to cell membrane antigens associated with human T-cell leukemia virus in patients with AIDS. Science (220):859-62, 1983.

3. Jaffe HW, Francis DP, McLane MF, Cabradilla C, Curran JW, Kilbourne BW, Lawrence DN, Haverkos HW, Spira TJ, Dodd RY, Gold J, Armstrong D, Ley A, Groopman J, Mullins J, Lee TH, Essex M: Transfusion-associated AIDS: serologic evidence of human T-cell leukemia virus infection of donors. Science (223):1309-12, 1984.

4. Lee TH, Coligan JE, Homma T, McLane MF, Tachibana N, Essex M: Human T-cell leukemia virus-associated membrane antigens: identity of the major antigens recognized after virus infection. Prac Natl Acad Sci (81):3856-60, 1984.

5. Gallo RC, Sarin PS, Gelman EP, Robert-Guroff M, Richardson E, Kalyanaraman VS, Mann D, Sidhu GD, Stahl RE, Zolla-Pazner S, Leibowitch J, Popovic M: Isolation of human T-cell leukemia virus in acquired immune deficiency syndrome (AIDS). Science (220):865-7, 1983.

6. Robert-Guroff M, Schubach J, Blayney DW, Kalyanaraman VS, Merino F, Sarngaharan MG, Clark JW, Saxinger WC, Blattner WA, Gallo RC: Seroepidemiologic studies on human T-cell leukemia/lymphoma virus, type I. In: Human T-cell leukemia/lymphoma virus. Eds. Gallo RC, Essex ME, Gross L. Cold Spring Harbor Laboratory, Cold Spring Harbor, New York, 1984.

7. Barre-Sinoussi F, Chermann J-C, Rey F, Nugeyne MT, Chamaret S, Gruest J, Dauguet C, Axler-Blin C, Vizenet-Brun F, Rouzioux C, Rozenbaum W, Montagnier L: Isolation of a T-lymphotropic retrovirus from a patient at risk for acquired immune deficiency syndrome (AIDS). Science (220):868-71, 1983.

8. Popovic M, Sarngadharan MG, Read E, Gallo RC: Detection, isolation and continuous production of cytopathic retroviruses (HTLV-III) from patients with AIDS and pre-AIDS. Science (220):497-500, 1983.

9. Gallo RC, Salahuddin SZ, Popovic M, Shearer GM, Kaplan M, Haynes BF, Palker TJ, Redfield R, Oleske J, Safai B, Foster P, Markham PD: Frequent detection and isolation of cytopathic retroviruses (HTLV-III) from patients with AIDS and at risk for AIDS. Science (220):500-2, 1984.

10. Schupbach J, Popovic M, Gilden RV, Gond MA, Sarngadharan MG, Gallo RC: Serological analysis of a subgroup of human T-lymphotropic retroviruses (HTLV-III) associated with AIDS. Science (224):503-5, 1984.

11. Sarngadharan MG, Popovic M, Bruch L, Schupbach J, Gallo RC: Antibodies reactive to human T-lymphotropic retroviruses (HTLV-III) in the serum of patients with AIDS. Science (224):506-8, 1984.

12. Evans AS, Yale J: Causation and disease: The Henle-Koch postulates revisited. Yale J. Biology and Mod. (49):175-195, 1976.

13. Kalyanaraman VS, Cabradilla CD, Getchell JP, Narayanan R, Braff EH, Chermann J-C, Barre-Sinoussi F, Montagnier L, Spira TJ, Kaplan J, Fishbein D, Jaffe HW, Curran JW, Francis DP: Antibodies to the core protein of the human retrovirus LAV in patients with acquired immunodeficiency syndrome and lymphadenopathy syndrome. Science (225):321-4, 1984.

14. Feorino PM, Kalyanaraman VS, Haverkos HW, Cabradilla CD, Warfield DT, Jaffe HW, Harrison AK, Gottlieb MS, Goldfinger D, Chermann J-C, Barre-Sinoussi F, Spira TJ, McDougal JS, Curran JW, Montagnier L, Murphy FA, Francis DP: Lymphadenopathy- associated virus (LAV) infection of a blood donor-recipient pair with acquired immunodeficiency syndrome (AIDS). Science (225):69-72, 1984.

15. Montagnier L, Chermann J-C, Barre-Sinoussi F, Chamaret S, Gruest J, Nugeyre MT, Rey F, Dauguet C, Axler-Biln C, Brun FV, Rouzioux C, Saimot G-A, Rozenbaum W, Gluckman JC, Klatzmann D, Vilmer E, Griscelli C, Foyer-Gazengel C, Brunet JB: A new human T-lymphotropic retrovirus: characterization and possible role in acquired immune deficiency syndrome. In: Human T-cell leukemia/lymphoma virus. Eds. Gallo RC, Essex ME, Gross L. Cold Spring Harbor Laboratory, Cold Spring Harbor, New York, 1984.

19

HUMAN RNA AND DNA ONCOGENIC VIRUSES AND THEIR IMPORTANCE IN TRANSMISSIBLE AND MALIGNANT DISEASES

GUY DE THE

Faculty of Medicine Alexis Carrel, Lyon, France

INTRODUCTION

The papers in this volume reflect both the importance of RNA and DNA oncogenic agents in human malignancies, as well as the growing evidence for the importance of growth factors and reactivation of onc-genes in human oncogenesis. While there is a present belief that sequential activation of onc-genes may well represent the final common pathway in oncogenesis, the importance of environmental infectious agents such as viruses should not be underestimated, as they represent environmental factors which can be traced at the molecular level in the organism, thus helping to unravel the molecular mechanism of tumorigenesis and to develop new ways for controlling certain human tumors.

This volume focuses on human retroviruses, stressing their importance in malignant and non-malignant human diseases. Both animal and human retroviruses share cytolytic and transforming potentialities on specific target cells. When these cells are responsible for the cell mediated immune response, their destruction may have importance from the public health viewpoint, as they may induce lethal immunodeficiencies. Their oncogenic potential may then be of lesser importance with regard to mortality. This is, in fact, the case for some retroviruses in cats, cows and non-human primates. Oncogenic DNA and RNA viruses also merit comparative study to appreciate their similarities and differences and thus better assess the best approach to control the associated tumors.

I would like to present a comparative evaluation from an epidemiological viewpoint of the different human viruses with oncogenic properties. Then, I shall present some recent results from our laboratory concerning the sero-epidemiology of HTLV-1.

COMPARATIVE EPIDEMIOLOGICAL EVALUATION OF HUMAN VIRUSES WITH ONCOGENIC PROPERTIES

Table 1 gives some characteristics of both RNA and DNA human viruses associated with spontaneous tumors in man. It is interesting to note that both the HTLV and HBV are geographically restricted, integrated in the cellular DNA and do induce severe acute diseases such as immunodeficiencies for HTLV or acute and active chronic hepatitis for HBV, diseases which in fact are responsible for many more deaths than the associated malignancies. It is worth remembering at this point that the number of HBV carriers in the world is estimated to be around 200 million.

In contrast, both the herpes and papillomaviruses are ubiquitous viruses, their integration in the cellular genome does not seem to be an obvious and regular event and both induce mild diseases (infectious mononucleosis and papillomas, respectively), which are not responsible for major death in any part of the world.

The question as to whether such viruses with oncogenic potential may represent the necessary and sufficient factor for some specific tumors should be answered differently for both groups of viruses. For the retro and hepdnaviruses the need for a co-factor is not obvious, although for HBV, it is believed that the aflatoxines (present in the diet of high risk areas) does play a critical role. In contrast, for the herpes and papillomaviruses, the need for co-factors is more obvious because these viruses are ubiquitous while the associated tumors are geographically very restricted. For the African Burkitt's lymphoma, hyperendemic malaria appears to depress specifically cell mediated immunity controlling the growth of EBV infected B lymphocytes (Moss et al, 1983), thus favouring the chance event of chromosomal translocation and onc-gene activation (Klein, 1979; Klein and Lenoir, 1982). For nasopharyngeal carcinoma, there are certainly factors other than the EBV involved in the development of this tumor, but no environmental factors have been yet proven to be etiologically associated with NPC, although certain food habits or traditional medicines may play a role (de The, 1982). For papillomaviruses, co-factors are not yet known, although Zur Hausen (1982) has proposed that the herpes type 2 could play an initiating role in a multistep carcinogenesis of cervical mucosa.

SEROEPIDEMIOLOGY OF HTLV IN THE FRENCH WEST INDIES

We have carried out sero epidemiological studies in the French West Indies to try and characterize the natural history of human retroviruses. In doing so, we came across two interesting observations. The first refers to the prevalence of HTLV-1 infection in Martinique and French Guiana. By testing 261 blood donors in Martinique and 135 blood donors in French Guiana, we observed a higher prevalence of HTLV-1 in Martinique than in French Guiana (see Table 2). We also investigated hematopoietic diseases in these areas for more than 18 months and did not come across any typical AIDS case in Martinique between January 1983 and January 1984. This suggests that these islands are not infected with HTLV-3 but are endemic for HTLV-1. The mode of transmission and epidemiological characteristics of both subgroups of viruses appear different and should be studied comparatively.

The second observation worth mentioning here refers to the difference in HTLV-1 prevalence among different ethnic groups present in the French Guiana. Along the Maroni River, in the area of Maripasoula, we observed that the Wayana Indians were not infected by HTLV-1 whereas the Black Bonis living nearby, and having little or no exchange with the Indians, had a high level of HTLV-1 infection, with 10% of adults having high antibody titers (Gessain et al, 1984). As seen in Table 2, the Haitians living in Cayenne have an intermediate prevalence rate comparable to that of the Dominican prostitutes. The Hmong who came in the last few years from Kampuchea are also infected at the same level as the Haitians or the Dominican prostitutes and the question of the origin of their infection remains unsolved. Were they infected in their homeland or after their emigration in the Carribean region?

The natural history of the human retroviruses and the characterization of their epidemiological characteristics is a matter of importance for understanding the associated diseases and for trying to control them possibly through vaccination. Therefore, we would like to implement an HTLV African sero epidemiological survey with the aim of determining the geographical distribution of the different subgroups of the HTLV family, their age prevalence, possibly their mode of transmission and to get data on the associated diseases. Such a survey could help to assess the situation with regard to the importance of such viruses as cause of immuno-deficiencies causing severe infectious diseases due either to viruses, bacteria or parasites.

Table 1: HUMAN VIRUSES WITH ONCOGENIC PROPERTIES

	Retroviruses HTLV family	Hepdnaviruses Hepatitis B virus (HBV)	Herpesviruses Epstein-Barr virus (EBV)	Papillomaviruses Human papilloma viruses 11 and 16 (HPV 11 and 16)
genome	diploid RNA 10^6 mw with integrated DNA provirus	10^3 DNA oncogenic when integrated	10^8 DNA usually not integrated	10^3 DNA integrated in tumorous lesions
epidemiological characteristics	geographically restricted	geographically restricted	ubiquitous virus	ubiquitous virus
associated human diseases	. immuno-deficiencies . acute T cell leukemia/lymphoma . non Hodgkin B lymphoma ?	. acute hepatitis . active chronic hepatitis . liver cell ca. 260,000 new cases/year	. infectious mononucleosis . polyclonal B cell proliferation . B cell lymphoma (Burkitt) . nasopharyngeal ca. 80,000 new cases/year	. papillomas (skin and mucosae) . condilomas . genital cancers 460,000 new cases/year carcinoma of the cervix alone
need of co-factor	?	aflatoxine (diet)	. hyperendemic malaria . chromosomal translocations and oncgene activat. (for Burkitt's lymph) . environmental co-factors for NPC - diet ?	HSV-2 as a co-factor ?
control of these viral associated proliferations	HTLV vaccine in the future ?	first and second generation HBV vaccine available	. EBV vaccine in prepar. . early diagnosis by IgA test and radiotherapy can control NPC	HPV vaccine ? problem with 28 diffe-rent HPV

Table 2: HTLV-1 ELISA ANTIBODIES IN FRENCH WEST INDIES

	N sera tested	BIOTECH ELISA R 5~8 +	R 8.1~15 ++	% +/++	% ++
MARTINIQUE					
Blood Donors	261	3	8	4.2	3
FRENCH GUIANA					
Blood Donors	135	1	1	1,5	0,7
Dominic. Prost.	66	3	3	9	4.5
Maripasoula	196	8	18	13	9.2
. Wayana Ind.	57	2	0	3.5	0
. Black Bonis	97	3	10	13.4	10.3
Haitians (Cayenne)	88	2	3	5.7	3,4
Hmongs (Cacao)	57	3	2	8.8	3.5

REFERENCES

1. Moss, D.J., Chan, S.H., Burrows, S.R., Chew, T.S., Kane, R.G., Staples, J.R. and Kunaratnam, N.: Epstein-Barr virus specific T cell response in nasopharyngeal carcinoma patients. Int. J. Cancer (32): 301-305, 1983

2. Klein, G. Lymphoma development in mice and humans: Diversity of initiation is followed by a convergent cytogenetic evolution. Proc. Natl. Acad. Sci. USA. (76): 2442. 1979

3. Klein, G. and Lenoir. G.: Translocations involving Ig-locus carrying chromosomes: a model for genetic transposition in carcinogenesis. Adv. Cancer Res. (37): 381-387. 1982

4. de-Thé, G. Epidemiology of Epstein-Barr virus and associated diseases. In: The Herpesviruses, vol. 1A, B. Roizman, ed. Plenum Press, New-York, pp. 25-103, 1982

5. Zur Hausen, H.: Human genital cancer: synergism between two virus infections or synergism between a virus infection and initiating events ? The Lancet, December 18, 1370. 1982

6. Gessain, A., Calender, A., Strobel, M., Lefait-Robin, R. and de-Thé, G. Hautre prévalence d'anticorps anti HTLV-1 chez les Boni, groupe d'origine africaine, isolé depuis le 18ème siècle en Guyane Française. C. R. Acad. Sci. Paris, in press

20

HUMAN T-CELL LEUKEMIA VIRUS (HTLV) ANTIBODIES IN MYCOSIS FUNGOIDES AND LEUKEMIAS AND LYMPHOMAS

B.I. SAHAI SRIVASTAVA AND MICHIKO KOGA

Roswell Park Memorial Institute, Buffalo, New York

1. INTRODUCTION

Except for mature T-cell leukemia/lymphoma, which is characterized by an aggressive course and poor prognosis, the antibodies to HTLV-1 antigens generally have not been found in patients with other leukemias from HTLV non-endemic areas of Japan, and infrequently have been present in mycosis fungoides/Sezary Syndrome (MF/SS) patients (1). The high incidence of HTLV antibodies in patients with acute leukemias (10%) compared to the normal healthy population (2%) in non-endemic areas of Japan was assumed to result from blood transfusions. The significance of HTLV antibodies in patients with leukemias/lymphomas other than mature T-cell leukemia/lymphoma from endemic areas of Japan has remained obscure due to the presence of HTLV antibodies in significant proportion of the healthy population. However, infection of not only T, but also B and non T/non B cells with HTLV (2), indicates that HTLV may not be strictly T-cell tropic, but that it could also infect any class of lymphocytes or stem cells of hematopoietic origin. Since the presence of HTLV in the healthy U.S. population is very rare {<1%}, we have examined U.S. patients with MF/SS and various leukemias/lymphomas for HTLV antibodies in serum/plasma and HTLV p-19 antigen expression by cells to assess the role of HTLV in these malignancies or its acquisition through blood products.

2. PROCEDURE

2.1. Materials and methods

2.1.1. Immunofluorescence (IF) assay for HTLV antibodies. Air-dried smears fixed in acetone-methanol (1:1) for 10 min. were used in indirect IF with fluorecein-conjugated rabbit antihuman IgG (α-chains) as the secondary reagent. Sera/plasma (examined at 1/10, 1/20, 1/40, 1/80, and 1/160 dilution) from patients, which reacted with HUT-102 and MT-2, but not with 16 HTLV negative cell types, were scored as HTLV-antibody positive. The antibody titers represent the lowest concentration of serum which specifically stained HUT-102 and MT-2 cells.

2.1.2. Immunofluorescence assay for HTLV p-19. Expression of HTLV p-19 was determined using air-dried leukocyte smears fixed for 10 min. in acetone-methanol (1:1), mouse monoclonal anti-HTLV p-19 at 1/600 dilution, and fluorecein-conjugated F $(ab^1)_2$ fragment sheep antimouse IgG heavy and light chains (free of cross reactions to human IgG) at 1/80 dilution. Appropriate irrelevant mouse monoclonal antibodies were used as controls.

2.1.3. Indirect enzyme-linked immunosorbent assay and titration. These procedures were carried out as described by Saxinger and Gallo (3), using zonal ultracentrifugation purified, detergent-disrupted whole HTLV for well coating with peroxidase-labelled goat-IgG antihuman IgG, o-phenylenediamine/H_2O_2, and measuring absorbance with Dynatech micro ELISA plate reader. Samples found positive in the screening test underwent absorption competition with cytosol preparations from phytohemagglutinin stimulated normal human lymphocytes, from HTLV producing cells, and from disrupted HTLV. Samples were scored positive if the difference between absorption with virus positive and negative cell preparations was at least 50% of the unabsorbed sera. Titre was determined by serial dilutions to a value that equalled the value of standard negative control sera.

3. RESULTS AND DISCUSSION

Before examining clinical samples, we established that a known HTLV antibody positive Japanese serum and anti-HTLV p-19 gave specific IF only with HTLV positive HUT-102 and MT-2 cells, but not with any of the 16 HTLV negative cells (CCRF-CEM, CCRF-HSB2, RPMI-8402, Peer, SKW-3, RPMI-8392; Ramos; Ruhl; REH; KM-3; NALM-16; KG-1; HL-60; U-937; K-562; phytohemagglutinin-stimulated normal lymphocytes) tested. HTLV antibody negative sera did not react with any cells.

HTLV positives are summarized by disease category in Table 1. The details on positive patients given in Table 2 indicate that about 25% of patients with MF/SS and 10% (Elisa assay) to 20% (immumofluorescence assay), with common forms of leukemias/lymphomas, had antibodies to HTLV. This is significantly higher than <1% HTLV antibody positivity observed in the healthy U.S. population. The leukocytes from patients

Table 1. HTLV positives by disease category in 108 subjects.

Disease category	No. positive/ No. tested HTLV-1 antibody IF assay	No. positive/out of HTLV antibody positive in IF assay: HTLV-1 antibody Elisa assay	HTLV-1 p-19 expression
Mycosis fungoides Sezary syndrome (MF/SS)	5/16	4[a]/5	1/5
Chronic myelogenous leukemia (CML)	3[b]/17	1/3	2/3
Acute myeloid leukemia (AML)	4/13	1/4	1/4
Acute lymphoblastic leukemia (ALL)	2/7	1/2	0/2
Lymphoma/lymphosarcoma	3/9	1/3	1/3
Hodgkin's disease	0/3	NT	NT
Hairy cell leukemia	0/3	NT	NT
Multiple myeloma	0/1	NT	NT
B-chronic lymphocytic leukemia (B-CLL)	0/6	NT	NT
T-chronic lymphocytic leukemia (T-CLL)	0/2	NT	NT
Other cancers	0/15	NT	NT
Normal	1[c]/16	0/1	NT

[a]Antibody activity specific for HTLV-1, but greater than 50% reduction could not be achieved after absorption with HTLV-1 antigens in 3/4 patients.

[b]2/3 positives were in blastic phase of CML.

[c]The positive subject with a titre of 80 is mother of CML patient No. 6 in Table 2; father was negative. Elisa assay was negative for both mother and father.

NT=Not tested.

Table 2. Mycosis fungoides/Sezary Syndrome and leukemia/lymphoma patients* (all caucasian except no. 8 black) found positive for HTLV antibodies by IF test using HUT-102 and MT-2 as target cells. Uncultured leukocytes from patients 4, 6, 8, 9, 17 were also positive for HTLV-p-19 antigen expression, whereas others were negative. Patients 6, 7, 10, 11, 12, 14, 15, had blood products infusions.

Patients Sex/Age		Diagnosis	HTLV Antibodies IF (titer)	Elisa (titer)
1.	M/68	MF	+(80)	+(7)
2.	M/67	MF	+(160)	-
3.	M/63	MF	+(40)	+(11)
4.	F/49	SS	+(80)	+(160)
5.	M/70	MF	+(40)	+(20)
6.	F/13	CML (Blastic at analysis)	+(80)	+(148)
7.	F/20	CML (Blastic at analysis)	+(160)	-
8.	M/37	CML (Chronic)	+(80)	-
9.	F/69	AML (Erythro-leukemia, M-6)	+(80)	+(550)
10.	M/72	Acute erythremia 2 yr later changing to Erythroleukemia	+(40)	-
11.	M/77	AMMOL M-4	+(20)	-
12.	F/67	AML, Mega-karyocytic	+(40)	-
13.	F/50	Lymphopro-liferative syndrome	+(80)	-
14.	M/67	Mixed lympho-histocytic stage IV	+(20)	-
15.	F/63	ALL FAB L-2	+(40)	+(34)
16.	M/7	c-ALL	+(40)	-
17.	F/62	Diffuse poorly differentiated lymphocytic lymphoma stage IV	+(40)	+(49)

*Plasma from patients obtained at several different occasions were positive for HTLV antibodies in IF test indicating persistence of these antibodies.

4, 6, 8, 9, and 17 in Table 2 were also positive for HTLV p-19 antigen which is expressed infrequently in uncultured cells. The IF reaction of HTLV positive patients' sera with HUT-102/MT-2 cells (Fig. 1) and of patients' leukocytes with anti-HTLV p-19 (Fig. 2) were characteristic of those given by known HTLV positive samples.

Among 17 HTLV antibody positives by the IF test, 8 were also positive in the Elisa assay, including 4 MF/SS patients and 1 patient each with CML-blastic, AML, ALL, and B-cell diffuse undifferentiated lymphoma. This discrepancy between the two assays could result from the greater sensitivity of the IF assay compared to the Elisa assay in which samples were scored positive only if the difference between absorption with HTLV positive and negative cell preparations was at least 50% of the unabsorbed sera. Moreover, the failure to obtain greater than 50% reduction on absorption with HTLV-1 antigens in 3/4 Elisa assay positive MF/SS patients could result from involvement of an HTLV variant virus. No MF/SS patients had received a blood transfusion. Among the 12 positives with leukemia/ lymphoma, 7 had received blood product transfusions, 5 had not, and at least 2 in each of these latter categories were also positive in the Elisa test. Therefore, blood transfusion, although a possibility for HTLV-antibody positivity in some cases, is negated for those patients who did not receive it. Alternatively, HTLV infection in common leukemia/ lymphoma patients, who are generally immunosuppressed, could represent a secondary or opportunistic infection; or HTLV or a variant virus may have some role in these malignancies but is expressed infrequently as in cutaneous T-cell lymphomas.

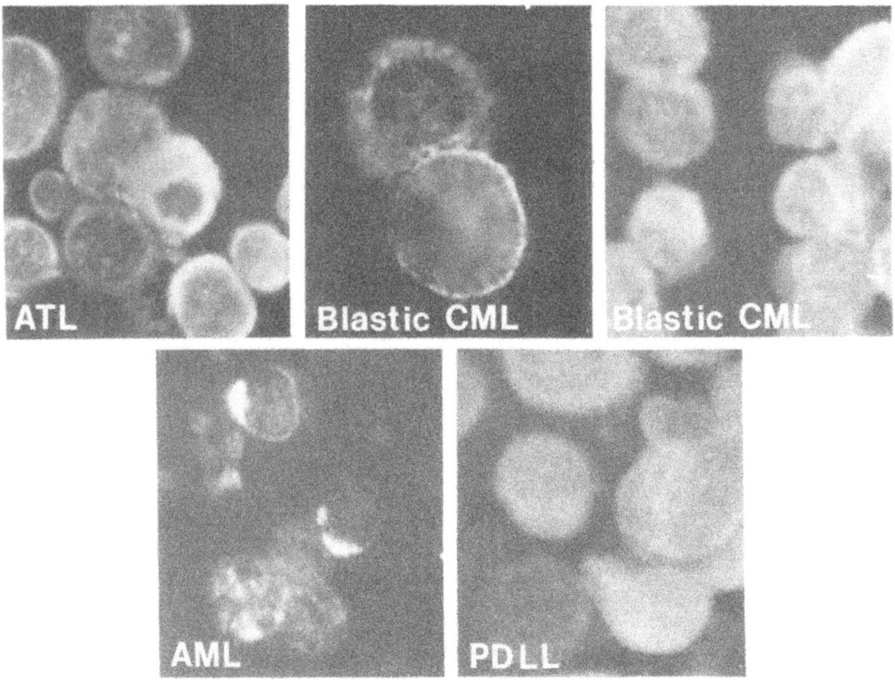

FIGURE 1. Immunofluorescence staining of HUT-102 cells using sera from Japanese ATL, blastic CML (patients #6, 7), AML (patient #9) and PDLL (patient #17) patients.

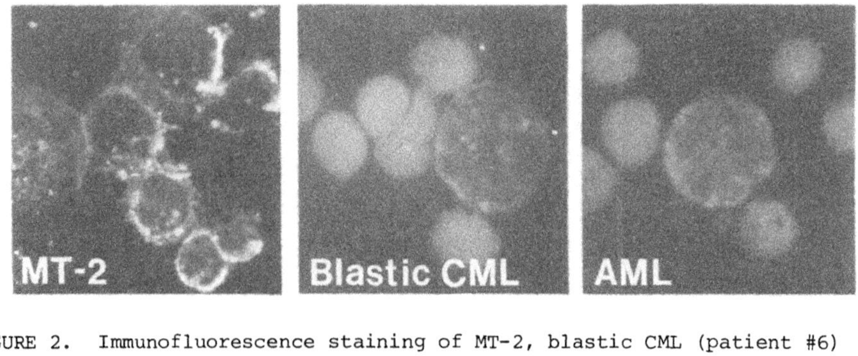

FIGURE 2. Immunofluorescence staining of MT-2, blastic CML (patient #6) and AML (patient #9) cells using HTLV-1 p-19 monoclonal antibodies.

REFERENCES

1. Yamamoto N, Matsumoto T, Koyanagi Y, Yuetsu T, Hinuma Y: Unique cell lines harbouring both Epstein-Barr virus and adult T-cell leukemia virus, established from leukemia patients. Nature (299):367-369. 1982.

2. Saxinger C, Gallo RC: Application of the indirect enzyme linked immunosorbent assay microtest to the detection and surveillance of human T-cell leukemia virus. Lab Invest (49):371-377. 1983.

3. Blattner WA, Robert-Guroff M, Kalyanaraman VS, Sarin P, Jaffe ES, Blayney DW, Zener KA, Gallo RC: Preliminary epidemiologic observations on a virus associated with T-cell neoplasia in man. In: Magrath IT, O'Conor CT, Ramot B (ed) Pathogenesis of leukemias and lymphomas. Raven Press, New York, 1984, pp. 339-348.

ACKNOWLEDGEMENTS

The authors wish to thank Drs. Miyoshi, Gallo, Sarin and Minowada for various materials. Elisa assays were carried out in Dr. Gallo's laboratory.

21

IMMUNOLOGIC FUNCTIONS AND THE PATHOGENESIS OF THE ACQUIRED IMMUNE DEFICIENCY SYNDROME (AIDS)

C. H. KIRKPATRICK, K. C. DAVIS, C. R. HORSBURGH, JR., P. E. RICKMANN, D. L. COHN, K. PENLEY, F. N. JUDSON AND B. S. DOBOZIN

Conrad D. Stephenson Laboratory for Research in Immunology, Department of Medicine, National Jewish Hospital and Research Center/NAC, and Denver Disease Control Service, Denver Department of Health and Hospitals, Denver, Colorado

1. INTRODUCTION

Since the syndrome was first reported in mid-1981 (1-3), over 5000 cases of AIDS have been reported in the United States. The majority of cases appear in homosexual or bisexual men, intravenous drug users, Haitian immigrants, and hemophiliacs (4), while lesser numbers of cases have occurred in recipients of blood transfusions (5) and among co-habitants of patients with AIDS (6). The epidemiologic evidence is most consistent with an etiologic role for a transmissible agent, probably a virus, and this has received strong support from recent serologic data (7-9).

Our studies are designed to examine the hypothesis that after encountering the etiologic agent(s) of AIDS, subjects who were clinically well and immunologically intact undergo progressive loss of cellular immune functions. Eventually their immunocompetence deteriorates to a point that they become susceptible to infections with opportunistic organisms such as *Pneumocystis carinii*, *Candida albicans* and *Mycobacterium avium-intracellulare* and to neoplasms such as Kaposi's sarcoma and non-Hodgkin's lymphoma. The recent discoveries of a virus that is tropic for T-lymphocytes of the helper phenotype are compatible with and supportive of this model (10-11).

By conducting serial prospective studies of immune functions of persons whose lifestyles or medical histories make them "at risk" for development of AIDS, we expect to be able to identify profiles of immune dysfunction that characterize persons with AIDS and to identify profiles of immune dysfunction and clinical characteristics that predict persons who are destined to develop AIDS. These latter studies may also establish the relationship between the generalized lymphadenopathy syndrome (GLS) (12) and susceptibility to AIDS and may allow us to identify critical immunologic abnormalities that are amenable to treatment.

2. PROCEDURE

2.1. Materials and methods

2.1.1 Subjects. The majority of participants in this study are homosexual or bisexual men who attend the clinics of the Denver Disease Control Service. These clinics provide medical care for sexually transmitted diseases for a significant portion of Denver's homosexual community. We have enrolled 61 asymptomatic homosexual men, and 30 homosexual men with the generalized lymphadenopathy syndrome (GLS) which is defined by the CDC as lymphadenopathy in two or more non-inguinal sites of three or more months duration (12). Within the GLS group, seven were considered as "symptomatic" because they had lost at least 10 pounds in weight and/or had had oral candidiasis. Thirty-one additional patients had AIDS (4); of these 12 had Kaposi's sarcoma, 14 had opportunistic infections and 5 had both Kaposi's sarcoma and opportunistic infections.

The control group consisted of 21 asymptomatic heterosexual subjects, aged 17 to 52 years; each of these persons denied membership in a group that is known to be at risk for AIDS.

2.1.2. Immunologic studies. The assays were selected to examine both quantitative and functional aspects of the immune system. The total numbers of T-lymphocytes and T-cells of the suppressor phenotype, helper phenotype or natural killer (NK) phenotype were enumerated using the Leu-1, Leu-2a, Leu-3a and Leu-7 monoclonal antibodies respectively (Beckton-Dickinson). The cells were counted with a FACS IV fluorescence activated cell sorter. In most assays, 9000-11000 cells of each phenotype were counted.

For examination of T-lymphocyte responses to specific antigens, tetanus toxoid, *Candida albicans* and tuberculin (PPD-S) were used. Mononuclear cells were separated from heparinized whole blood with Hypaque-Ficoll, washed and suspended at a density of 250,000 lymphocytes per ml in RPMI 1640 containing 5 percent homologous human serum and the appropriate concentrations of antigen. After six days of culture, the cells were labelled with tritiated thymidine, harvested and the radioactivity was counted. The stimulation index (SI) was calculated as the log of the mean counts per minute (cpm) by antigen-stimulated cells minus the log of the mean cpm of the same cells in the absence of antigen. Skin-test responsive healthy subjects have S.I.'s of three or greater.

T-lymphocyte responses to non-specific mitogens were assessed with phytohemagglutinin and concanavalin A. The studies were conducted in a similar manner except that the cultures were labelled and harvested on day 3. Responses by patients' cells were considered to be normal if they were $\geq$50 percent of the cpm by cells from the normal control subject on the same day.

Interleukin-2 (IL-2) was produced by incubation of 10^6 mononuclear cells in 1 ml of RPMI 1640 with 5% pooled human serum, 5×10^{-5}M 2-mercaptoethanol, and 1 ug of PHA. Supernatants were harvested at 48 hrs. IL-2 was assayed by the method of Gillis et al (13) using HT-2 cells, an IL-2 dependent murine cell line. Serial 1:2 dilutions of the supernatant or IL-2 standard (kindly provided by Drs. John Kappler and Philippa Marrack) were aliquoted into microtiter plates. Four x 10^3 HT-2 cells were added to each well. The wells were harvested at 24 hours after being pulsed with ^{3}H-thymidine during the final six hours. Results were expressed as the $\log_2$ of the dilution of supernatant that allowed 50% of maximal thymidine incorporation (ED_{50}).

2.1.3. Study design. The healthy homosexual men and men with GLS were seen approximately every six months at which time a questionnaire including demographic data, past medical histories, sexual practices, histories of illicit drug use and a review of systems was completed. A physical examination was done and blood was drawn for the laboratory analyses. When possible, AIDS patients were studied when they were clinically stable and not receiving chemotherapy.

2.2. Statistics. Laboratory data were collected and analyzed by patient group (i.e. AIDS, GLS, etc.) using a one-way analysis of variance by both the Tukey (14) and Scheffe (14) tests. Our softward programs distinguish significance at $p<0.05$. IL-2 titers were compared with the Mann-Whitney U test.

3. RESULTS

3.1 Immunologic profiles of patients with AIDS. The most striking immunologic abnormalities were seen in patients with AIDS. Within this group, the patients with AIDS and Kaposi's sarcoma (AIDS/KS) had somewhat less severe immune defects than persons with AIDS and opportunistic infections (AIDS/OI) or AIDS patients with both opportunistic infections and Kaposi's sarcoma (KS/OI). For example, only 3 of 12 AIDS/KS patients were lymphopenic while 11 of 14 AIDS/OI and KS/OI patients were lymphopenic (Figure 1). The mean lymphocyte counts of

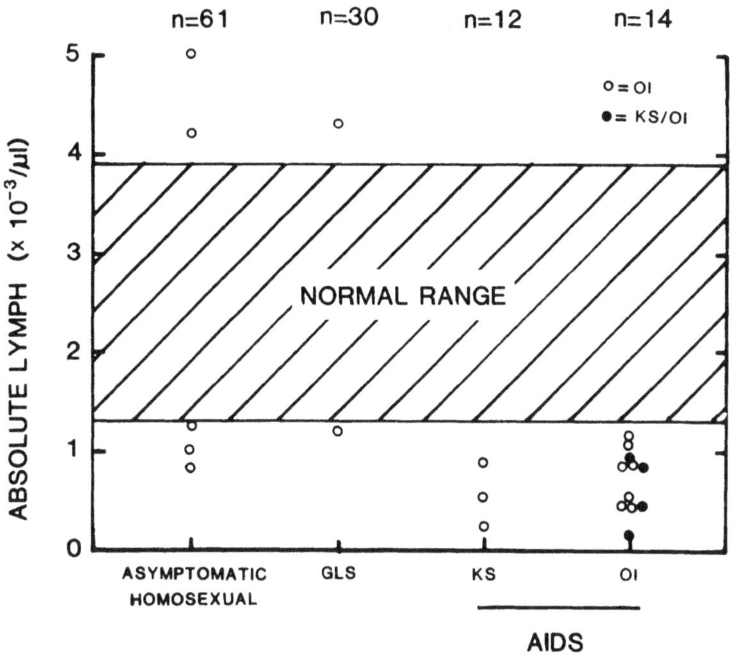

Figure 1. Absolute lymphocyte numbers in asymptomatic homosexual men, homosexual men with the generalized lymphadenopathy syndrome (GLS), and patients with AIDS with Kaposi's sarcoma (KS), AIDS with opportunistic infections (o) and AIDS with both KS and OI (•). The asymptomatic homosexual men and GLS subjects were not different from the heterosexual controls, but the absolute lymphocyte counts of the AIDS population was significantly lower ($p < 0.05$).

the AIDS population was significantly lower than the heterosexual controls, asymptomatic homosexual men and the GLS subjects ($p < 0.05$).

Studies of lymphocyte phenotypes further illustrated the nature of the immunologic abnormalities. The Leu-1-positive cells (total mature T-lymphocytes) were subnormal in 8 of 12 AIDS/KS patients and 13 of 14 AIDS/OI and KS/OI patients (Figure 2). The mean T-cell counts in each of the AIDS populations was significantly ($p < 0.05$) lower than the heterosexual and homosexual control populations and the GLS group. In most instances this was due to loss of cells of the helper phenotype (Leu-3a-positive cells) with the numbers of these cells being moderately to markedly reduced in 9 patients with AIDS/KS and severely reduced in 13 of the AIDS/OI and KS/OI group (Figure 3). The values for each of the AIDS groups was significantly ($p < 0.05$) lower than the control groups and GLS subjects.

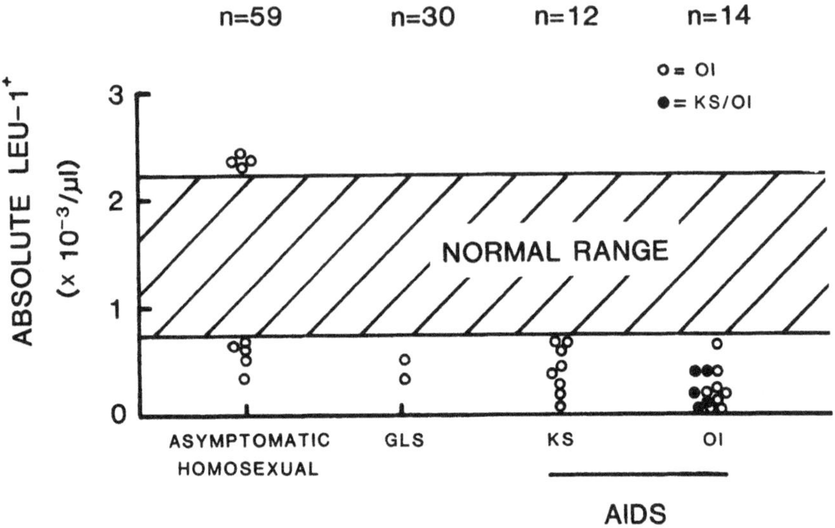

Figure 2. Total mature T-lymphocytes (Leu-1$^+$ cells) in the study populations. There were no differences in T-cell numbers of the heterosexual controls, asymptomatic homosexuals or GLS subjects, but each of these groups was significantly ($p < 0.05$) greater than the AIDS/KS, AIDS/OI and KS/OI groups.

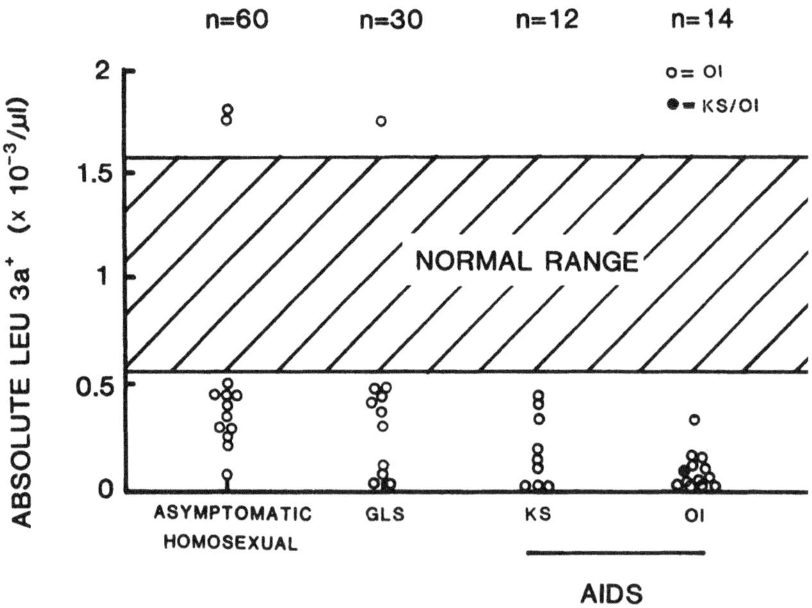

Figure 3. Helper (Leu-3a$^+$) T-lymphocyte counts in the study populations. Note the marked reduction in helper cells in the AIDS/OI and KS/OI groups. All AIDS groups were significantly ($p < 0.05$) lower than the control or GLS groups.

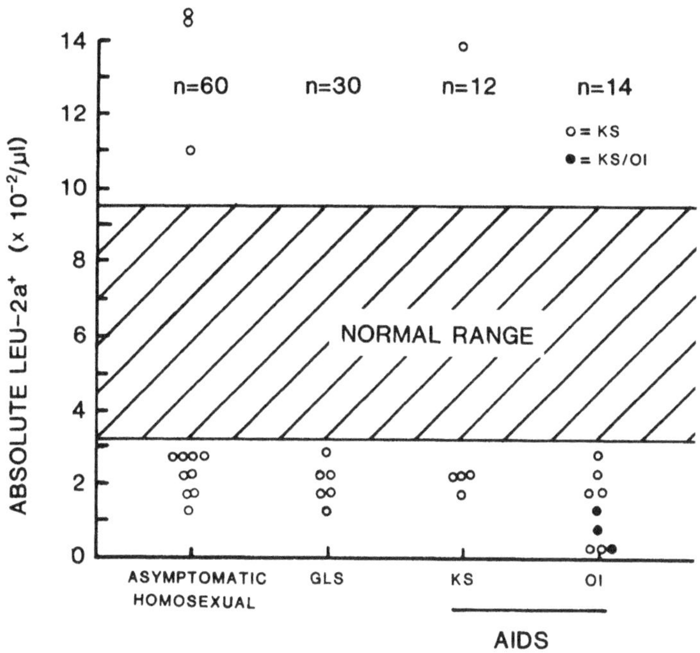

Figure 4. Suppressor (Leu-2a$^+$) T-lymphocytes in the study populations. Although many AIDS/OI and KS/OI patients had subnormal numbers of cells of this phenotype, there were no significant differences between any of the populations.

In contrast, lymphopenia of the suppressor phenotype (Leu-2a$^+$) was less common in AIDS/KS patients, and while present in 9 of 14 AIDS/OI and KS/OI patients it was less severe (Figure 4). Abnormal ratios of helper cells to suppressor cells (3a/2a) are very sensitive but rather non-specific findings in AIDS patients. As shown in Figure 5, 11 of 13 AIDS/KS patients had abnormal 3a/2a ratios, and this value was abnormal in 17 of 18 AIDS/OI and KS/OI patients. Each of the AIDS groups was significantly ($p < 0.05$) less than the heterosexual and homosexual controls.

Cells of the natural killer (NK) (Leu-7-positive) phenotype were abnormally low in only 2 of 12 AIDS/KS patients, and three other AIDS/KS patients had abnormally high values. These cells were modestly reduced in 9 of 13 AIDS/OI and KS/OI subjects. There were no differences in cells of the NK phenotype in any of our populations. Assays of NK activity have not been done.

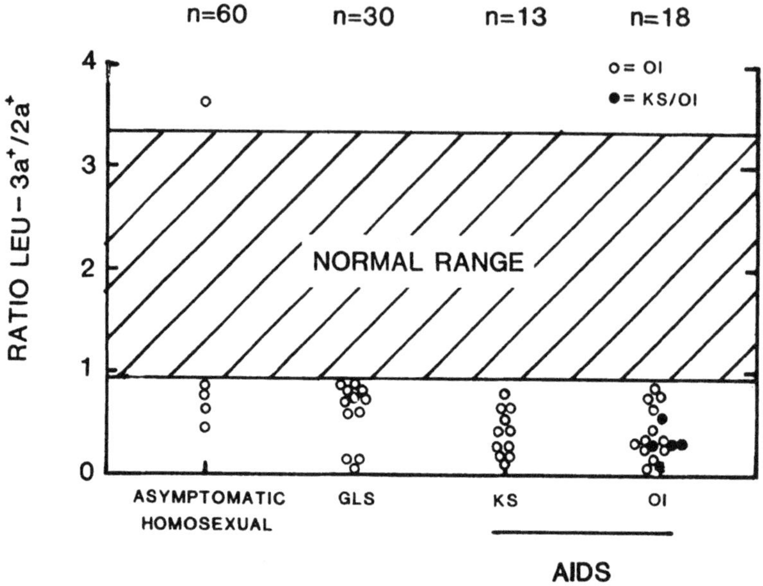

Figure 5. Ratios of helper T-cells (Leu 3a$^+$) to suppressor T-cells (Leu-2a$^+$). The asymptomatic homosexual and heterosexual groups were not different from one another. However, both the GLS group and all AIDS groups had significantly ($p < 0.05$) lower ratios than the control groups.

Table 1. Responses to concanavalin-A by persons with AIDS or GLS and control groups.

Group	Number with subnormal responses/number studied*
Asymptomatic homosexual	16/61 (26%)
GLS	13/30 (43%)
AIDS/KS	4/12 (33%)
AIDS/OI and KS/OI	10/19 (53%)

*Subnormal responses are defined as values < 50 percent of healthy heterosexual subject studied on the same day.

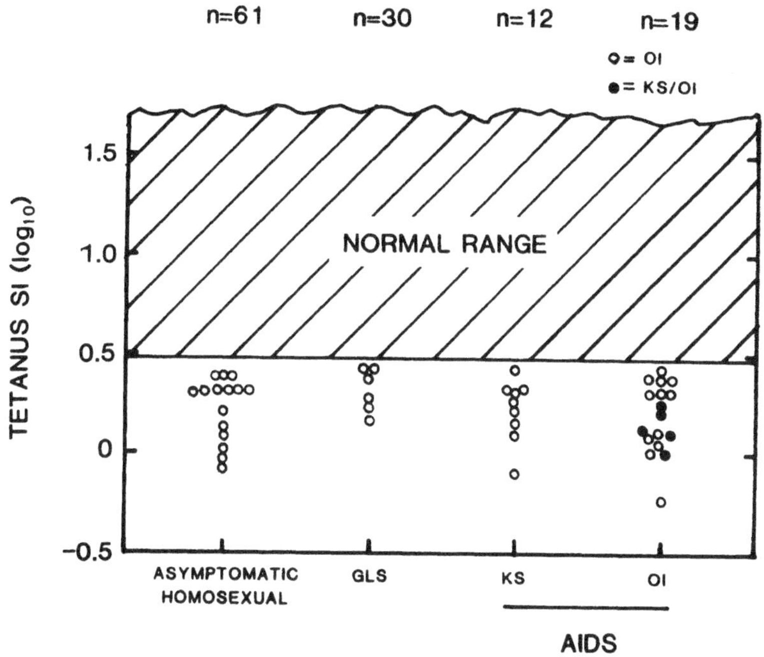

Figure 6. Thymidine incorporation responses by tetanus toxoid-stimulated peripheral blood mononuclear cells. The results are expressed as the stimulation index (SI) which is the log of mean cpm by antigen-stimulated cells minus the log of mean cpm by unstimulated cells. Normal cells give a value of ≥ 3. Note significant ($p < 0.05$) reductions in the AIDS patients.

T-lymphocyte proliferation responses to antigens such as tetanus toxoid is due to replication of T-helper cells (15). Nine of 12 AIDS/KS patients and 17 of 19 AIDS/OI and KS/OI patients showed subnormal T-cell proliferation responses to this antigen (Figure 6) and the mean S.I. of each of the AIDS populations was significantly less than the controls and GLS subjects ($p < 0.05$). Mitogens such as concanavalin-A stimulate growth of all T-cells (15), but this response is non-specific. In general, abnormalities of responses to mitogens only occur in diseases with profound dysfunction of the T-lymphocyte system. Only 4 of 12 AIDS/KS patients, but 10 of 19 AIDS/OI and KS/OI patients had subnormal responses to concanavalin A (Table 1).

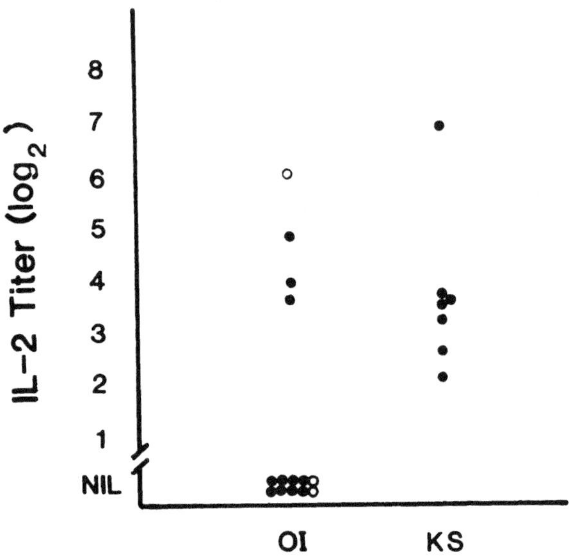

Figure 7. Production of interleukin-2 by PHA-activated cells from patients with AIDS. Note IL-2 production by AIDS/KS patients. Eight AIDS/OI patients (o) and 2 KS/OI (•) patients failed to produce detectable amounts of IL-2.

Interleukin-2 (IL-2) is an essential second signal for proliferation of T-lymphocytes in response to antigens and mitogens (16). Thus, failure to produce interleukin-2 could be a mechanism for impaired T-cell responses. In fact, our studies disclosed that production of IL-2 was abnormally low in many patients with AIDS/OI and KS/OI, but was normal in AIDS patients with KS alone (Figure 7).

3.2. Immunologic profiles of healthy homosexual men and persons with GLS. Lymphopenia was not a common finding in our populations of asymptomatic homosexual men or persons with GLS (Figure 1). The mean value of peripheral blood lymphocytes in both of these groups was significantly ($p < 0.05$) greater than in patients with AIDS (2382 cells/ul and 2204 cells/ul versus 1404 cells/ul). The absolute numbers of T-lymphocytes (Leu-1-positive cells) (Figure 2) and cells of the helper phenotype (Leu-3a-positive cells) (Figure 3) in the asymptomatic homosexual men and the GLS patients were not significantly different from the heterosexual controls, but these subjects had significantly more T-cells and T-helper cells than the AIDS patients ($p < 0.05$). However, Figure 3 also illustrates the heterogeneity of these two groups. Eleven asymptomatic homosexual men (18%) and 10 men with GLS (33%) had numbers of helper T-cells that were less than the normal range. Whether these subjects are at greater risk for development of AIDS than subjects with normal numbers of helper T-cells will be determined by future studies.

The number of suppressor cells (Leu-2a-positive cells) was higher in GLS (569 ± 255 cells/ul) and AIDS/KS (524 ± 358 cells/ul) patients and lower in KS/OI (291 ± 283 cells/ul) patients, but none of these differences achieved statistical significance.

When the ratios of T-helper cells to T-suppressor cells (Leu-3a/Leu-2a) were compared, the GLS patients had significantly lower values than the asymptomatic homosexuals and the heterosexual controls ($p < 0.05$) (Figure 5).

The number of Leu-7-positive (NK) cells were not different in any of the study groups.

Even though the means of the SI's of T-cell responses to tetanus toxoid or concanavalin A for asymptomatic homosexual men and GLS subjects were not different from the heterosexual controls, there was striking heterogeneity in these groups. For example, 16 of the 61 asymptomatic homosexuals and 13 of 30 GLS subjects had subnormal T-cell responses to concanavalin A (Table 1), and 15 asymptomatic homosexuals and 6 GLS subjects had subnormal responses to tetanus toxoid (Figure 5). These subjects deserve close monitoring to see if these abnormalities represent early changes in immune functions that are prodromata of AIDS.

Interleukin-2 production by cells from asymptomatic homosexual men was equal to that of normal subjects. All but four GLS patients produced detectable amounts of IL-2, but the titer of IL-2 produced by symptomatic GLS patients was significantly ($p < 0.01$) greater than that of asymptomatic GLS patients. Since IL-2 production is a consequence of T-cell activation (16), these observations may indicate activation by the same factors or agents that are responsible for production of the symptoms.

4. DISCUSSION

There is now impressive virologic (10,11) and serologic (7-9) evidence that AIDS is caused by a retrovirus, and that this virus is tropic for T-lymphocytes of the helper phenotype (7,9-11). Presumably, infection with this virus is responsible for depletion of cells of the cellular immune system with development of profound immune deficiency and susceptibility to infections with a variety of opportunistic organisms and to neoplasms such as Kaposi's sarcoma and non-Hodgkin's lymphoma. The mechanisms through which the virus induces injury to the immune system are unknown. One possibility is a lytic infection that primarily affects T-helper cells. However, many AIDS patients have severe depletion of lymphocytes of all phenotypes as well as cells of the natural killer phenotype. These data may indicate that the virus can infect other cells, or that the infection impairs or suppresses production or maturation of cells of other phenotypes. An interesting, but untested, hypothesis is that viral infection impairs expression of antigen recognition units on T-cells. This effect has been noted in expression of Class I histocompatibility antigens by adenovirus 12-transformed rat cells and is associated with impaired production of specific mRNA for the Class I heavy chain (17). Conceivably, infections of human T-cells with the etiologic agent of AIDS could impair expression of antigens such as T-3 or other components of the T-cell receptor for antigen (18), but this possibility has not been examined.

Our studies have shown profound defects of cell mediated immunity in patients with AIDS. They have also shown that patients with AIDS and Kaposi's sarcoma have fewer and less severe immune defects than patients with AIDS and opportunistic infections. These differences are most striking in measurements of total T-cells and helper T-cells and in functional responses to antigens and mitogens and production of interleukin-2. It is possible that the differences are caused by the opportunistic infections. However, they persist for many months after resolution of clinically apparent infections. Thus, these data may indicate fundamental differences in immune functions that affect host defenses against certain infections and neoplastic diseases.

In contrast to studies by others (19,20), we did not find major immunologic abnormalities in asymptomatic homosexual men. The other studies were conducted in New York and Los Angeles, cities in which AIDS was recognized in 1981. In contrast, the first case of AIDS in a homosexual man in Denver was diagnosed in August, 1982. This may indicate that our studies were begun prior to development of immunologic abnormalities by persons who are currently incubating the disease, but who are asymptomatic. Serologic studies for exposure to the etiologic agents are currently in progress and should help answer this possibility. A trivial explanation, that our patient population is significantly different from those in other cities, seems unlikely in view of the fact that our subjects were recruited from a clinic for sexually-transmitted diseases that traditionally has provided care for the more promiscuous members of the community.

ACKNOWLEDGEMENTS

This research was supported by USPHS Grant CA-35006. The authors are indebted to Terrilee Day, Lynn Greenberg, Debbie Leto, Terri McFarland and Chaim Urbach for excellent technical assistance and to Mrs. Billie Wilson for preparation of the manuscript.

References

1. Gottlieb MS, Schroff R, Schanker HM, Weisman JD, Fan PT, Wolf RA, Saxon A: Pneumocystis carinii pneumonia and mucosal candidiasis in previously healthy homosexual men: evidence of a new acquired cellular immunodeficiency. New Engl J Med (305):1425-1430, 1981.
2. Masur H, Michelis MA, Greene JB, Onorato I, Vande Stouwe RA, Holzman RS, Gormser G, Brettman L, Lange M, Murray HW, Cunningham-Rundles S: An outbreak of community-acquired Pneumocystis carinii pneumonia: initial manifestation of cellular immune dysfunction. New Engl J Med (305): 1431-1438, 1981.
3. Siegel FP, Lopez C, Hammer GS, Brown AE, Kornfeld SJ, Gold J, Hassett J, Hirschman SZ, Cunningham-Rundles C, Adelsberg BR, Darham DM, Seigal M, Cunningham-Rundles S, Armstrong D: Severe acquired immunodeficiency in male homosexuals manifested by chronic Herpes simplex lesions. New Engl J Med (305):1439-1444, 1981.
4. Selik RM, Haverkos HW, Curran JW: Acquired immune deficiency syndrome (AIDS) trends in the United States. Am J Med (76):493-500, 1984.
5. Curran JW, Lawrence DN, Jaffe H, Kaplan J, Zyla LD, Chamberland M, Weinstein R, Lui K-J, Schonberger LB, Spira TJ, Alexander WJ: Acquired immunodeficiency syndrome (AIDS) associated with transfusions. New Engl J Med (310):69-75, 1984.
6. Harris C, Small CB, Klein RS, Friedland GH, Moll B, Emeson EE, Spigland I, Steigbigel NH: Immunodeficiency in female sexual partners of men with the acquired immunodeficiency syndrome. New Engl J Med (308):1181-1184, 1983.
7. Sarngahharan MG, Papovic M, Bruch L, Schupbach J. Gallo RC: Antibodies reactive with human T-lymphotropic retrovirus (HTLV-III) in the serum of patients with AIDS. Science (224):506-508, 1984.

8. Brun-Vezinet F, Rouzioux C, Barre-Sinoussi F, Klatzmann D, Saimot AG, Rozenbaum W, Chistol D, Gluckmann JC, Montagnier L, Chermann JC: Detection of IgG antibodies to lymphadenopathy-associated virus in patients with AIDS or lymphadenopathy syndrome. Lancet (1):1253-1256, 1984.
9. Safai B, Sarngadharan MG, Groopman JE, Arnett K, Papovic M, Sliski A, Schupbach J: Seroepidemiological studies of human T-lymphotropic retrovirus type III in acquired immunodeficiency syndrome. Lancet (1):1438-1440, 1984.
10. Barre-Sinoussi F, Chermann JC, Rey F, Nugeyre MT, Chamaret S, Gruest J, Dauguet C, Axler-Blin C, Vizinet-Brun F, Rouzioux C, Rozenbaum W, Montagnier L: Isolation of a T-lymphocytropic retrovirus from a patient at risk for acquired immune deficiency syndrome (AIDS). Science (220):868-871, 1983.
11. Papovic M, Sarngadharan MG, Read E, Gallo RD: Detection, isolation and continuous production of cytopathic retroviruses (HTLV-III) from patients with AIDS and pre-AIDS. Science (224):497-500, 1984.
12. Centers for Disease Control: Persistent, generalized lymphadenopathy among homosexual males. MMWR (31):249-251, 1982.
13. Gillis S, Ferm MM, Ou W, Smith KA: T-cell growth factor: parameters of production and a quantitative microassay for activity. J Immunol (120):2027-2032, 1978.
14. Kim J-O, Kahout FJ: Analysis of variance and covariance: subprograms, ANOVA and one way. In: Nie NH, Hull CH, Jenkins JG, Steinbrenner K, Bent DH (eds) SPSS. Statistical Package for the Social Sciences. Second Edition, McGraw-Hill, New York, 1975, pp 426-428.
15. Schlossman SF, Reinherz EL: Human T-cell subsets in health and disease. Springer Sem Immunopathol (7):9-18, 1984.
16. Gillis S: Interleukin-2: biology and biochemistry. J Clin Immunol (3):1-13, 1983.
17. Schrier PI, Bernards R, Vaessen RTMJ, Houweling A, van der Eb AJ: Expression of class I major histocompatibility antigens switched off by highly oncogenic adenovirus 12 in transformed rat cells. Nature (305):771-775, 1983.
18. Weiss A, Wiskocil RL, Stobo JD: The role of T3 surface molecules in the activation of human T-cells: a two-stimulus requirement for IL-2 production reflects events occurring at pretranslational level. J Immunol (133):123-128, 1984.
19. Kornfeld H, Vande Stouwe RA, Lange M, Reddy MM, Grieco MH: T-lymphocyte subpopulations in homosexual men. New Engl J Med (307):729-731, 1982.
20. Detels R, Fahey JL, Schwartz K, Greene RS, Visscher BR, Gottlieb MS: Relationship between sexual practices and T-cell subsets in homosexually active men. Lancet (1):609-611, 1983.

22

EXPERIMENTAL STUDIES OF THE PATHOGENESIS OF FELINE LEUKEMIA VIRUS INFECTION

EDWARD A. HOOVER

Department of Pathology, Colorado State University, Fort Collins, Colorado

Feline leukemia virus (FeLV) infection is transmissible by contact exposure, by oral-nasal or parenteral inoculation, and by congenital exposure of outbred cats to FeLV. The susceptibility *vs* resistance of cats to FeLV is determined by early containment *vs* amplification of retroviral replication in target hemolymphatic cells. The course of these pivotal early events is age-dependent, macrophage-dependent, and corticosteroid-sensitive. Either of two host-virus relationships ensue in cats exposed to FeLV: (a) progressive infection characterized by persistent viral replication in hemolymphatic and epithelial cells, persistent viremia, minimal anti-viral immune response, and a high risk of subsequent disease, or (b) regressive infection characterized by transient retroviral replication in hemolymphatic cells, abrogation of viremia, and a low incidence of subsequent disease. Some regressively infected cats harbor persistent latent FeLV infection in certain hemolymphatic cells. Such residual non-productive FeLV infections may be reactivated, transmitted congenitally, or be involved in the genesis of virus-negative leukemias. Although less notorious than leukemogenesis, it is the cytosuppressive disease syndromes which constitute the predominant pathogenic manifestations of FeLV infection in cats.

Transmission of FeLV

Experimental studies (1-10), confirming investigations have shown that efficient transmission of the feline retrovirus requires close social contact facilitating relatively direct oral-nasal transfer of virus to mucosal surfaces or the use of common feeding utensils, confirming investigations of cats infected with FeLV in Nature (11-14). Salivary secretions from viremic cats contain concentrations of infectious virus equivalent to those in plasma (12,15-17). Viral infectivity is extinguished rapidly under conditions of dessication at room temperature (18). Although FeLV replicates in urinary and intestinal mucosal epithelium, viral infectivity is preserved poorly in urine and feces (17).

FeLV infection is transmissable by oronasal, subcutaneous, and intraperitoneal inoculation. The latter appears most sensitive. Oronasal administration of at least 100 focus forming units (ffu) (19) of FeLV-Rickard strain appears necessary to provoke an antibody response and a minimum of 1000 ffu are required to elicit viremia in adult (6-month or older) specific-pathogen-free (SPF) cats (20).

FeLV Strain and Age-Related Resistance

Although comparative investigations of the biologic activity of naturally occurring feline retroviruses have been limited, studies employing limited numbers of age-matched SPF cats infected with equivalent infectious doses of several FeLV isolates have demonstrated substantial variation in the virulence and pathogenicity of feline retrovirus (8,21,Table 1). Demonstration of pathogenicity may require use of sensitive hosts (e.g. newborn kittens) and may reveal additional pathogenic properties of the phenotypic mixture of viruses in most inocula. Some FeLV isolates have minimal disease-inducing capacity demonstrable by experimental transmission. An important relationship between disease inducing proclivity and FeLV subgroup classification as determined by viral interference reflecting polymorphism in viral envelope gp70 and probably variation in viral cytotropism (22-26). Most notable to date is the association of subgroup C viruses with erythroid progenitor cell ablation and consequent induction of aplastic anemia (27-29).

The natural resistance of cats to a standard (10^5 ffu) exposure to FeLV is minimal in the period from birth to weaning age (≤8 weeks) unless passive material antibody is transferred in colostrum (30,31)(8, Table 1).

Table 1. Virus strain and age of cat as determinants of the pathogenicity of FeLV isolates under experimental conditions

FeLV Isolate and Disease In Original Cat[a]	Age of Inoculated SPF Cat			Resultant Disease
	Newborn	8 Weeks	>4 Months	
Rickard (Thymic lymphoma)	100[b]	85	11	Thymic lymphoma
K-T(Lymphoma and anemia)	100	NT[c]	16	Anemia
W2041 (Lymphatic leukemia)	100	83	0	Anemia
U5516 (Anemia)	100	100	67	Anemia
S2727 (Anemia)	100	NT	NT	Anemia
X852 (No disease)	100	NT	0	None[d]
DQ (Thymic lymphoma)	100	100	56	Immuno-deficiency syndrome

[a] Tissue homogenates containing from 5 X 10^4 to 1 X 10^5 focus forming units (19)
[b] Percent of cats developing persistent viremia (n for each group = 4-20)
[c] Not tested
[d] No clinical, hematologic, or histologic abnormalitites after >2 years

Age-related resistance to FeLV in naive cats develops between 2 and 6 months of age, by which time FeLV susceptibility approximates that of adult cats (8). Autologous FeLV resistance can be abrogated by treatment with corticosteroids (32), silica (33), methylnitrosourea (34) (and presumably other immunomodulators) during the period of early host-virus interactions when either curtailment or amplification of retroviral replication transpires (35,36).

A direct correlation exists between the age-related susceptibility of cats to FeLV infection _in vivo_ and the permissiveness of feline macrophages (MØ) to productive FeLV infection _in vitro_ (33). Although phagocytic capacities of isolated MØ from 8 week-old *vs* 6-month-old SPF cats are equivalent, the mean FeLV susceptibility of MØ from kittens is fivefold that of adult cats (33). Moreover, adrenal corticosteroid treatment, which enhances the susceptibility of adult cats to FeLV *in vivo*, likewise enhances the permissiveness of adult cat MØ to FeLV *in vitro* to approximate that of kittens (33)(Table 2).

Table 2. Effect of hydrocortisone on the permissiveness of isolated, cultured macrophages from adult cats *vs*. kittens to FeLV-R infection *in vitro*

Number of cats	Mean age of cats (mo.)	Hydrocortisone concentration (M)	FeLV infectivity ($ffu/10^6$ MØ[a])	FeLV enhancement index
12	2	0	721	184
12	2	10^{-6}	132,742	
12	9	0	330	534
12	9	10^{-6}	176,346	

[a]mean cell-free + cell-associated virus assayed 7 days after *in vitro* infection with FeLV-R

Thus, age-related resistance to FeLV is linked to MØ resistance to productive FeLV infection and correlates with initial restriction of viral replication in lymphoreticular tissues (35,36).

Early FeLV-Target Cell Interactions and Resultant Virus-Host Relationships

Experiments with SPF cats inoculated with standard (10^5 ffu) doses of FeLV-Rickard (R) have established that within 6 weeks after viral exposure, either of two major host-virus relationships evolve, i.e. (a) progressive infection characterized by productive infection of systemic hemolymphatic cells, persistent viremia, and minimal anti-FOCMA and antiviral immune response or (b) regressive infection characterized by early curtailment of viral replication in hemolymphatic cells, transient or absent viremia, and substantial antiviral immune response (8,35,36). Further studies established that the early pathogenesis of progressive FeLV-R infection in cats involved sequential viral replication in: (1) macrophages and germinal center lymphocytes in tonsils and local lymph nodes (Figs. 1,2), (2) small numbers of circulating mononuclear leukocytes (cell-associated viremia), (3) lymphoreticular cells of systemic lymphoid tissues, (4) bone marrow megakaryocytes and myelo-monocytic progenitor cells (Fig. 3), (5) circulating platelets and neutrophils (marrow-origin viremia), and (6) mucosal and glandular epithelia with viral excretion (Fig. 4)(35,36).

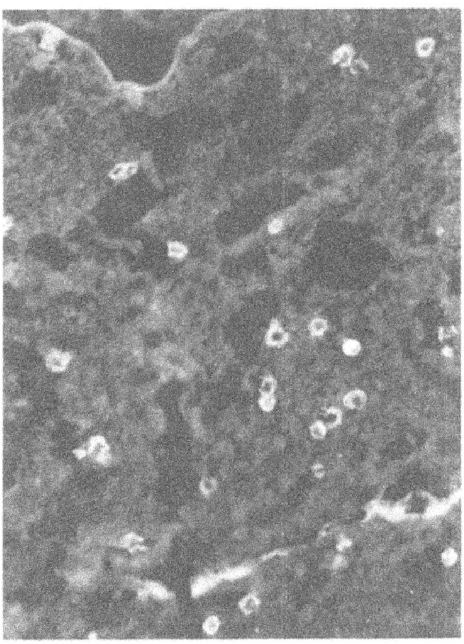

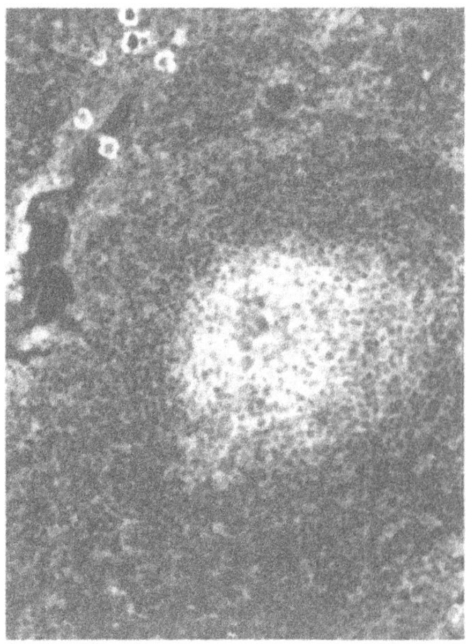

FIGURE 1 (left). Initial stage of FeLV in an experimentally infected cat. Cytoplasmic p27 antigen in scattered sinusoidal macrophages of the pharyngeal lymph node. Fixed, paraffin-embedded section indirect immunofluorescence.

FIGURE 2 (right). Phase of initial FeLV amplification in regional lymphoid tissues. Typical focus of FeLV replication in follicular lymphocytes of lymph node.

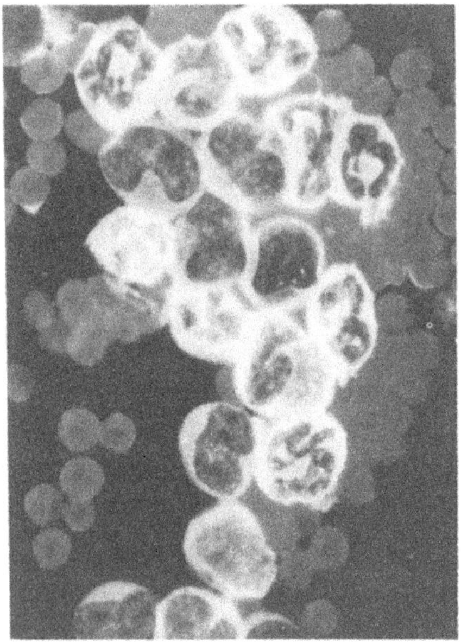

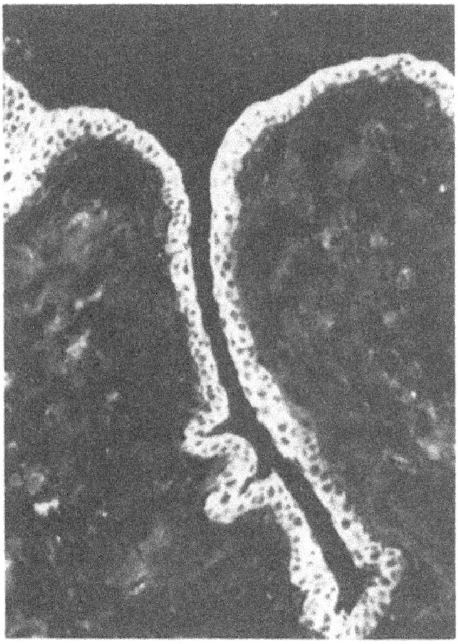

FIGURE 3 (left). Phase of productive FeLV infection in systemic hemolymphatic cells and onset of marrow-origin viremia. FeLV p27 in bone marrow myeloid progenitor cells.

FIGURE 4 (right). Extensive FeLV infection of mucosal epithelium of the urinary bladder during the phase of epithelial dissemination and viral excretion. (from ref. 36).

The establishment of marrow-origin persistent viremia precedes by weeks to years the onset of anti-proliferative (cytopathic) or proliferative (neoplastic) disease. Although regressive, immunizing FeLV infections are not associated with proven pathogenic consequences, up to 60% of regressor cats harbor latent integrated in marrow myelomonocytic progenitor cells and a Staphlococcus protein A-responsive populations of nodal lymphoreticular cells (62). Furthermore, convincing epidemiologic evidence has been presented for a potential role of latent, integrated FeLV in the genesis virus-negative lymphosarcoma in naturally infected cats (38).

Preleukemic Changes

Lymphomagenic FeLV isolates (such as FeLV-R) transform predominantly T cells after latent periods of 3 to >18 months (2,7,8). Preleukemic events in infected cats include: atrophy of the thymus (3,7,39,40)(Fig. 5), impairment of cell mediated immunity (39,41) and T helper cell dependent humoral antibody responses (42,43), redistribution of certain lymphoid cells subsets (37) and eventual clonal proliferation of T lymphoblasts arising within the atrophoid thymus (40,41a) (Fig. 6).

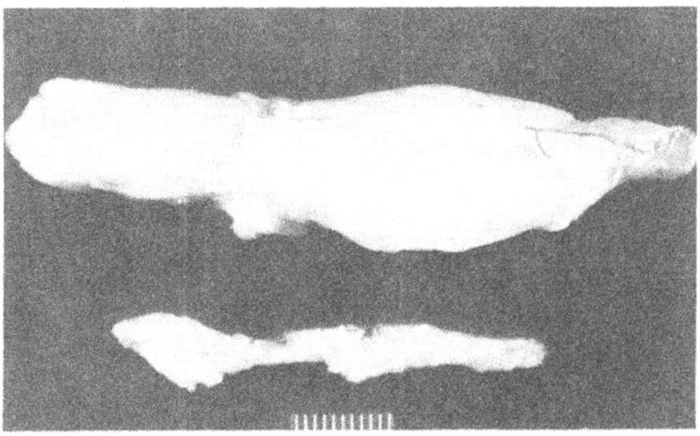

FIGURE 5. Preleukemic thymic atrophy. Thymus from inoculated cat (bottom) vs age-matched control cat (top) 7 weeks after inoculation of leukemogenic FeLV-R. (from ref 39).

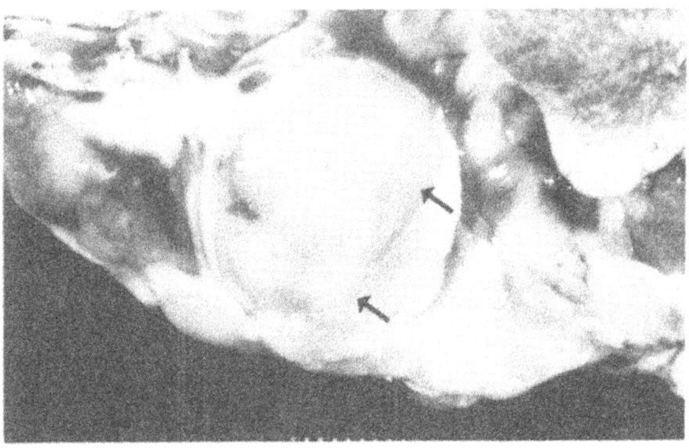

FIGURE 6. T-cell lymphomagenesis. Early T-cell lymphoma (arrows) arising from the atrophied thymus of a cat inoculated with FeLV-R.

In vivo and *in vitro* studies of the interactions of FeLV-R with hemolymphatic cells indicate preleukemic viral tropism for nodal follicular B cells, a minority subset of T lcells, and marrow megakaryocytic and myelomonocytic progenitor cells (37). Thus, the target cells for preleukemic FeLV replication and eventual neoplastic transformation are divergent.

The mechanism by which FeLV mediates lymphomagenesis is not known. Recent evidence suggests that in at least a portion of virus-producing T cell lymphomas transduction generation of MCF-like recombinant viruses and/or rearrangement of the protoncogene *myc* in the process of FeLV provirus integration may be relevant to leukemogenesis involving feline T lymphoblasts (44-46).

Aplastic Anemia

FeLV-induced aplastic anemia was transmitted initially by serial passage of FeLV-KT other field isolates in neonatal cats (27-29,47) and subsequently in corticosteroidtreated weanling or adult cats (48-50) (Fig. 7).

FIGURE 7.

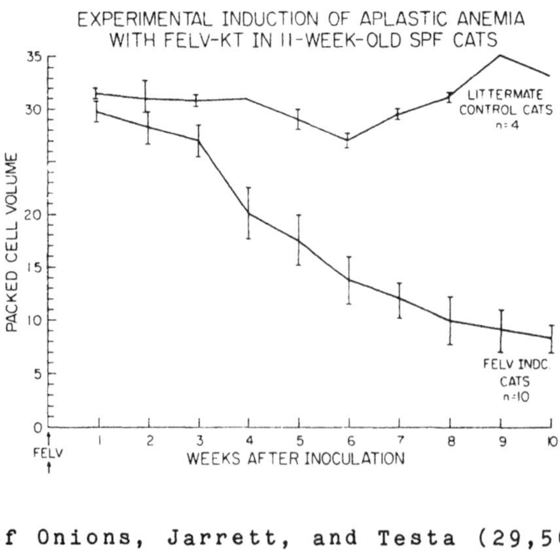

The work of Onions, Jarrett, and Testa (29,50) has shown that FeLV aplastic anemia is induced preferentially by subgroup C viruses. Moreover, the FeLV-C-Sarma isolate has been molecularly cloned by Mullins (51a) and shown to retain its erythrosuppressive proclivity *in vivo* and *in vitro* (52, Tables 3,4).

The pathogenesis of FeLV aplastic anemia appears to involve cytopathic viral deletion of early erythroid progenitor cells, which are recognized as burst-forming units erythroid (BFU-e) in clonigenic bone marrow colony-forming cell culture assays in methylcellulose medium (50,51,53). The rapid, selective, and inexorable erythrosuppressive activity of anemogenic FeLV has been demonstrated after *in vivo* and *in vitro* exposure of normal marrow BFU-e progenitors to infectious virus (Tables 3,4).

Table 3. *In vivo* FeLV strain-specific ablation of bone marrow erythroid progenitor cell proliferation

Erythropoietic Index	Days After Inoculation of Cats[a]						
	8	14	19	27	33	40	57
BFU-e[b]	89[d]	60	46	15	4	5	ND
CFU-e[c]	120[d]	110	69	40	15	ND	ND
Hematocrit	97[d]	99	98	78	75	54	28

[a]=7 FeLV-KT infected and 7 age-matched control cats
[b]Burst-forming units-erythroid (day 11 after culture in methylcellulose medium)
[c]Colony-forming units-erythroid (day 5 after culture in methylcellulose medium)
[d]All data expressed as percent of control mean

Table 4. *In vitro* FeLV strain-specific ablation of bone marrow erythroid progenitor cell proliferation

Erythropoietic Index	Inoculum			
	Normal Spleen Extract	FeLV-KT Spleen Origin	mcFeLV-S[a] Culture Origin	FeLV-R Spleen Origin
BFU-e[b]	150[d]	21	27	130
CFU-e[c]	110	92	84	94

[a]Molecularly cloned FeLV-Sarma, subgroup C
[b]Burst-forming units-erythroid (day 11 after culture in methylcellulose medium
[c]Colony-forming units-erythroid (day 5 after culture in methylcellulose medium
[d]Data expressed as percent of parallel non-infected marrow cell cultures

Although the molecular mechanism of FeLV-C-mediated suppression of erythropoiesis is not known, selective tropism for erythroid precursor cells or enhanced genomic replication and resultant excessive unintegrated proviral copies in erythroid progenitor cells are principal candidates.

FeLV-C erythrocytopathic activity probably reflects recombination within the env gene or U3 LTR region. Recent evidence suggests that FeLV subgroup C viruses are in fact recombinants that may arise in hemolymphatic cells and may specify a membrane protein related to FOCMA-L (53-55).

The recent work of Wellman et al (56) has shown that the lymphocyte-suppressive FeLV envelope protein p15E purified from FeLV-KT effects a dramatic, dose-dependent suppression of normal feline marrow CFU-e proliferation. Whether the anti-proliferative action of p15E is specific for anemogenic FeLV strains or is a general property of this hydrophobic membrane-interactive protein is an important question. Infectious FeLV-A or-B subgroup viruses also have been shown to produce transient impairment of erythrogenesis *in vivo* and to suppress proliferation of normal feline CFU-e *in vitro* (57). Ablation of erythropoiesis *in vivo* and abatement of primitive BFU-e progenitor cells however, has yet to be associated with non-subgroup C FeLV's.

Immunodeficiency Syndrome

Feline acquired immunodeficiency syndrome (FAIDS) probably is the most catholic and significant pathogenic manifestation of FeLV infection encountered under experimental (1,7,39-41) and natural (58) conditions. The occurrence of thymo-lymphoid depletion in experimental FeLV transmission experiments has been recognized for 13 years (1,7). Impairment in cell mediated immune functions (39,41), dramatic depletion of T or both T and B cell regions in lymphoid tissues (1,7,40-41a)(Fig. 8), debilitative weight loss, and severe opportunistic infections (Figs. 9,10) characterize FAIDS.

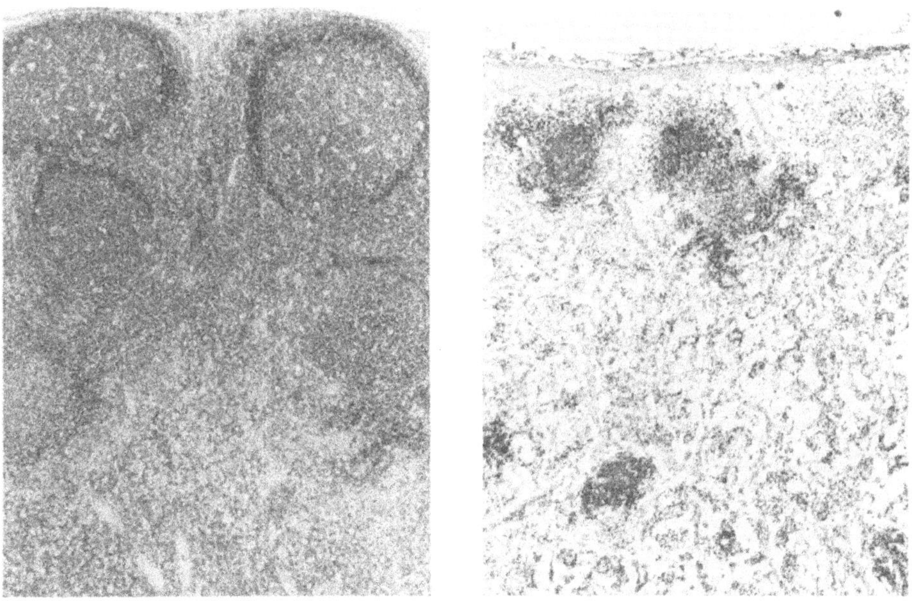

FIGURE 8. Experimentally induced feline acquired immunodeficiency syndrome. Severe paracortical (T cell) and cortical (B cell) depletion in mesenterid lymph node of a cat with experimentally induced immunodeficiency syndrome (right) *vs* the mesenteric node of a normal cat (left).

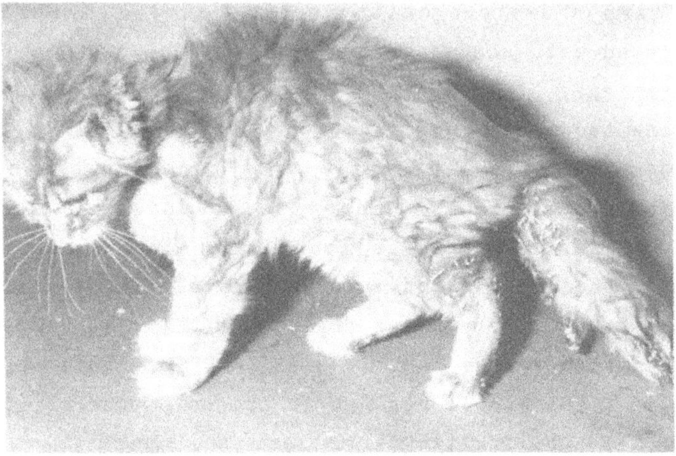

FIGURE 9. Experimentally induced feline acquired immunodeficiency syndrome. Typical clinical manifestations are weight loss, diarrhea, weakness and opportunistic infections.

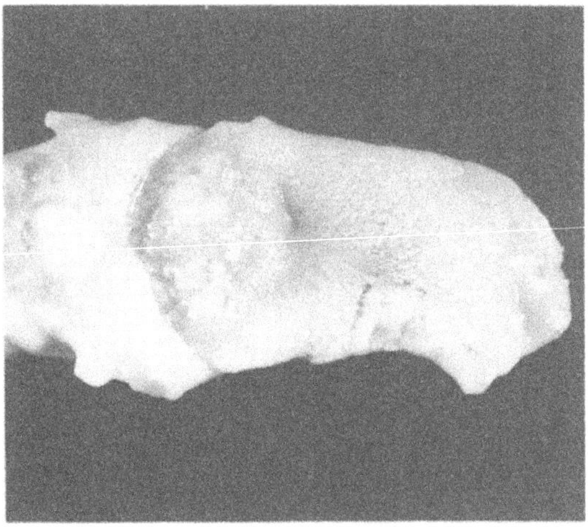

FIGURE 10. Experimentally induced feline acquired immunodeficiency syndrome: Opportunistic infection: Tongue of an affected cat bearing mycotic, necrotizing lesions (arrows) indicative of oral "thrush".

In recent experiments employing serial passage of one FeLV isolate in SPF cats, we have derived a potent FAIDS-inducing strain of FeLV (59). The specific lymphoid cell subset deletion and the molecular mechanism responsible for the immunodeficiency disease elicited by this FeLV strain, as with the erythrosuppressive FeLV isolates, await elucidation.

Embryonic Mortality and Covert Congenital Infection

That FeLV may exhibit tropism for and cytopathic effects on the placenta and embryo were first suggested by the clinical observations of Cotter *et al* (60) identifying the relationship between FeLV viremia and reproductive failure in female cats. Previously, by Chapman *et al* (61) had reported that incubation of hamster embryos with FeLV prior to transfer into receptive uteri interfered with embryonic development. Finally, the finding of Rojko *et al* (62) that latent feline retrovirus was detectable in cultured hemolymphatic tissues of some fetuses or post-natal kittens from queens harboring latent FeLV in bone marrow suggested that regressively infected immune queens may transmit latent FeLV infection transplacentally.

We investigated the potential for congenital retrovirus infection by breeding female SPF cats with either productive or latent FeLV infection to non-infected males. These experiments established that although conception and early embryogenesis proceed normally in viremic pregnant cats, embryonic mortality and placental involution ensued in most pregnancies (78%)(Fig. 11)(63).

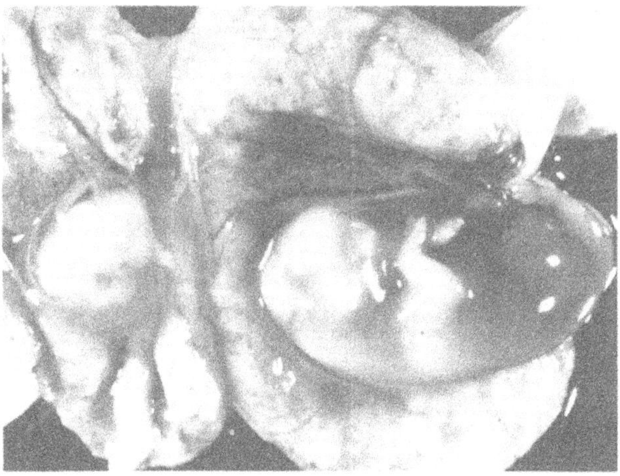

FIGURE 11. FeLV-induced embryonic mortality. Two fetuses and corresponding placentas from a viremic pregnant cat demonstrate asynchronous arrest in fetal development.

Conversely, neither fetal mortality nor overt viral infection were observed in 7 latently infected pregnant cats. However, in 42% of fetuses, low levels of latent FeLV were reactivated by *in vitro* culture. In none of 5 regressor queens in which no latent was detectable, was latent retrovirus detected in fetuses. These results identify an additional cytopathic property of FeLV and provide further evidence for transplacental transfer of latent ecotropic retrovirus infection in mammals.

FeLV Latency and Reactivation

Some cats that develop regressive immunizing FeLV infections retain latent FeLV in marrow myeloid progenitor cells (62). Latent FeLV is reactivatable by *in vitro* by culture of bone marrow of *in vivo* by chronic administration of adrenal corticosteroids. Latent FeLV has been detectd in from marrow myelomonocytic progenitors and staphlococcus protein A-responsive cells in lymph nodes of regressor cats as well as from marrow myelomonocytic cells of cats bearing FeLV-negative neoplasms, and kittens born to dams harboring latent FeLV infection (62). Antibody and cell-mediated reactivity was demonstrated in regressor cats against autologous marrow cells after reactivation of latent FeLV in these target cells by *in vitro* culture (62).

The incidence of latency in cats that experience transient regressive infection after FeLV exposure undoubtedly varies substantially with the infecting virus strain and dose. It appears that establishment of latency requires that curtailment of viral replication in predicated upon progression of infection to the stage of amplification in systemic hemolymphatic tissues (36,37). Cats which restrict FeLV infection at the level of regional lymphoid or mucosal tissues by contrast, do not harbor latent FeLV. Of 17 regressor cats studied by Jarrett and Madewell (64), latent FeLV was recoverable from 10 cats after 20 weeks and from 5 of these cats after 88 weeks. It is probable, therefore, that the duration of FeLV latency in hemopoietic cells varies directly with both the magnitude of the original marrow progenitor cell infection, the immaturity of the hemopoietic cell population infected, and, potentially, the infecting virus strain. It is likely, therefore, that in some cats all clones of latently infected committed myeloid cells undergo extinction via differentiation and emigration from the marrow (clonal extinction).

The epidemiologic studies of Hardy *et al* (39) indicate an association of previous FeLV exposure with FOCMA-bearing, FeLV-negative lymphosarcomas and suggest an etiologic relationship between latent FeLV genomes and leukemogenesis in FeLV-negative cats. Direct evidence for FeLV proviral integration in virus-negative lymphoma, however, remains lacking (65,66). Virus-negative lymphomas have not been produced by experimental inoculation of cats with FeLV, although these experiments are tethered by obvious logistical difficulties. However, Rickard *et al* (67) reported induction of FeLV-negative lymphoproliferative disease in fetal dogs inoculated with FeLV-R. Additionally, de Noronha *et al*. (68) observed one case of FeLV-negative lymphoma in a cat in which injection of passive viral gp70 antibody was used to abrogate FeLV infection early after viral inoculation. In a similar experiment employing cats inoculated with anemogenic FeLV-KT and treated with polyclonal feline immune serum, we have observed one instance of FeLV-negative aplastic anemia (69). The pathogenenic significance of FeLV latency, therefore, remains a cogent subject which awaits further investigation.

In conclusion, experimental investigations of FeLV in outbred cats, illustrate both overt and covert virus-host relationships associated with cytoproliferative and cytopathic diseases. Data obtained with the feline retrovirus system has provided a link between the highly expressed retroviruses of inbred chickens and mice and the highly repressed retroviruses of wild mice, cattle, sheep, horses, macaques, gibbon apes, and man.

REFERENCES:

1. Jarrett WF, Martin WB, Crighton GW, Dalton RG, Stewart MF: Leukemia in the cat. Transmission experiments with leukemia (lymphosarcoma). Nature (London)(202):566-567, 1965.

2. Rickard CG, Post JE, Noronha F, Barr LM: A transmissible virus-induced lymphocytic leukemia of the cat. J Natl Cancer Inst (42):987-1014, 1969.

3. Anderson LJ, Jarrett WF, Jarrett O: Leukemia virus infection of kittens: mortality associated with atrophy of the thymus and lymphoid depletion. J Natl Cancer Inst (47):807-817.

4. Mackey LJ, Jarrett WFH, Jarrett O, Laird HM: An experimental study of leukemia in cats. J Natl Cancer Inst (48):1663-1670.

5. Theilen GH, Dungworth DL, Kawakami T, Munn RJ, Ward JM, Harrold JB: Experimental induction of lymphosarcoma in the cat with "C"-type virus. Cancer Res (30):401-403, 1970.

6. Gardner MB, Arnstein P, Rongey RW, Estes JD, Sarma P, Rickard CG, Huebner RJ: Experimental transmission of feline fibrosarcoma to cats and dogs. Nature (London) (226):807-809, 1970.

7. Hoover EA, McCullough B, Griesemer RA: Intranasal transmission of feline leukemia. J Natl Cancer Inst (9):973-983, 1972.

8. Hoover EA, Olsen RG, Hardy WD Jr., Schaller JP, Mathes LE: Feline leukemia virus infection: age-related variation in response of cats to experimental infection. J Natl Cancer Inst (5):365-369, 1976.

9. Hoover EA, Olsen RG, Hardy WD Jr., Schaller JP: Horizontal transmission of feline leukemia virus under experimental conditions. J Natl Cancer Inst (58):443-444, 1977.

10. Jarrett W, Jarrett O, Mackey L, Laird HM, Hardy WD Jr., Essex M: Horizontal transmission of leukemia virus and leukemia in the cat. J Natl Cancer Inst (51):833, 1973.

11. Hardy WD Jr., Old LJ, Hess PW, Essex M, Cotter SM: Horizontal transmission of feline leukemia virus. Nature (London)(244):266-269, 1973.

12. Hardy WD Jr., Hess PW, MacEwen EG, McClelland AJ, Zuckerman EE, Essex M, Cotter SM, Jarrett O: Biology of feline leukemia virus in the natural environment. Cancer Res (36):582-588, 1976.

13. Essex M, Cotter SM, Hardy WD Jr., Hess P, Jarrett W, Jarrett O, Mackey L, Laird H, Perryman L, Olsen RG, Yohn DS: Feline oncornavirus-associated cell membrane antigen. IV. Antibody titers in cats with naturally occurring leukemia, lymphoma, and other diseases. J Natl Cancer Inst (55):463-467, 1975.

14. Essex M, Cotter SM, Sliski AH, Hardy WD Jr., Stephensen FU, Aaronson SA, Jarrett O: Horizontal transmission of feline leukemia virus under natural conditions in a feline leukemia cluster household. Int J Cancer (19): 90-96, 1977.

15. Gardner MB, Rongey RW, Jonson EY, DeJournett R: C-type tumor virus particles in salivary tissue of domestic cats. J Natl Cancer Inst (47):561-568.

16. Hoover EA, Olsen RG, Mathes LE, Schaller JP: Relationship between feline leukemia virus antigen expression in blood and bone marrow and viral infectivity in blood, bone marrow, and saliva of cats. Cancer Res (37):3707-3710, 1977.

17. Francis DP, Essex M, Hardy WD Jr:. Excretion of feline leukemia virus by naturally infected pet cats. Nature (London) (269):252-254, 1977.

18. Francis DP, Essex M, Gayzagian D: Feline leukemia virus survival under home and laboratory conditions. J Clin Microbiol (9):154-156, 1979.

19. Fischinger PJ, Blevins CS, Nomura S: Simple quantitative assay for both xentropic murine leukemia and ecotropic feline leukemia viruses. J Virol (14):177-179, 1974.

20. Hoover EA, Quackenbush SL, Gasper PW: Unpublished data.

21. Hoover EA, Rojko JL, Olsen RG: Pathogenesis of Feline Leukemia Virus Infection. In: Olsen RG (eg) Feline leukemia. CRC Press, Boca Raton, Florida, 1980, pp. 32-51.

22. Sarma PS, Log T: Subgroup classification of feline leukemia and sarcoma viruses by viral interference and neutralization tests. Virology (54):160-169, 1973.

23. Sarma PS, Log T, Skuntz S, Krishman S, Burkley K: Experimental horizontal transmission of feline leukemia viruses of subgroups A,B, and C. J Natl Cancer Inst (60):871-874, 1978.

24. Jarrett O, Laird HM, Hay D: Determinants of the host range of feline leukemia viruses. J Gen Virol (20):169-175, 1973.

25. Jarrett O, Hardy WD Jr., Golder MC, Hay D: The frequency of occurrence of feline leukemia virus subgroups in cats. Int J Cancer (21)334-337, 1978.

26. Jarrett O, Russel PH: Differential growth and transmission in cats of feline leukemia viruses of subgroups A and B. Int J Cancer (21):466, 1978.

27. Hoover EA, Kociba GJ, Hardy WD Jr., Yohn DS: Erythroid hypoplasia in cats inoculated with feline leukemia virus. J Natl Cancer Inst (53):1271-1276, 1974.

28. Mackey L, Jarrett W, Jarrett O, Laird HM: Anemia associated with feline leukemia virus infection in cats. J Natl Cancer Inst (54):209-217, 1975.

29. Onions DO, Jarrett O, Testa N, et. al.: Selective effect of feline leukemia virus on early erythroid precursors. Nature (296):156-158, 1982.

30. Essex M, Klein G, Snyder SP, Harrold JB: Antibody to oncornavirus-associated cell membrane antigen in neonatal cats. Int. J. Cancer (8):384-390, 1971.

31. Hoover EA, Schaller JP, Mathes LE, Olsen RG: Passive immunity to feline leukemia: Evaluation of immunity from dams naturally infected and experimentally vaccinated. Infect Immun (16):54-59, 1977.

32. Rojko JL, Hoover EA, Mathes LE, Krakowka S, Olsen RG: Influence of adrenal corticosteroids on the susceptibility of cats to feline leukemia virus infection. Cancer Res (38):3789-3791, 1979.

33. Hoover EA, Rojko JL, Wilson PL, Olsen RG: Determinants of susceptibility and resistance to feline leukemia virus: I. Role of Macrophages. J Natl Cancer Inst (67):889-898, 1981.

34. Schaller JP, Mathes LE, Hoover EA, Koestner A, Olsen RG: Increased susceptibility to feline leukemia virus infection in cats exposed to methylnitrosourea. Cancer Res (38):996-998, 1978.

35. Rojko JL, Hoover EA, Mathes LE, Krakowka S, Olsen RG: Pathogenesis of experimental feline leukemia virus infection. J Natl Cancer Inst (63):759-768, 1979.

36. Hoover EA, Rojko JL, Olsen RG: Host-virus interactions in progressive vs. regressive feline leukemia virus infection cats. In: Cold Spring Harbor Conference on Cell Proliferation, Vol 7, Cold Spring Harbor, New York. 1980, pp 86-95.

37. Rojko JL, Hoover EA, Finn BL, et. al.: Determinants of susceptibiligy and resistance to feline leukemia virus: II. Susceptibility of feline lymphocytes to productive infection. J. Natl. Cancer Inst. (67):899-910, 1981.

38. Hardy WD Jr, McClelland AJ, Zuckerman EE, Snyder HW Jr, MacEwen EG, Francis D, Essex M: Development of virus nonproducer lymphosarcomas in pet cats exposed to FeLV. Nature (288):90, 1980.

39. Perryman LE, Hoover EA, Yohn DS: Immunologic reactivity of the cat: Immunosuppression in experimental feline leukemia. J. Natl Cancer Inst (49):1357-1365, 1972.

40. Hoover EA, Perryman LE, Kociba GJ: Early lesions in cats inoculated with feline leukemia virus. Cancer Res (33):145-152, 1973.

41. Cockerell GL, Hoover EA, Krakowka S, Olsen RG, Yohn DS. Lymphocyte mitogen reactivity and enumeration of circulating B- and T-cells during feline leukemia virus infection in the cat. J Natl Cancer Inst (57):1095-1099, 1976.

41a. Cockerell GL, Krakowka S, Hoover EA, Olsen RG, Yohn DS: Characterization of feline T-and B-lymphocytes and identification of an experimentally induced T-cell neoplasm in the cat. J. Natl. Cancer Inst. (57):907, 1976.

42. Mathes LE, Olsen RG: Immunobiology of Feline Leukemia Virus Disease, In: Olsen RG (ed) Feline Leukemia, Olsen RG (ed) CRC Press, 1981, pp. 77-88.

43. Trainin Z, Ungar-Waron H, Essex M: Suppression of the Humoral Antibody Response in Natural Retrovirus Infections. Science (220):858-859, 1983.

44. Neil JC, Hughes D, McFarlane R, Wilkie NM: Transduction and rearrangement of the myc gene by feline leukaemia virus in naturally occurring T-cell leukaemias. Nature (308):814-820, 1984.

45. Levy LS, Gardner MB, Casey JW: Isolation of a feline leukaemia provirus containing the oncogene myc from a feline lymphosarcoma. Nature (308):853-856, 1984.

46. Mullins JI, Brody DS, Binari RC Jr, Cotter SM: Viral transduction of c-myc gene in naturally occurrine feline leukaemias. Nature (308):856-858, 1984.

47. Boyce JT, Hoover EA, Kociba GJ, Olsen RG: Feline Leukemia Virus-Induced Erythroid Aplasia. In Vitro Hemopoietic Culture Studies. Exp. Hematol. (9):990-1001, 1981.

48. Gasper PW, Hoover EA: Feline leukemia virus-induced aplastic anemia: The sequence of antiproliferative events. Exp Hematol 11 (suppl), (14):153, 1983.

49. Kociba GJ, Hoover EA, Sciulli VM, Olsen RG: Feline leukemia virus-induced erythroid aplasia: Corticosteroid enhancement in vivo and FeLV suppression of erythroipoiesis in vitro. In: Yohn DS and Blakeslees JR (eds) Advances in comparative leukemia research 1981, Elsevier, New York 1981, pp. 211-212.

50. Gasper PW, Hoover EA: Feline leukemia virus strain specific abatement of erythroid burst forming units (BFU-e). Leuk Rev Int (1):71-72, 1983.

51. Testa NG, Onions D, Jarrett O, Frassoni F, Eliason JF: Haemopoietic colony formation (BFU-e, GM-CFC) during the development of pure red cell hypoplasia induced in the cat by feline leukaemia virus. Leuk Res (7):103-15, 1983.

51a. Mullins JI: Personal communication, 1984.

52. Gasper PW, Hoover EA, Dornsife RE, Mullins JI: Cytopathic depletion of erythroid burst forming progenitor cells by anemogenic feline leukemia viruses (FeLV). Proc. International Conference on RNA Tumor Viruses in Human Cancer, June 10-14, 1984.

53. Snyder HW, Singhal MC, Zuckerman EE, Jones FR, Hardy WD Jr: The feline oncornavirus-associated cell membrane antigen (FOCMA) is related to, but distinguishable from, FeLV-C gp70. Virology (131):315-327, 1983.

54. Vedbrat SS, Rasheed S, Lutz H, Gonda MA, Ruscetti S, Gardner MB, Prensky W: Feline oncornavirus-associated cell membrane antigen: a viral and not a cellularly coded transformation-specific antigen of cat lymphomas. Virology (124):445-461, 1983.

55. Hardy WD Jr, Zuckerman EE, Markovich R, Singhal M, Snyder HW Jr.: Correlation of FOCMA and FeLV-C neutralizing antibodies in pet cats. Proc IVth Int FeLV Meeting, Dec. 11-16, 1983, pp 53.

56. Wellman ML, Kociba GJ, Lewis MG, Mathes LE, Olsen RG: Inhibition of erythroid colony-forming cells by a MW 15,000 protein of feline leukemia virus. Cancer Res (44):1527-1529, 1984.

57. Rojko JL, Cheney CM, Kociba GJ, Mathes LE, Olsen RG: Infectious feline leukemia virus depresses erythrogenesis in vitro. Leuk Rev Int (1):129-130, 1983.

58. Hardy WD Jr: Immunopathology induced by the feline leukemia virus. Springer Semin Immunopathol (5):75-106, 1982.

59. Hoover EA, Quackenbush SL: Unpublished data, 1984.

60. Cotter SM, Hardy WD Jr, Essex M: Association of feline leukemia virus with lymphosarcoma and other disorders in the cat. J. Am Vet Med Assoc (166):449-454, 1975.

61. Chapman AL, Weitlauf HM, Bopp W: Effect of feline leukemia virus on transferred hamster fetuses. J Natl Cancer Inst (52):583-586, 1974.

62. Rojko JL, Hoover EA, Quackenbush SL, Olsen RG: Reactivation of latent feline leukemia virus infection. Nature (298):385-388, 1982.

63. Hoover EA, Rojko JL, Quackenbush SL: Congenital feline leukemia virus infection. Leuk Rev Int (1):7-8, 1983.

64. Jarrett O, Madewell BR, Pacitti A: Latent FeLV infection in the bone marrow of naturally infected cats. Proc. IVth Int FeLV Meeting. Dec. 12-16, 1983, pp 74.

65. Casey JW, Roach A, Mullins JI, Bauman Burck K, Nicholson M, Gardner MB, Davidson N: The U3 portion of feline leukemia virus DNA identifies horizontally acquired proviruses in leukemic cats. Proc Natl Acad Sci USA (78):7778-7782, 1981.

66. Wong Stall F, Koshy R, Gallo RC: Feline leukemia virus genomes associated with the domestic cat: a survey of normal and leukemic animals. In: Essex M, Todaro G, Zur hausen H (eds) Viruses in naturally occurring cancers. Cold Spring Harbor Laboratory, New York, 1980, pp 635-640.

67. deNoronha F, Schafer W, Essex M, Bolognesi D: Influence of antisera to oncornavirus glycoprotein (gp71) on infections of cats with feline leukemia virus. Virology (85):617-621, 1978.

68. Hoover EA, Quackenbush SL, Gasper PW: Unpublished data, 1984.

69. Rickard CG, Post JE, Noronha F, Barr LM: Interspecies infection by feline leukemia virus: Serial cell-free transmission in dogs of malignant lymphomas induced by feline leukemia virus. In: Dutcher RM and Chieco-Bianchi L (eds) Unifying concepts of leukemia. Karger, Basel, 1973, pp 102-112.

23

FELINE LEUKEMIA AND SARCOMA VIRUSES

WILLIAM D. HARDY, JR.
Memorial Sloan Kettering Cancer Center, New York, New York 10021

INTRODUCTION

There are an estimated 40 million pet cats in the United States and approximately 2%, or 1 million cats, are infected with the feline leukemia virus (FeLV) (1). The virus is spread contagiously among pet cats and is the most frequent killer of cats among infectious disease microorganisms (1-4). FeLV causes both proliferative (neoplastic) and degenerative (blastopenic) diseases in cats living in household conditions (2,3). More FeLV-infected pet cats develop degenerative diseases than develop neoplastic diseases (1). Of all the retroviruses, the biology of FeLV has been most completely elucidated.

VIROLOGY

The cat has two major groups of retroviruses, the endogenous and exogenous viruses (Table 1).

Endogenous retroviruses

The RD-114 virus is an endogenous xenotropic retrovirus that has not been associated with any feline disease (5,6). The virus is closely related to the baboon endogenous virus (BaEV) and, although the virus does not replicate in cats, multiple complete proviral copies are present in all cat cells (7,8).

Endogenous FeLV-related sequences

The cellular DNA of healthy uninfected pet cats also contains sequences that are partially homologous with the exogenous contagiously transmitted FeLV

(9,10). There are 8 to 12 discrete copies of endogenous FeLV-related sequences arranged in a non-tandem fashion in the cat genome (11). The endogenous FeLV sequences have a large deletion in the *gag-pol* region and a smaller deletion in the *env* region making the sequences 4 kbp compared to the 8.5 to 8.7 kbp genome of infectious FeLV (12). Due to the large genomic deletions, the endogenous FeLV sequences are not inducible as infectious viral particles (12,13). However, the endogenous FeLV sequences may recombine with infectious FeLV to form FeLV with a recombinant *env* gene, similar to the leukemogenic MCF MuLVs of mice (14,15).

Table 1

FELINE RETROVIRUSES

Type of Virus	Characteristics
Endogenous Viruses	
RD-114	Xenotropic- does not replicate in cats no known disease association
Endogenous FeLV-related sequences	Cannot be induced to replicate as virus
Exogenous Viruses	
FeLVs	
Subgroup A	Ecotropic- found in all infected cats
Subgroup B	Amphotropic- found in 50% of infected cats
Subgroup C	Amphotropic- found rarely, less than 1%
Defective FeLV-*myc* recombinant proviruses	Found in 14% of FeLV-infected thymic LSAs
FeSVs	
10 well characterized isolates to date	Recombinants between FeLV and cellular oncogenes

Exogenous infectious FeLVs

The three FeLV subgroups, A, B, and, C are distinguished by their gp70 molecules (16,17). FeLV-A is ecotropic since it has the most restricted host range and grows almost exclusively in cat cells (16,17). FeLV-A has been found in all infected cats either alone (50%), in combination with FeLV-B (49%), or as a mixture with FeLV-B and FeLV-C (1%) (18,19). FeLV-B is amphotropic, has the widest host range and can infect cat, mink, hamster, dog, pig, cow, monkey and human cells (16,17). The nucleotide sequences of the *env* genes of FeLV-B and a Moloney MuLV MCF virus show striking homology (23). This suggests that FeLV-B may arise from recombination of FeLV-A and endogenous *env* sequences. FeLV-C is also amphotropic but has an intermediate host range. Although there is no clear association of any subgroup of FeLV with any specific disease, one strain of FeLV-A has induced mainly thymic lymphosarcomas (LSAs) and several isolates of FeLV-C have induced erythroid hypoplasia (20-22).

Defective FeLV-*myc* recombinant proviruses

Defective FeLV proviruses containing the *myc* oncogene have been found in the DNA of 8 of 58 (14%) pet cats with FeLV-positive thymic LSAs (24-26). The *myc* sequences were found to be encapsidated in helper infectious FeLV (24). These findings suggest that oncogene containing defective retroviruses may occur more frequently than was previously thought and that these viruses may be transmitted contagiously. However, it is not clear what, if any, relationship these defective *myc*-containing proviruses have to the etiology of feline LSAs.

Latent FeLV

FeLV can persist in a latent state in mononuclear cells of the bone marrow of immune cats that have rejected the virus (27). Latent FeLV can be reactivated *in vivo* from the bone marrow cells by treating such cats with corticosteroids or by stimulating bone marrow cultures *in vitro* with corticosteroids or *Staphylococcus aureus* Cowan I. However, reactivation of latent FeLV has not been shown to occur without experimental stimulation in immune pet cats living in households.

Feline sarcoma viruses

Feline sarcoma viruses (FeSVs) are replication defective acute transforming retroviruses that possess oncogenes (v-oncs), acquired through recombination of the FeLV genome with single copy cellular c-onc (protooncogenes) genes (28-30). FeSVs induce neoplasms in a short latent period and transform cells of various species in vitro. To date there are 10 well characterized FeSV isolates (Table 2). Seven different oncogenes have been transduced by FeSVs: v-fes, v-fms, v-sis, v-abl, v-fgr, v-rasK, and v-kit. The gene order in the FeSVs characterized to date is 5'-gag-onc-env-3' (8).

Table 2

FELINE SARCOMA VIRUSES

FeSV Isolate		v-onc	Protein Product	Protein Kinase
Snyder-Theilen	ST-FeSV	fes	$P85^{gag-fes}$	+
Gardner-Arnstein	GA-FeSV	fes	$P95^{gag-fes}$	+
Hardy-Zuckerman 1	HZ1-FeSV	fes	$P96^{gag-fes}$	+
Susan-McDonough	SM-FeSV	fms	$gp170^{gag-fms}$	-
Hardy-Zuckerman 5	HZ5-FeSV	fms	ND	-
Parodi-Irgens	PI-FeSV	sis	$P76^{gag-sis}$	-
Gardner-Rasheed	GR-FeSV	fgr	$P70^{gag-fgr}$	+
Hardy-Zuckerman 2	HZ2-FeSV	abl	$P98^{gag-abl}$	+
Noronha-Youngren	NY-FeSV	rasK	ND	ND
Hardy-Zuckerman 4	HZ4-FeSV	kit	$P80^{gag-kit}$	-

ND= not determined

v-fes FeSVs: ST-, GA-, and HZ1-FeSVs. The fes oncogene is the most prevalent retroviral oncogene and is found in 3 FeSVs and 5 avian sarcomas viruses (ASVs) (8). The three FeSVs possessing v-fes are the Snyder-Theilen (ST), Gardner-Arnstein (GA), and Hardy-Zuckerman 1 (HZ1) isolates (31-34). The fps sequences of the Fujinami ASV are homologous with the fes sequences of the cat FeSVs (35,36). The gag-fes product of the FeSV genomes exhibit a tyrosine-specific protein kinase activity (37).

v-fms FeSVs: SM- and HZ5-FeSVs. Two FeSVs possess the v-fms oncogene which, to date, has only been found in FeSVs. The two FeSV isolates containing v-fms are the Susan McDonough (SM) and the Hardy-Zuckerman 5 (HZ5)-FeSVs (29,38-40). Unlike other transforming proteins, the v-fms protein products are extensively glycosylated (41).

Other v-onc containing FeSVs. Five other FeSV isolates have been found to contain v-oncs other than v-fes and v-fms. The Hardy-Zuckerman 2 (HZ2)-FeSV has the v-abl oncogene that is homologous to the v-abl of the Abelson MuLV (33,42). The v-abl oncogene of the Abelson MuLV induces B-, T-, and myeloid tumors in mice whereas v-abl in the HZ2-FeSV induces sarcomas. The Parodi-Irgens (PI)-FeSV possesses the v-sis oncogene that is homologous to the v-sis of the simian sarcoma virus (SSV) (43,44). PI-FeSV and SSV sis sequences are in different contexts in their viral genomes (43). Recently the sis oncogene has been shown to encode a protein that has extensive homology with platelet-derived growth factor (PDGF), a growth factor produced in platelets which stimulates fibroblast proliferation in healing wounds (45-47).

The v-onc of a new FeSV, the Noronha-Youngren (NY)-FeSV is homologous to the v-rasK of the Kirsten sarcoma virus (48). Two other FeSVs, the Gardner-Rasheed (GR) and the Hardy-Zuckerman 4 (HZ4)-FeSV, possess unique oncogenes, v-fgr and v-kit respectively (49-52).

The cat appears to be a unique species from which acute transforming viruses, FeSVs, are commonly isolated. To date, FeSVs have transduced 7 different oncogenes, 3 of which are unique to FeSVs. Since there are an estimated 1 million FeLV-infected cats in the United States today, it is likely that many more FeSVs will be isolated, some of which may possess new oncogenes.

The observation that many oncogenes have been transduced by retroviruses from different species suggests that the number of oncogenes is limited.

EPIDEMIOLOGY

Large epidemiological studies of the occurrence of FeLV, using an immunofluorescent antibody (IFA) test, have been done in the U.S. and Europe (1,4,18,53-55). These studies showed that the virus is transmitted contagiously among cats and that 28% of exposed healthy cats are persistently infected (4,18). However, 42% of exposed cats become immune to the virus and the remaining 30% become neither persistently infected nor immune (1,18). In contrast to multiple cat pet households, less than 1% of stray cats are infected with the virus (1). Approximately 10 to 20% of persistently infected pet cats develop LSA whereas more far more infected cats die of the immunosuppressive effects of the virus than develop LSA (1,4,18).

The spread of FeLV among cats can be prevented by detecting infected carrier cats and removing them from contact with other cats (58). When all cats are negative for FeLV in two consecutive tests, done 3 months apart, the cats in the household are considered free of the virus. This IFA test and removal program has reduced the spread of FeLV 40 fold in those households where infected cats are removed from contact with uninfected cats compared to households that did not remove infected cats (58). The FeLV test and removal program is presently used by veterinarians throughout the world to prevent the spread of this virus.

IMMUNOLOGY

The fate of an FeLV-exposed cat depends on its immune response to the viral gp70, virus neutralizing (VN) antibody, and to the FeLV-induced tumor-specific feline oncornavirus associated cell membrane antigen (FOCMA). Cats with 1:10 or greater VN antibody titers are resistant to FeLV infection and cats with 1:32 or greater FOCMA antibody titers are resistant to the development of LSA, but are not resistant to the development of FeLV degenerative diseases (1,18,56,57). Both VN and FOCMA antibody are found mainly in cats living in FeLV-infected exposure households (18,19). Few, if any FeLV-infected cats have detectable free FeLV-A or -B VN antibody.

FELINE ONCORNAVIRUS ASSOCIATED CELL MEMBRANE ANTIGEN (FOCMA)

FOCMA was initially described as an antigen on the cell membranes of cultured feline LSA cells (59). Cats with high titers of FOCMA antibody are resistant to FeLV-induced LSAs (18,57). FOCMA is found on the cell membranes of all feline T-and B-LSA cells irrespective of their FeLV status and on FeLV-induced erythroid and myeloid leukemia cells (56,60). In contrast, FOCMA is absent from normal feline lymphoid and myeloid cells, even those replicating FeLV-A and -B (56). Thus, FOCMA is an FeLV-induced tumor-specific antigen. The expression of FOCMA on FeLV-negative LSA cells indicates that FOCMA is a marker of FeLV leukemogenesis.

The FOCMA molecule has been characterized as a protein of 70,000 dalton molecular weight which, by peptide mapping, is different from the gp70 molecules of FeLV-A and -B (60-62). Recent studies have found that FOCMA is related to, but distinguisable from FeLV-C gp70 (61,62). Since FeLV-C is rarely (<1%) detected in infected cats, FOCMA may be a variant of FeLV-C gp70 induced through recombination of contagiously transmitted FeLV-A with endogenous FeLV-C related sequences.

FELV DISEASES

FeLV replicates in rapidly dividing cells and can produce proliferative (neoplastic) and degenerative (blastopenic) diseases in these cells (Table 3).

Table 3

Feline Leukemia Virus Diseases

Cell Type	Proliferative Diseases (Neoplastic)	Degenerative Diseases (Blastopenic)
Lymphocytes	Lymphosarcoma	Thymic atrophy Lymphopenias Feline acquired immune deficiency syndrome (FAIDS)
Bone Marrow Cells:		
Primitive mesenchymal cell	Reticuloendotheliosis	------
Erythroblast	Erythremic myelosis	Erythroblastosis
	Erythroleukemia	Erythroblastopenia Pancytopenia
Myeloblast	Granulocytic leukemia	Myeloblastopenia
Megakaryocyte	Megakaryocytic leukemia	Thrombocytopenia
Fibroblast	Myelofibrosis	------
Osteoblast	Medullary osteosclerosis	------
	Osteochondromatosis	------
Kidney	-----	FeLV immune complex glomerulonephritis
Uterus	-----	Abortions and resorptions
Fibroblasts,skin	FeSV-induced multicentric fibrosarcomas	-----

The most frequent clinical consequence of FeLV infection is not the development of LSA but is the severe immunosuppression which leads to development of secondary opportunistic infections and death (1,63).

Lymphoid diseases

Lymphosarcoma. Pet cats have the highest incidence of naturally occurring LSA of any animal with 200 cases occurring per 100,000 cats at risk (1). Most feline LSAs are T-cell tumors (56). Seventy per cent of cats with LSA are infected with FeLV whereas 30% are FeLV-negative. In contrast to FeLV-positive LSAs, FeLV-negative LSAs do not have infectious FeLV nor FeLV-antigens, occur in older cats (over 7 years of age), and are usually B-cell in origin (56,64). However, both FeLV-positive and -negative LSAs have FOCMA expressed on their cell membranes (56). In a large epidemiological survey, we found that FeLV-negative cats with LSA have the same degree of exposure to FeLV as do FeLV-positive LSA cats (64). Recently, FeLV has been reactivated from the bone marrow cells, but not from the LSA cells, of cats with FeLV-negative LSAs (27). This finding is direct evidence for the etiologic association of FeLV in FeLV-negative LSAs.

Degenerative lymphoid diseases. FeLV replicates in feline lymphoid cells and often induces severe depletion and dysfunctions of these cells. Thymic atrophy is a degenerative lymphoid disease of T-cells of the thymus of kittens (63,65). The virus causes depletion of thymic lymphocytes resulting in a deficient cellular immune system and death from secondary infections. Lymphoid atrophy occurs in FeLV-infected adult cats and leads to lowered resistance to infectious agents and to the frequent occurrence of secondary opportunistic diseases.

Feline acquired immune deficiency syndrome (FAIDS)

FeLV-infected cats often develop immune cell deficiencies characterized by drastic reduction of lymphocytes and neutrophils, cutaneous anergy, reduced T-cell blastogenic responsiveness and impaired antibody production (63,66-68). More pet cats die from FeLV-induced FAIDS than die from neoplastic diseases (63).

The mechanism by which FeLV causes FAIDS is not understood, but several possibilities exist: 1) FeLV may cause cell lysis by budding from the cell membrane, 2) FeLV p15E has been shown to decrease *in vitro* blast transformation by 45 to 92% (69) and free p15E in the plasma of viremic cats may thus be immunosuppressive and, 3) circulating immune complexes (CICs) are immunosuppressive and CICs composed of whole infectious FeLV, FeLV gp70, p27, p15, and p15E have been detected in FeLV-infected cats (63,70).

There are numerous similarities between FeLV-induced FAIDS and human AIDS (71). Both syndromes are characterized by lymphopenias, reduced lymphocyte blastogenesis, cutaneous anergy, reduced numbers of T-cells, impaired antibody response and the occurrence of secondary infectious diseases. FAIDS is caused by a T-cell tropic retrovirus and human AIDS is caused by a variant of the T-cell tropic human T-cell leukemia virus, HTLV-III (72).

Erythroid diseases

FeLV replicates in nucleated erythroid cells in the bone marrow and can induce neoplastic or degenerative erythroid diseases (2,53,73,74).

Erythroid neoplastic diseases. FeLV rarely causes erythremic myelosis and erythroleukemia in infected cats (74,75). Acute leukemia viruses, similar to the acute avian leukemia viruses, may be the etiologic agents of these feline diseases.

FeLV-induced anemias. Erythroid degenerative diseases, anemias, occur far more frequently in infected cats than do erythroid neoplastic diseases (74,75). Three types of FeLV-induced anemias occur: 1) erythroblastosis (regenerative anemia), 2) erthroblastopenia (non-regenerative anemia) and, 3) pancytopenia (73,74). Non-fatal transient regenerative anemias have been experimentally induced by FeLV-A whereas several FeLV-C isolates have induced fatal non-regenerative anemias (22,76).

Myeloid diseases

FeLV replicates in all myeloid cells, neutrophils, basophils, and eosinophils, in the bone marrow and causes neoplastic and degenerative diseases of these cells (53,73).

Myeloproliferative diseases. FeLV-induced neoplastic myeloid disease include reticuloendotheliosis, neutrophilic leukemia, myelofibrosis, and osteosclerosis. These diseases occur only rarely in infected cats.

Myeloid degenerative diseases. A specific FeLV-induced myeloblastopenia syndrome occurs more commonly than do myeloproliferative diseases. In this disease there is severe erosion of the epithelium of the intestinal mucosa of the small bowel and a panleukopenia (73, 74). Cats with this disease die of secondary infections which enter through the intestinal lesions.

Other FeLV diseases

FeLV induces abortions and resorptions in some persistently infected pregnant queens (73,74). The virus has also been associated with a neurologic syndrome that is similar to the neurologic syndrome observed in amphotropic MuLV-infected wild mice (53,,74,). In addition, as in AKR and NZB mice, some FeLV-infected cats develop immune complex glomerulonephritis where FeLV antigens, IgG and complement are deposited in the glomeruli (63,73,74,77).

FeSV fibrosarcomas

Fibrosarcomas account for between 6-12% of cat tumors (28,30). FeSVs rarely induce multicentric fibrosarcomas in young cats (average age 3 years) whereas the more common solitary fibrosarcomas that occur in older cats (average age 10 years) are not caused by FeSVs. FeSV-induced fibrosarcomas are usually poorly differentiated tumors and are more invasive than the non-FeSV-induced fibrosarcomas. There are no reports of clusters of FeSV-induced fibrosarcomas in multiple cat households which suggests that FeSVs arise *de novo* in FeLV-infected cats and thus are probably not transmitte contagiously.

REFERENCES

1. Hardy WD Jr : The feline leukemia virus. J Am Animal Hosp Asso (17):951-976, 1981.

2. Hardy WD Jr : Feline Retroviruses. *In*: Klein, G. (ed) Advances in Vira Oncology. Raven Press, New York, in press.

3. Essex M : Feline leukemia and sarcoma viruses. *In*: Klein, G (ed) Vira Oncology. Raven Press, New York, 1980, pp.205-229.

4. Hardy WD Jr, Old LJ, Hess PW, Essex M, Cotter S : Horizonta transmission of feline leukaemia virus. Nature (244):266-269, 1973.

5. McAllister RM, Nicolson M, Gardner MB, Rongey RW, Rasheed S, Sarma PS Huebner RJ, Hatanaka M, Oroszlan S, Gilden RV, Kabigting A, Vernon L : RD 114 comparison with feline and murine type C viruses released from R cells. Nature (242):75-78, 1973.

6. Sarma PS, Tsing J, Lee YK, Gilden RV : Viruses similar to RD114 virus i cat cells. Nature (224):56-59, 1973.

7. Benveniste RE, Todaro GJ : Homology between type-C viruses of variou species as determined by molecular hybridization. Proc. Natl. Acad. Sc (70):3316-3320, 1973.

8. Todaro GJ, Tevethia S, Melnick J : Isolation of an RD-114 related type- virus from feline sarcoma virus-transformed baboon cells. Intervirolog (1):399-404, 1974.

9. Benveniste RE, Sherr CJ, Todaro GJ : Evolution of type C viral genes Origin of feline leukemia virus. Science (190):886-888, 1975.

10. Okabe H, Twiddy E, Gilden RV, Hatanaka M, Hoover EA, Olsen RG : FeLV related sequences in DNA from a FeLV-free cat colony. Virolog (69):798-801,1976.

11. Koshy R, Wong-Staal F, Gallo RC, Hardy WD Jr, Essex M : Distribution c feline leukemia virus DNA sequences in tissues of normal and leukemi domestic cats. Virology (99):135-144, 1979.

12. Soe LH, Devi BG, Mullins JI, Roy-Burman P : Molecular cloning ar characterization of endogenous feline leukemia virus sequences from a ca genomic library. J Virol (46):829-840, 1983.

13. Okabe H, DuBuy J, Gilden RV, Gardner MB : A portion of the felir leukemia virus genome is not endogenous in cat cells. Int J Cance (22):70-78, 1978.

14. Hartley JW, Wolford NK, Old LJ, Rowe WP : A new class of murine leukem virus associated with development of spontaneous lymphomas. Proc Na

Acad Sci (74):789-792, 1977.

15. Hardy WD Jr : A new package for an old oncogene. Nature (308): 775, 1984.

16. Sarma PS, Log T : Subgroup classification of feline leukemia and sarcoma viruses by viral interference and neutralization tests. Virology (54):160-169, 1973.

17. Jarrett O, Laird HM, Hay D : Determinants of the host range of feline leukaemia viruses. J Gen Virol (20):169-175, 1973.

18. Hardy WD Jr, Hess PW, MacEwen EG, McClelland AJ, Zuckerman EE, Essex M, Cotter SM, Jarrett O : Biology of feline leukemia virus in the natural environment. Cancer Res (36):582-588, 1976.

19. Jarrett O, Hardy WD Jr, Golder MC, Hay D : The frequency of occurrence of feline leukemia virus subgroups in cats. Int J Cancer(21):334-337, 1978.

20. Rickard CG, Post JE, Noronha F, Barr LM : A transmissible virus-induced lymphocytic leukemia of the cat. J Natl Cancer Inst (42):987-1014, 1969.

21. Hoover EA, Kociba GJ, Hardy WD Jr, Yohn DS : Erythroid hypoplasis in cats inoculated with feline leukemia virus. J Natl Cancer Inst (53):1271-1276, 1974.

22. Onions D, Jarrett O, Testa N, Frassoni F, Toth S : Selective effect of feline leukaemia virus on early erythroid precursors. Nature (296):156-158, 1982.

23. Elder JH, Mullins JI : Nucleotide sequence of the envelope gene of Gardner-Arnstein feline leukemia virus B reveals unique sequence homologies with a murine mink cell focus-forming virus. J Virol 46:871-880, 1983.

24. Neil JC, Hughes D, McFarlane R, Wilkie NM, Onions DE, Lees G, Jarrett O : Transduction and rearrangement of the _myc_ gene by feline leukaemia virus in naturally occurring T-cell leukaemias. Nature (308):814-820, 1984.

25. Levy LS, Gardner MB, Casey JW : Isolation of a feline leukaemia provirus containing the oncogene _myc_ from a feline lymphosarcoma. Nature (308):853-856, 1984.

26. Mullins JI, Brody DS, Binari RC Jr, Cotter SM : Viral transduction of _c-myc_ gene in naturally occurring feline leukaemias. Nature (308):856-858, 1984.

27. Rojko JL, Hoover EA, Quackenbush SL, Olsen RG : Reactivation of latent feline leukaemia virus infection. Nature (298):385-388, 1982.

28. Besmer P : Acute transforming feline retroviruses. Curr Top Microbiol and Immunol (107):1-27, 1983.

29. Frankel AE, Gilbert JH, Porzig KJ, Scolnick EM, Aaronson SA : Nature and distribution of feline sarcoma virus nucleotide sequences. J Virol (30):821-827, 1979.

30. Hardy WD Jr. : The biology and virology of the feline sarcoma viruses. In: Hardy WD Jr, Essex M, McClelland AJ (eds) Feline Leukemia Virus. Elsevier, New York, 1980, pp 79-118.

31. Snyder SP, Theilen GH : Transmissible feline fibrosarcoma. Nature (221):1074-1075, 1969.

32. Gardner MB, Arnstein P, Rongey RW, Estes JD, Sarma PS, Rickard CF, Huebner RJ : Experimental transmission of feline fibrosarcoma to cats and dogs. Nature (226):807-809, 1970.

33. Hardy WD Jr, Zuckerman E, Markovich R, Besmer P, Snyder HW : Isolation of feline sarcoma viruses from pet cats with multicentric fibrosarcomas. In: Yohn DS, Blakeslee, JR (eds) Advances in Comparative Leukemia Research 1981, Elsevier, North Holland, 1982, pp 205-206.

34. Snyder HW Jr, Singhal MC, Zuckerman EE, Hardy WD Jr : Isolation of a new feline sarcoma virus (HZ1-FeSV): Biochemical and immunological characterization of its translation product. Virology (132):205-210, 1984.

35. Fujinami A, Inamoto K : Ueber geschwulste bei japanischen haushuhnern insbesondere uber einen transplantablen tumor. Zeitschr F Krebsforsch (14):94-119, 1914.

36. Shibuya M, Hanafusa T, Hanafusa H, Stephenson JR : Homology exists among the transforming sequences of avian and feline sarcoma viruses. Proc Natl Acad Sci USA (77):6536-6540, 1980.

37. Snyder HW Jr : Biochemical characterization of protein kinase activities associated with transforming gene products of the Snyder-Theilen and Gardner-Arnstein strains of feline sarcoma virus. Virology (117):165-172, 1982.

38. McDonough SK, Larsen S, Brodey RS, Stock ND, Hardy WD Jr : A transmissible feline fibrosarcoma of viral origin. Cancer Res (31):953-956, 1971.

39. Hardy WD Jr, Zuckerman EE, Besmer P, Markovich R, George PC, Lederman L, Snyder HW Jr : Isolation of a new feline sarcoma virus HZ5-FeSV containing the v-fms oncogene. manuscript in preparation.

40. Besmer P, George PC, Snyder HW Jr, Zuckerman EE, Lederman L, Hardy WD Jr: Characterization of the v-fms oncogene from a new feline sarcoma virus, HZ5-FeSV. manuscript in preparation.

41. Anderson SJ, Furth M, Wolff L, Ruscetti SK, Sherr CJ : Monoclonal antibodies to the transformation specific glycoprotein encoded by the feline retroviral oncogene v-fms. J Virol (44):696-702, 1982.

42. Besmer P, Hardy WD Jr, Zuckerman EE, Bergold P, Lederman L, Snyder HW Jr : The Hardy-Zuckerman 2-FeSV, a new feline retrovirus with oncogene homology to Abelson-MuLV. Nature (303):825-828, 1983.

43. Besmer P, Snyder HW Jr, Murphy JE, Hardy WD Jr, Parodi A : The Parodi-Irgens feline sarcoma virus and simian sarcoma virus have homologous

oncogenes, but in different contexts of the viral genomes. J Virol (46):606-613, 1983.

44. Irgens K, Wyers M, Moraillon A, Parodi A, Fortuny V : Isolement d'un virus sarcomatogene feline a partir d'un fibrosarcome spontane du chat: etude du pouvoir sarcomatogene in vivo.C R Acad Sci Paris(276):1783-1786,1973.

45. Doolittle RF, Hunkapiller MW, Hood LE, Devare SG, Robbins KC, Aaronson SA, Antoniades HN F : Simian sarcoma virus onc gene, v-sis, is derived from the gene (or genes) encoding a platelet-derived growth factor. Science (221):275-277, 1983.

46. Robbins KC, Antoniades HN, Devare SG, Hunkapiller MW, Aaronson SA : Structural and immunological similarities between simian sarcoma virus gene product(s) and human platelet-derived growth factor. Nature (305):605-608, 1983.

47. Waterfield MD, Scrace GT, Whittle N, Stroobant P, Johnsson A, Wasteson A. Westermark B, Heldin C-H, Huang JS, Deuel TF : Platelet-derived growth factor is structurally related to the putative transforming protein $p28^{sis}$ of simian sarcoma virus. Nature (304):35-39, 1983.

48. Noronha F, Youngren SD : Unpublished observation.

49. Rasheed S, Barbacid M, Aaronson S., Gardner MB : Origin and biological properties of a new feline sarcoma virus. Virology (117):238-244, 1982.

50. Naharro G, Dunn CY, Robbins KC : Analysis of the primary translational product and integrated DNA of a new feline sarcoma virus, GR-FeSV. Virology (125):502-507, 1983.

51. Hardy WD Jr, Zuckerman EE, Besmer P, Markovich R , Murphy JE, Lader E, George PC, Lederman L, Snyder HW Jr : Isolation of a new feline sarcoma virus, HZ4-FeSV, containing a unique oncogene v-kit. manuscript in preparation.

52. Besmer P, Murphy JE, Lader E, George PC, Snyder HW Jr, Zuckerman EE, Lederman L Hardy WD Jr : Characterization of a unique oncogene, v-kit, from a new feline sarcoma virus, HZ4-FeSV. manuscript in preparation.

53. Hardy WD Jr, Hirshaut Y, Hess P : Detection of the feline leukemia virus and other mammalian oncornaviruses by immunofluorescence. In : Dutcher, RM, Chieco-Bianchi L (eds) Unifying Concepts of Leukemia, Karger, Basel, 1973, pp 778-799.

54. Gardner MB, Brown JC, Charman HP, Stephenson JR, Rongey RW, Hauser DE, Diegmann F, Howard E, Dworsky R, Gilden RV, Huebner RJ : FeLV epidemiology in Los Angeles cats: Appraisal of detection methods. Int J Cancer (19):581-589, 1977.

55. Weijer K, Daams JH : The control of lymphosarcoma/leukaemia and feline leukaemia virus. J Small An Pract (19):631-637, 1978.

56. Hardy WD Jr, Zuckerman EE, MacEwen EG, Hayes AA, Essex M : A feline leukaemia virus- and sarcoma virus-induced tumour-specific antigen. Nature

(270):249-251, 1977.

57. Essex M, Sliski A, Cotter SM, Jakowski RM, Hardy WD Jr Immunosurveillance of naturally occurring feline leukemia. Scienc (190):790-792,1975.

58. Hardy WD Jr, McClelland AJ, Zuckerman EE, Hess PW, Essex M, Cotter SM MacEwen EG, Hayes AA : Prevention of the contagious spread of felin leukaemia virus and the development of leukaemia in pet cats. Natur (263):326-328, 1976.

59. Essex M, Klein G, Snyder SP, Harrold JB : Correlation between humora antibody and regression of tumours induced by feline sarcoma virus. Natur (233):195-196, 1971.

60. Snyder HW Jr, Hardy WD Jr, Zuckerman EE, Fleissner E : Characterization o a tumour-specific antigen on the surface of feline lymphosarcoma cells Nature (275):656-658, 1978.

61. Snyder HW Jr , Singhal MC, Zuckerman EE, Jones FR, Hardy WD Jr : Th feline oncornavirus-associated cell membrane antigen (FOCMA) is relate to, but distinguishable from, FeLV-C gp70. Virology (131):315-327, 198

62. Vedbrat SS, Rasheed S, Lutz H, Gonda MA, Ruscetti S, Gardner MB, Prensky : Feline oncornavirus-associated cell membrane antigen: A viral and not cellularly coded transformation-specific antigen of cat lymphomas Virology (124):445-461, 1983.

63. Hardy WD Jr : Immunopathology induced by the feline leukemia virus. In Klein G (ed) Springer Semin Immunopathol. Springer-Verlag, New York, 198 pp75-105.

64. Hardy WD Jr, McClelland AJ, Zuckerman EE, Snyder HW, Jr, MacEwen EG Francis D, Essex M : Development of virus non-producer lymphosarcomas i pet cats exposed to FeLV. Nature (288):90-92, 1980.

65. Anderson LJ, Jarrett WFH, Jarrett O, Laird HM : Feline leukemia-viru infection of kittens: Mortality associated with atrophy of the thymus an lymphoid depletion. J Natl Cancer Inst (47):807-817, 1971.

66. Perryman LE, Hoover EA, Yohn DS : Immunologic reactivity of the cat Immunosuppression in experimental feline leukemia. J Natl Cancer In (49):1357-1365, 1972.

67. Cockerell GL, Hoover EA : Inhibition of normal lymphocyte mitogeni reactivity by serum from feline leukemia virus-infected cats. Cancer R (37):3985-3989, 1977.

68. Trainin Z, Wernicke D, Ungar-Waron H, Essex M : Suppression of the humora antibody response in natural retrovirus infections. Science (220):858-85 1983.

69. Mathes LE, Olsen RG, Hebebrand LC, Hoover EA, Schaller JP : Abrogation c lymphocyte blastogenesis by a feline leukemia virus protein. Natur (274):687-689, 1978.

70. Snyder HW Jr, Jones FR, Day NK, Hardy WD Jr : Isolation and characterization of circulating feline leukemia virus-immune complexes from plasma of persistently infected pet cats removed by ex vivo immunosorption. J Immunol (128):2726-2730, 1982.

71. Hardy WD Jr : Feline leukemia virus as an animal retrovirus model for the human T-cell leukemia virus. In: Gallo RC, Essex M, Gross L (eds) Human T-Cell Leukemia/Lymphoma Viruses. Cold Spring Harbor Laboratory, New York, 1984, pp 35-43.

72. Gallo RC, Salahuddin SZ, Popovic M, Shearer GM, Kaplan M, Haynes BF, Palker TJ, Redfield R, Oleske J, Safai B, White G, Foster P, Markham PD : Frequent detection and isolation of cytopathic retroviruses (HTLV-III) from patients with AIDS and at risk for AIDS. Science (224):500-503, 1984.

73. Hardy WD Jr : Feline leukemia virus non-neoplastic diseases. J Am Animal Hosp Assoc (17):941-949, 1981.

74. Hardy WD Jr : Feline leukemia virus diseases. In: Hardy WD Jr, Essex M, McClelland AJ (eds) Feline Leukemia Virus. Elsevier, New York,1980, pp3-31.

75. Hardy WD Jr : Hematopietic tumors of cats. J Am Animal Hosp Assoc (17):921-940, 1981.

76. Mackey LJ, Jarrett W, Jarrett O, Laird H : Anemia associated with feline leukemia virus infection in cats. J Natl Cancer Inst (54):209-217, 1975.

77. Jakowski RM, Essex M, Hardy WD Jr, Stephenson JR, Cotter SM : Membranous glomerulonephritis in a household of cats persistently viremic with feline leukemia virus. In: Hardy, WD Jr, Essex M, McClelland AJ (eds) Feline Leukemia Virus. Elsevier, New York, 1980, pp 141-149.

24

BOVINE LEUKEMIA VIRUS: PAST, PRESENT AND FUTURE

A. BURNY[·•], C. BRUCK[•], D. COUEZ[•], J. DESCHAMPS[•], J. GHYSDAEL[•], D. GREGOIRE[•], R. KETTMANN[·•], M. MAMMERICKX[+] and D. PORTETELLE[·•°]

• Departement of Molecular Biology, University of Brussels,
. Faculty of Agronomy, Gembloux
+ National Institute for Veterinary Research, Uccle, Belgium.

N. RICE and R. STEPHENS
LBI-Frederick Cancer Research Facility, National Cancer Institute, Frederick, Maryland, USA

R. GILDEN
PRI-Frederick Cancer Research Facility, National Cancer Institute, Frederick, Maryland, USA

INTRODUCTION

Enzootic bovine leukemia has been perceived as an infectious cancer since about 50 years. Appearance of tumor cases has been linked to introduction, in a naïve herd, of animals coming from a "tumor case„ herd and experimental transmission experiments easily showed that an agent was indeed most probably involved. The exact nature of the agent remained elusive until 1969, when Miller and coworkers (1) observed virus particles in short term cultures of lymphocytes from animals in persistent lymphocytosis, a condition frequently associated with increased risk of leukemia. Since 1969, the virus itself, its host-range and mode of propagation, its interactions with the host and ways of leukemogenesis, ... have been the subject of intense investigation. The nucleotide sequence of several BLV proviruses is now known, thus allowing deep insight to be gained into virus integration and expression and hypotheses to be put forward about putative modes of action. Times are now ripe and the tools are available to undertake a detailed analysis of the chain of events that starts at infection and ends with full blow of the tumor phase. It had been observed, already in 1972 (2), that BLV behaved as a separate entity from the then known retroviruses. Since the discoveries of the HTLVs, viruses spread among humans and primates, the BLV-HTLV family has acquired new and versatile members; some induce leukemias and lymphomas, others cause immunodeficiency. Studies of the virus - cell interplay will enlighten our views about cell differenciation and should teach us why the cell response to virus infection can be as different as cell death or immortalization and transformation.

BLV PROVIRUS

<u>BLV provirus-structure</u> (3, 4, 5, 6, 7)

As is the rule for all proviruses, BLV provirus contains the viral genes flanked by long terminal repeat (LTR) sequences. The latters are covalently linked to cell DNA when the provirus is integrated in the host cell genome. The total length of BLV proviral DNA amounts to about 9,000 base pairs. Restriction maps have been published for the FLK-BLV isolate, a Belgian and a Japanese cloned proviruses. As expected, the maps derived from the FLK-BLV isolate and the Japanese isolate are very similar, due to the fact, that the Japanese clone was from an Holstein cow. The Belgian isolate showed some variations especially in the gag and pol gene regions. Such observations do not necessarily mean that protein sequences vary significantly from one BLV variant to another. Indeed, comparison of p12 amino acid sequence of FLK-BLV with nucleotide sequence of the Belgian BLV clone stresses the point that variations among BLV strains are minimal and thus reemphasizes the significance of the observed kinship between the $p12_s$ of BLV and HTLV (8 - 10).

<u>DNA sequence analysis</u>

Most of the BLV provirus from the FLK and the Belgian isolates have been sequenced so far with the hope that a detailed characterization of the genome and the comparison between different isolates would yield clues to the mechanism of leukemogenesis.

<u>Sequence of LTR from the Belgian tumor - derived BLV provirus clone</u> (11). Sequencing of LTRs was a high priority prerequisite as it has been repeatedly (12 - 16) suspected that the U_3 region of LTR plays a key role in leukemogenesis by a number of viruses.

The sequence is shown in fig. 1. The size of U_3 is still uncertain. U_3 might start at the TG pair at position -305 or at the TC pair at position -215. U_3 contains a number of direct and inverted repeats, characteristic features of DNA regions involved in regulation of transcription. The R region is 234 bp long, a value very similar to that found for HTLV-I LTR (R = 228 bp).

A.

```
-471           G AATTCGAGCT GCCCCTTATC CAAACGCCCG GCCTGTCTTG  -431
-430 GTCTGTCCCC GCGATCGACC TATTCCTAAC CGGTCCCCCT TCCCCATACG  -381
-380 ACCGGTTACA CGTGTGGTCC AGTCCTAAGG CCTTACAACG CTTCCTCCAT  -331
            Z DNA
-330 GACCCTACGC TCACCTGGTC AGAATTGGTT GCTAGCGGGA AACTAAGACT  -281
                                                1
-280 TGATTCACCC TTAAAATTAC AGCTGTTAGA AAATGAATGG CTCTCCCGCC  -231
                           5'LTR
-230 TTTTTTGAGG GGGAGTCATT TGTATGAAAG ATCATGCAGG CCTAGCGCCG  -181
            PBS+       IR          2       Z DNA          3
-180 CCACCGCCCC GTAAACCAGA CAGAGACGTC AGCTGCCAGA GAAGCTGCTG  -131
          3          2              4           4
-130 ACGGCAGCTG GTGGTCAGAA TCCCCGTACC TCCCCAACTT CCCCTTTCCC   -81
                5              5
 -80 GAAAAATCCA CACCCTGAGC TGCTGACCTC ACCTGCTGAT AAATTAATAA   -31
                                  U3 | 5'CAP
 -30 AATGCCGGCC CTGTCGAGTT AGCGGCACCA GAAGCGTTCT CCTCCTGAGA    20
  21 CCCTAGTGCT CAGCTCTCGG TCCTGAGCTC TCTTGCTCCC GAGACCTTCT    70
  71 GGTCGGCTAT CCGGCAGCGG TCAGGTAAGG CAAACCACGG TTTGGAGGGT   120
 121 GGTTCTCGGC TGAGACCGCC GCGAGCTCTA TCTCCGGTCC TCTGACCGTC   170
 171 TCCACGTGGA CTCTCTCTCT TGCCTCCTGA CCCCGCGCTC CAAGGGCGTC   220
                R
 221 TGGCTTGCAC CCGCGTTTGT TTCCTGTCTT ACTTTCTGTT TCTCGCGGCC   270
                LH                                  3'LTR
 271 CGCGCTCTCT CCCTCGGCGC CCTCTAGCGG CCAGGAGAGA CCGGCAAACA   320
     CELL       L'H                                    IR
 321 ACAAAGCACT GGACATGACT TAGAGACTGA ACAACAACCA TCTTGAGGIG   370
 371 GCAGGTGGGC AGGTTTATAA GAAGCACATT GGTTTGAATT C            411
```

B.

```
                             45
          TGCAGGGGGGGGGGGGAGCTCTCTTGCTCCCGAGACCTT......
                             5'LTR 321
......GCGGCCAGGAGAGACCCGCAAACAATTGGGGGCTCGTCCGGGATT
                              IR           PBS-
```

FIGURE 1.

A computer-assisted search was used to look for homologous sequences in BLV-LTR and LTRs of Moloney leukaemia virus, simian sarcoma virus, Rauscher leukaemia virus, gibbon ape leukaemia virus, baboon endogenous virus and HTLV-I. No significant homology was revealed between these LTRs, indicating that genetic drift occurs within these structures, even if signals for transcription are present in all of them.

Sequence of the gene for envelope glycoprotein gp51 (17). The sequence of the env gene has been located by comparison of the translated DNA sequence with amino acid sequence data on purified gp51 and gp30 (18). Gp51 is predicted to contain 268 amino acids. It shows distant but nonetheless statiscally significant homology to HTLV-I gp51.

Sequence of the gene for transmembrane protein (g)p30 (17). The sequence coding for (g)p30 is the 3' part of the open reading frame that contains the information for gp51 at its 5' part. The DNA regions coding for the respective envelope proteins have been delineated, using the N-terminal amino acid sequence data of purified proteins (18). By this approach, (g)p30 is predicted to contain 214 amino acids and shows structural features typical of type C viral transmembrane proteins. A two dimensional model of protein folding valid for HTLV-I envelope proteins has been presented by Haseltine (pers. commun.). From the data obtained in our study (17) it can be inferred that BLV and HTLV-I envelope proteins have very similar three-dimensional configurations.

Sequence of the px region (17). BLV provirus contains a region of 1817 base pairs between the presumptive terminator of the env gene (3' side of (g)p30) and the 5' end of U_3, when the limits of LTR are taken as proposed by Couez et al. (11). This sequence contains two open reading frames : one in one frame (potential protein = 128 amino acids) and the second one in a second frame (potential protein = 154 amino acids). RNA processing involving a spliced on initator methionine could increase the size of the potential proteins considerably. Some remarkable similarities between the BLV and HTLV sequences in this region have been noted (17). Intensive search is going on to identify the putative proteins product. Is it at all related to the 18,000 MW protein seen by Ghysdael _et al_. (19) in _in vitro_ translation experiments of viral RNAs ? What role does it play as a candidate involved in leukemogenesis by BLV ?

Integration site of the provirus (20, 21). As already mentioned above, it seems well established that tumor induction by BLV is not related to the site at which the provirus is found in the fully developed tumor, unless activation of many oncogenes can lead to the neoplastic state. The latter possibility being a remote one, we encline to think that a viral product is required to start the transformation process. In contrast, maintenance of the tumor stage does not seem to require presence nor expression of the provirus.

BLV PROTEINS

Core proteins

The virus contains gag, pol and env genes and a px region. It has been proposed that 4 proteins are encoded in the gag gene region. They are designated p15, p10, p24 and p12 (22-25).

_p15_. Two different p15 molecules seem to exist in BLV, as illustrated by gel electrophoresis data (23, 26, 27). P15 is a basic protein and was identified as the major virus phosphoprotein. Chemical cross-linking experiments have located p15 in the vicinity of membrane lipids but also close to viral RNA (23). It has also been observed that BLV p15 is myristilated and hypothesized that myristilation of p15 might be relevant to the phenomenon of transformation (25). In the gag sequence, p15 is the first protein at the NH_2 terminus of the gag precursor.

_p10_. This is a highly basic protein with DNA binding capacity (28). It is found in homologous dimers (p10-p10) and heterologous complexes (p10-p15) after cross linking. A lower molecular weight has been sometimes attributed to this molecule. This puzzling situation will soon be clarified by protein and DNA sequencing data.

_p24_. It is the major core protein of BLV called in the early literature the ether-resistant antigen (22). It has been characterized in detail and partially sequenced (29, 30). Its relatedness to HTLV-I p24 is striking. Monoclonal antibodies have been raised against two different epitopes (Bruck et al., unpublished). P24 exists as homologous dimers and complexes to p10.

p12 is the RNA binding protein. It has been sequenced and its primary sequence compared to the corresponding DNA. This is a proline rich protein as expected. The presence of two stop codons at the 3' end of the sequence indicates that p12 is on the carboxyl side of the gag protein. As seen above, p12 exists as homologous dimers and complexed to RNA in native viral particles.

Envelope proteins

Glycoproteins 51 and 30 are the major envelope protein and the transmembrane protein respectively. They are synthesized as a single glycosylated precursor of MW = 72,000, Pr 72^{env} (19, 31, 32). It has been suggested that gp51 is a cleavage product of a larger molecule of MW = 60,000 (18). From amino acid (18) and nucleotide sequence data (17), it was found that gp51 has 268 amino acids and (g)p30, 214. The cleavage site between both proteins is an arginine as observed in other virus systems (17).

HTLV-I and BLV gp51s display a number of similarities in amino acid sequence and thus three dimensional configuration. The two transmembrane proteins show 36 % identities in an alignment requiring 6 gaps. More distant relatedness is also seen between BLV (g)p30 and both murine leukemia virus p15E and Rous sarcoma virus gp36.

Knowing the entire sequence of BLV gp51 will allow identification of the three biologically crucial epitopes (F, G, H) of the protein (33-35). Moreover, BLV variants have been identified which carry mutations affecting F, G or H. DNA sequence analysis of these variants and comparison with the sequence presented here should allow to correlate the presence of specific amino acids with regions of defined function and/or three dimensional structure.

CONCLUSIONS

Considered since a number of years as an enigma, the mode of action of BLV is probably coming out of the dark. It is felt that the px region of the provirus encodes a protein whose action is critical for cell transformation. We seem to be confronted with a new type of transforming agent. The virus probably carries a function directly involved in transformation but still induces a chronic leukemia. The choice is left between two possibilities: (1) Cell transformation is not a rare event but transformed cells are eliminated by the immune system of the host. (2) Cell transformation is a rare event. The function fulfilled by px is necessary but not sufficient for cell transformation. Uncovering the mechanism involved already appears as a tantalizing adventure that will lead more and more deeply in the intricacies of cell differentiation.

The data harvested from the studies on gp51 have important implications for the design of a BLV vaccine. The repeated observation that passive antibodies to BLV structural proteins efficiently protect the calf or the lamb from infection by the administered virus has proved that vaccination should be feasible. Analysis of bovine and ovine immune sera has shown that protective sera contain immunoglobulins reactive against epitopes F, G and H of BLV gp51, the same three epitopes that apparently play a role in the biological activities of the virus (infectivity and syncytia induction). The polysaccharide moiety of gp51 plays a critical role in determining the native structure of crucial epitopes. It follows that design of an efficient long lasting BLV vaccine is not an easy task. It requires the large scale production of defined and adequately folded epitopes of gp51. It has been suggested (P. Fischinger, pers. commun.) that some epitopes of (g)p30 could be ad hoc determinants (interspecies determinants) to be used in vaccine trials, especially considering their highly conserved structure. This has obviously to be tested in the forthcoming future.

A third and immediate outcome of BLV research has to do with epidemiology. The design of a very specific, sensitive, fast and cheap ELISA test has allowed large scale surveys in the cattle population. Pools of as many as eighty sera can be analyzed as a single assay. The presence of only one positive serum can be detected. Accurate and easy testing is a major part in any sanitation program in veterinary medicine. The data obtained in this part of the work show that BLV infection can be detected and controled, a major step toward elimination of enzootic bovine leukemia.

Finally, our previous observation that BLV can be infectious to rabbits and induce lymphopenia should be reconsidered in view of the involvement of members of the BLV family in induction of the acquired immuno-deficiency syndrome.

The accumulating results encountered in BLV and HTLV research confirm that both viruses are related and probably derive from a common ancestor. Any progress made in one system may be used in the other; they cross-feed continuously. BLV research is not only rewarding for itself and profitable to animal health, it also provides valuable observations to be used in human medicine in relation to HTLV-induced diseases.

ACKNOWLEDGEMENTS

This work was made financially possible in Belgium by the generous support of the Fonds Cancérologique de la Caisse Générale d'Epargne et de Retraite. CB, DC and RK are fellows of FNRS. DG holds a fellowship from IRSIA.

The work at Frederick was carried out under NCI contract.

REFERENCES

1. Miller J.M., Miller L.D., Olson C. and Gillette K.G.: Virus-like particles in phytohaemagglutinin-stimulated lymphocyte cultures with reference to bovine lymphosarcoma. J. Nat. Cancer Inst.(43):1297-1305, 1979.
2. Ferrer J.F.: Antigenic comparison of bovine type-C virus with murine and feline leukemia viruses. Cancer Res.(32):1871-1877, 1972.
3. Kettmann R., Couez D. and Burny A.: Restriction endonuclease mapping of linear unintegrated proviral DNA of bovine leukemia virus. J. Virol.(38):27-33, 1981.

4. Deschamps J., Kettmann R. and Burny A.: Experiments with cloned complete tumor-derived bovine leukemia virus information prove that the virus is totally exogenous to its target animal species. J. Virol.(40): 605-609, 1981.

5. Kashmiri S.V.S., Mehdi R. and Ferrer J.F.: Molecular cloning of covalently closed circular DNA of bovine leukemia virus. J. Virol.(49):583-587, 1983.

6. Kashmiri S.V.S., Mehdi R. and Ferrer J.F.: Molecular cloning of covalently closed circular DNA of bovine leukemia virus. J. Virol.(49):583-587, 1984.

7. Sagata N., Ogawa Y., Kawamura J., Onuma M., Izawa H. and Ikawa Y.: Molecular cloning of bovine leukemia virus DNA integrated into the bovine tumor cell genome. Gene (26):1-10, 1983.

8. Copeland T.D., Morgan M.A. and Orozzlan S.: Complete amino acid sequence of the nucleic acid binding protein of bovine leukemia virus. FEBS Letters (156):37-40, 1983a.

9. Copeland T., Oroszlan S., Kalyanaraman V.S., Sarngadharan M.G. and Gallo R.C.: Complete amino acid sequence of human T-cell leukemia virus structural protein p15. FEBS Letters (162): 390-395, 1983b.

10. Burny A., Bruck C., Cleuter Y., Couez D., Dekegel D., Deschamps J., Ghysdael J., Gilden R.V., Kettmann R., Marbaix G., Mammerickx M. and Portetelle D.: Leukemogenesis by bovine leukemia virus. In: Mechanisms of viral leukemogenesis vol.1, eds J. Goldmann and O. Jarrett, Edinburgh, Churchill Livingstone. 1976,pp.229-260.

11. Couez D., Deschamps J., Kettmann R., Stephens R., Gilden R. and Burny A.: Nucleotide sequence analysis of the long terminal repeat of integrated bovine leukemia provirus DNA and of adjacent viral and host sequences. J. Virol.(49):615-620, 1984.

12. Czernilofsky A.P., De Lorbe W., Swanstrom R., Varmus H.E., Bishop J.M., Fischer E. and Goodman H.M.: The nucleotide sequence of an untranslated but conserved domain at the 3' end of the avian sarcoma virus genome. Nucl. Ac. Res.(8):2967-2984, 1980.

13. Robinson H.L., Blais B.M., Tsichlis P.L. and Coffin J.M.: At least two regions of the viral genome determine the oncogenic potential of avian leukosis viruses. Proc. Nat. Acad. Sci. U.S.A.(79):1225-1229, 1982.

14. Tsichlis P.N. and Coffin J.M.: Recombinants between endogenous and exogenous avian tumor viruses: role of the C region and other portions of the genome in the control of replication and transformation. J. Virol.(33):238-249, 1980.

15. Lenz J., Celander D., Crowther R.L., Patarca R., Perkins D.W. and Haseltine W.A.: Determination of the leukemogenicity of a murine retrovirus by sequences within the long terminal repeat. Nature (308):467-470, 1984.

16. Chen I.S.Y., McLaughlin J. and Golde D.W.: Long terminal repeats of human T-cell leukemia virus II genome determine target cell specificity. Nature (309):276-279, 1984.

17. Rice N.R., Stephens R.M., Couez D., Deschamps J., Kettmann R., Burny A. and Gilden R.V.: The nucleotide sequence of the env gene and post-env region of bovine leukemia virus. Virology, in press, 1984.

18. Schultz A.M., Copeland T.D. and Oroszlan S.: The envelope proteins of bovine leukemia virus: purification and sequence analysis. Virology (135), in press, 1984.

19. Ghysdael J., Kettmann R. and Burny A.: Translation of bovine leukemia virus virion RNAs in heterologous protein-synthesizing systems. J. Virol.(29):1087-1098, 1979.

20. Kettmann R., Deschamps J., Couez D., Claustriaux J.J., Palm R. and Burny A.: Chromosome integration domain for bovine leukemia provirus in tumors. J. Virol.(47):146-150, 1983.

21. Grégoire D., Couez D., Deschamps J., Heuertz S., Hors-Cayla M.C., Szpirer J., Szpirer C., Burny A., Huez G. and Kettmann R.: Different bovine leukemia virus-induced tumors harbor the provirus in different chromosomes. J. Virol.(50): 275-279, 1984.

22. Burny A., Bruck C., Chantrenne H., Cleuter Y., Dekegel D., Ghysdael J., Kettmann R., Leclercq M., Leunen J., Mammerickx M. and Portetelle D.: Bovine leukemia virus : molecular biology and epidemiology. In: Viral Oncology, ed G. Klein. New York, Raven Press, 1980, pp. 231-289.
23. Uckert W., Wunderlich V., Ghysdael J., Portetelle D. and Burny A.: Bovine leukemia virus (BLV)- A structural model based on chemical crosslinking studies. Virology (133):386-392, 1984.
24. Morgan M.A., Copeland T.D. and Oroszlan S.: Structural and antigenic analysis of the nucleic acid binding proteins of bovine and feline leukemia viruses. J. Virol.(46):177-186, 1983.
25. Schultz A.M. and Oroszlan S.: Myristylation of gag-onc fusion proteins in mammalian transforming retroviruses. Virology (133):431-437, 1984.
26. Prachar J. and Hlubinova K. (1980). Glycoprotein and protein composition of BLV. Neoplasma (27):669-674, 1980.
27. Uckert W., Westermann P. and Wunderlich V.: Nearest neighbor relationship of major structural proteins within bovine leukemia virus particles. Virology (121):240-250, 1982.
28. Long C.W., Henderson L.E. and Oroszlan S.: Isolation and characterization of low molecular-weight DNA-binding proteins from retroviruses. Virology (104):491-496, 1980.
29. Gilden R.V., Long C.W., Hanson M., Toni R., Charman H., Oroszlan S., Miller J.M. and Van der Maaten M.J.: Characterization of the major internal protein and RNA-dependent DNA polymerase of bovine leukemia virus. J. Gen. Virol.(29:305-314, 1975.
30. Oroszlan S., Copeland T.D., Henderson L.E., Stephenson J.R. and Gilden R.V.: Amino-terminal sequence of bovine leukemia virus major internal protein: Homology with mammalian type C virus p30s. Proc. Nat. Acad. Sci. U.S.A. (76):2996-3000, 1979.

31. Bruck C., Rensonnet N., Portetelle D., Cleuter Y., Mammerickx M., Burny A., Mamoun R., Guillemain B., Van der Maaten M.J. and Ghysdael J.: Biologically active epitopes of bovine leukemia virus glycoprotein gp51: their dependence on protein glycosylation and genetic variability. Virology. in press, 1984.

32. Mamoun R.Z., Astier T., Guillemain B. and Duplan J.F.: Bovine lymphosarcoma: expression of BLV-related proteins in cultured cells. J. Gen. Virol.(64):1895-1905, 1983.

33. Bruck C., Mathot S., Portetelle D., Franssen J.D., Herion P. and Burny A.: Monoclonal antibodies define eight independent antigenic sites on the bovine leukemia virus envelope glycoprotein gp51. Virology (122):343-352, 1982a.

34. Bruck C., Portetelle D., Burny A. and Zavada J.: Topographical analysis by monoclonal antibodies of BLV-gp51 epitopes involved in viral functions. Virology (122): 353-362, 1982b.

35. Bruck C., Portetelle D., Mammerickx M., Mathot S. and Burny A.: Epitopes of bovine leukemia virus glycoprotein gp51 recognized by sera of infected cattle and sheep. Leukaemia Res.(8): in press, 1984.

25

A NEW MESSENGER RNA EXPRESSED BY BOVINE LEUKEMIA VIRUS INFECTED CELLS

R.Z. MAMOUN*. T .ASTIER-GIN* R. KETTMANN** J. DESCHAMPS**

N. REBEYROTTE*. B.J. GUILLEMAIN*

*INSERM U. 117, 229 crs de l'Argonne 33076 Bordeaux. France

**ULB. Dép. Chimie Biologique.1640 Rhode-Ste-Genèse. Belgique.

SUMMARY

The bovine leukemia virus (BLV) is the aetiological agent of the enzootic form of bovine lymphosarcoma. Because the mechanism of tumor induction is unknown we performed an analysis of the viral messenger RNAs expressed in cultured bovine cells of different origins i.e. from enzootic or sporadic tumourous tissues normal cells infected or not with BLV and the reference FLK-BLV cells. We also investigated BLVs of different origins

In addition to the two expected viral mRNAs (i.e. 9.0Kb genomic RNA and 5.1Kb env RNA) we detected the expression of a 2.1Kb mRNA which is also specific of BLV infected cells.

The use of clonal small BLV-DNA probes representative of the BLV genome led us to define the regions of the provirus from which these mRNAs were originating. It was found that the smallest mRNA corresponded to the transcription of pX termed sequences located in between the env gene and the 3' end of the BLV provirus.

1. INTRODUCTION

The bovine leukemia virus (BLV). an exogenous competent retrovirus, is known to be the aetiological agent of the enzootic form of the B type cell bovine leukemia (1, 2. 3. 4. 5. 6). The provirus is found integrated in the tumor cells in which it remains unexpressed (6, 7). An interesting feature is that in regions of endemic BLV-infection, only a small fraction of BLV-infected animals develops preclinical signs of leukemia (persistent lymphocytosis) and among these, not all finally become leukemic (see for a review 8). This suggests that cell transformation is a rare event involving either a proviral modification or a specific interaction between viral and cellular sequences.

Previous investigations (9) showed that at least one to four copies of the viral information are integrated in the cellular genome. It was also observed that in tumor cells, the provirus is frequently deleted (25 %) and when this occurs it concerns systematically the 5' end moiety. This may be taken as an indication of a major role of the 3' side end of the BLV genome in the tumoral process.

The models known to be applicable for virus leukemogenesis cannot explain cell transformation after BLV infection. Indeed, (i) because BLV sequences are entirely exogenous, the "MCF" mechanism is excluded for such virus arise at least partialy via recombination between endogenous proviral sequences (ii) a viral coded oncogene is not implicated because proviral sequences encountered in tumor cells do not have any homology with normal cell sequences (10) and furthermore no evidence of onc" or onc" bearing viral proteins specific of the tumor state could be detected by immunoprecipitation techniques (11) and (iii) the downstream promotion (12) of an "onc" cellular gene in the tumor does not seem to be likely for BLV does not integrate at specific chromosomal sites or regions (13, 14) and no viral LTR containing cellular mRNA is synthetized (15).

All these findings also apply to the recently described human T-cell leukemia virus HTLV (16 17) and thus the bovine system is quite appropriate as an experimental model. Interestingly the analysis of the sequence at the 3' end of the <u>env</u> gene of both HTLV and BLV revealed the existence of open reading frames the putative product of which was tentatively called pX and which could play an important role in tumor genesis.

In these conditions to investigate the BLV-induced leukemogenic process, the expression of the virus seems to be required · this is why we developed <u>in vitro</u>, from bovine lymphoid tumors. a number of cell lines which express BLV (11, 18).

We report here an analysis of BLV mRNAs encountered in <u>in vitro</u> cultured cells which shows that in addition to the genomic (9.0 Kb) and env (5.1 Kb) RNAs an additional mRNA (2.1 Kb) is also transcribed from a region of the BLV genome located immediately at the 5' side of the 3' LTR.

2. MATERIAL AND METHODS

Animals

LB44 LB59 2412, 3010 and 3894 were referral cases of bovine lymphosarcomas.

Cells

The exact origin and BLV status of the cells used in this study are presented in table 1. Bovine leukaemic lymphocytes (Ly) and lymph nodes (gg) lymphomatous kidney (K), normal cornea (C) and normal embryo spleen cells (BESP) were established as permanent cultures as described previously (18). The foetal lamb kidney cells chronically infected with the bovine leukaemia virus, FLK-BLV, were kindly supplied by Dr M.J. Van Der Maaten and Dr J.M. Miller (19) (National Animal Disease Laboratory, U.S. Department of Agriculture, Ames, Iowa, U.S.A.). BLV from LB59-Ly cells were used to infect BESP cells (referred as BESP-LB59). All these cell lines were maintained as monolayers in RPMI 1629 culture medium supplemented with 10 % heat inactivated foetal calf serum, 4 ng/ml 2-mercaptoethanol, 100 units/ml penicillin and 100 μg/ml streptomycin.

Detection of RNA expression

RNA was extracted in TNE buffer (0.01 M Tris pH 7.9 0.1 M Nacl 0.001 M EDTA) containing 0.5 % SDS and 0.5 % Macaloid three times with phenol chloroform saturated in TNE. Poly(A)$^+$RNA was selected on [Oligo (dT)]-cellulose and denaturated either with the glyoxal (20) or with the methylmercuric hydroxide (21). Size separations (2 to 5 μg of RNA) were carried out by electrophoresis on 1.2 % agarose gels. The RNAs were transfered (Northern blotting) on diazo-benzyloxymethyl paper and then hybridized with (^{32}P)labeled DNA probes. Conditions of hybridization and washing were performed as described by Maniatis (22) but the temperature of hybridization was 37°C.

BLV fragment probes were subclones of the 8.3 Kb SaCI clone containing the BLV information, except for 104 bases missing because

Table 1

CELLULAR ORIGIN OF THE POLY (A^+) RNAs ANALYSED BY BLOT HYBRIDIZATION

CULTURED NORMAL CELLS		
	3010 C	: normal corneal cells from lymphosarcomatous cow # 3010
	3894 C	: normal corneal cells from lymphosarcomatous cow # 3894
CULTURED NORMAL CELLS IN VITRO INFECTED WITH BLV		
	FLK BLV	: foetal lamb kidney cells
	BESP LB59	: bovine embryo spleen cells
CULTURED TUMOR CELLS WITH NO BLV EXPRESSION		
	2412 Ly	: leukemic leukocytes from sporadic bovine lymphosarcoma # 2412
	LB44K	: lymphomatous kidney from enzootic bovine lymphosarcoma # LB44
CULTURED TUMOR CELLS WITH BLV EXPRESSION		
	LB59Ly	: leukemic leukocytes from enzootic bovine lymphosarcoma # LB59
	3010gg	: leukemic lymph node from enzootic bovine lymphosarcoma # 3010
	3894gg	: leukemic lymph node from enzootic bovine lymphosarcoma # 3894 (with very low BLV expression)
NON CULTURED TUMOR CELLS		
	T3010	: leukemic leukocytes from enzootic bovine lymphosarcoma # 3010

Figure 1 : Localisation of the probes used in this study.
(S : SaCI, P : PstI, B : BamHI, Bg : BglII,
X : XbaI, E : EcoRI)

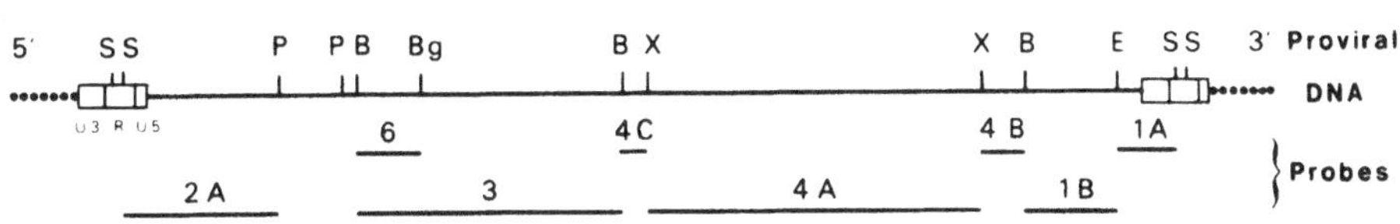

the LTR of this virus contains two SaCI sites (10). This was performed using the pBR322 and pAT153 plasmids. Restriction of the cloned BLV DNAs were generated by the specific restriction endonucleases digestions as specified in figure 1. Each fragment was further purified by preparative agarose gel electrophoresis. DNAs were labeled by nick-translation in the presence of (^{32}P)dCTP($\sim$600 Ci/mM) from New England Nuclear using 5 U of DNA polymerase according to Maniatis (22). A (^{32}P)c-DNA representative probe (c-DNArep) was prepared by the reverse transcriptase method using purified 35 S BLV RNA of the FLK-BLV strain. Probes were isolated from triphosphates by centrifugation through Sephadex G-50. The final specific activity was about 10^8 cpm/ μg.

3. RESULTS

Hybridization of poly(A)$^{\pm}$RNA from BLV infected cells with BLV c-DNArep.

Poly(A)$^+$RNA were prepared from a non cultured tumor (T3010), three BLV infected cultured tumor cells (LB59Ly, 3010 gg. 3894 gg). non BLV infected cultured tumor cells (LB44K), normal (3894c, 3010c). in vitro BLV infected normal cells (FLK-BLV, BESP-LB59) and non BLV infected cultured tumor cells from a sporadic tumor case (2412Ly). After size separation and Northern blotting, the RNA was hybridized with c-DNA representative of the BLV contained in FLK-BLV cells (c-DNArep). The pattern of hybridization presented in figure 2 shows that the two classical retroviral mRNAs i.e. the gag-pol mRNA (9.0kb) and the env mRNA (5.1kb) are present only in BLV producing cells. One can also notice the presence of bands corresponding to contaminant 28 S and 18 S ribosomal rRNAs. The presence of such contaminants which could have masked other RNA species led us to conduct the same type of experiment but using cloned probes.

Hybridization of messenger RNAs with cloned 3' end BLV DNA probes

The 1A probe (figure 1) represents the 3'end sequence located between EcoRI and SaCI sites and including the entire U3 and the first 45 bases of the R region. Figure 3 shows a representative pattern indicating a clear hybridization in infected cells of not only the expected 9.0 kb and 5.1 kb mRNAs but of also a 2.1 kb mRNA specie. Such a result is evocative of the avian lymphoma model in which

Figure 2 : c-DNArep probe.

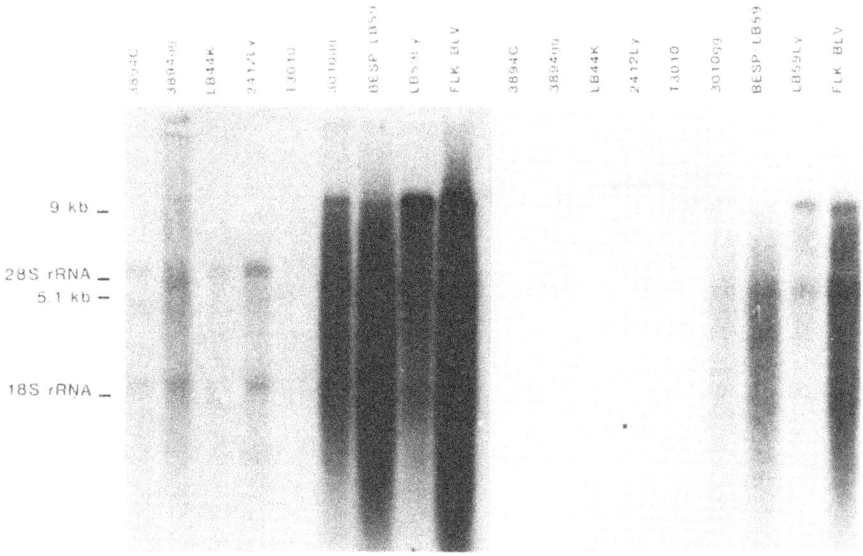

Figure 3 : lA probe.

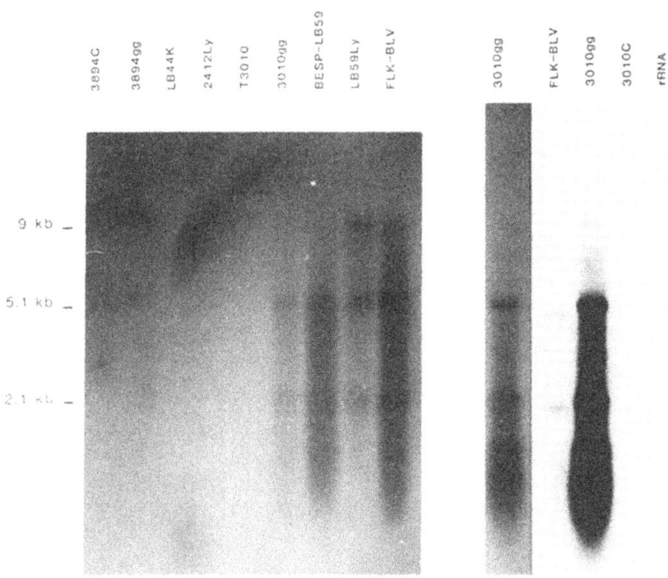

Figure 4 : 1B probe.

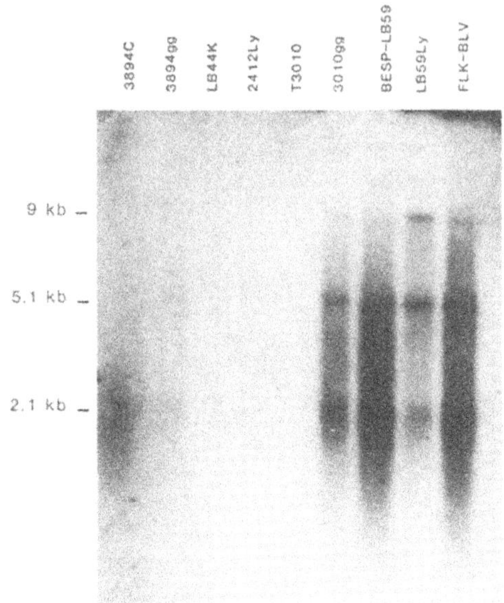

Figure 5 : 4B probe.

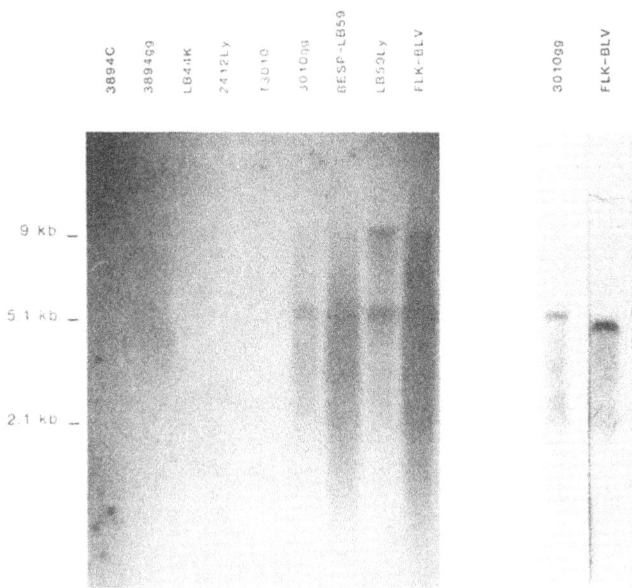

Figure 6

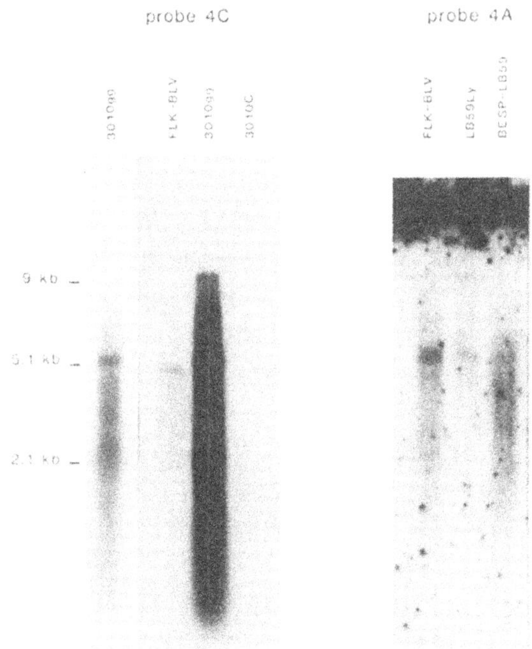

Figure 7

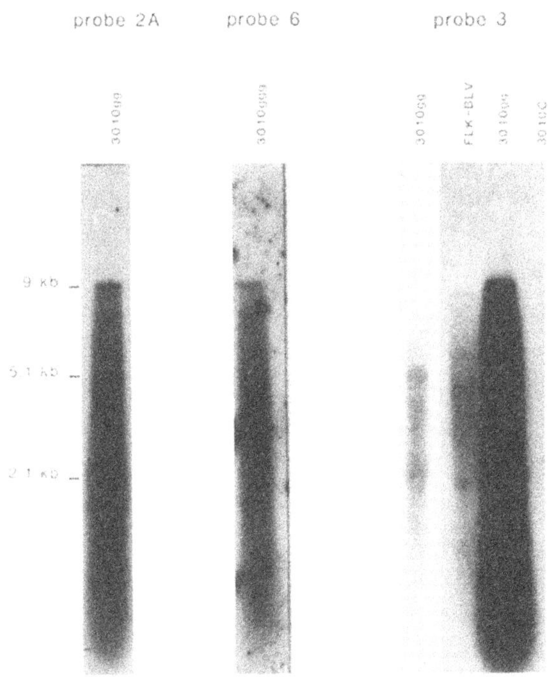

cellular mRNAs often contain viral sequences originating from the 3' end of the viral genome. However this does not seem to be applicable in the BLV system, indeed although BLV has no specific integration site, the size of the small mRNA observed in these experiments remains constant (2.1 kb) whatever its cell origin. Furthermore, the sole contribution of the 45 bases of the R region cannot explain the clear hybridization observed at this size. Thus we undertook the same investigations but using a fragment probe (1B), one kb distal from the R region (figure 1) Again, as shown in figure 4 all BLV producing cells presented the same pattern indicating that such a transcript (2.1 kb) does not originate from a LTR downstream promotion of cellular sequences.

Hybridization of messenger RNAs with other cloned BLV subgenomic DNA probes

Hybridizations were then performed with the 4B probe (figure 1) located just upstream the 1B probe (defined by XbaI - BamHI restriction endonuclease sites). With the same transfer (figure 5) one can see essentialy the putative *env* mRNA (5.1 Kb) in addition to the genomic 9.0 Kb mRNA. Noteworthy no 2.1 Kb mRNA was visualized, indicating that such a mRNA is coded by sequences lying in between the LTR SacI site and the next upstream BamHI site.

When the same blots were tested with the 4A or 4C probes (figure 6) representative of the *env* gene and located immediatly upstream of the 4B (figure 1) the same results were obtained as with the 4B probe.

In the following experiments we used (see figure 1) a *gag* specific probe (2A), a *pol* specific probe (6) and a *pol-env* probe (3). As shown in figure 7, only one band corresponding to a 9.0 Kb mRNA was observed with the two former probes. Such a result indicates that this mRNA corresponds to the *gag-pol* mRNA. In contrast, in addition to the 9.0 Kb mRNA, two faint bands were obtained with probe 3 corresponding to 5.1 and 2.1 Kb. Because the 5.1 Kb mRNA is dimly recognized, this suggest that only a small portion located at the 3' end of the probe contains sequences of the 5' end of the *env* gene. As a 2.1 Kb mRNA is also dimly recognized, this RNA should contain sequences of the 5' end of the *env* gene.

Comparison of the mRNA species recognized in cells of different origins

All these hybridizations were also performed with mRNAs originating from normal, non-BLV infected, cells (3010c, 3894c). No hybridization could be observed confirming the viral nature of the mRNAs described above. The same findings and the same conclusions hold true for cells of a sporadic lymphosarcomatous cow (2412Ly) or from non-BLV infected cells derived from an enzootic lymphosarcomatous cow (LB44K). The known absence of BLV expression in tumor cells which was previously assessed by hybridizations using full length probes was also confirmed with T3010 cells. In addition, these results were extended for the 2 1Kb mRNA.

Note : All experiments performed with mRNAs of cells infected with BLVs of lymphosarcomatous animals gave hybridizations corresponding to the three same sizes. It is noticeable that the three mRNAs detected in FLK-BLV cells, known to contain a BLV isolate originating from a non tumorous cow, were of a smaller size than reported above.

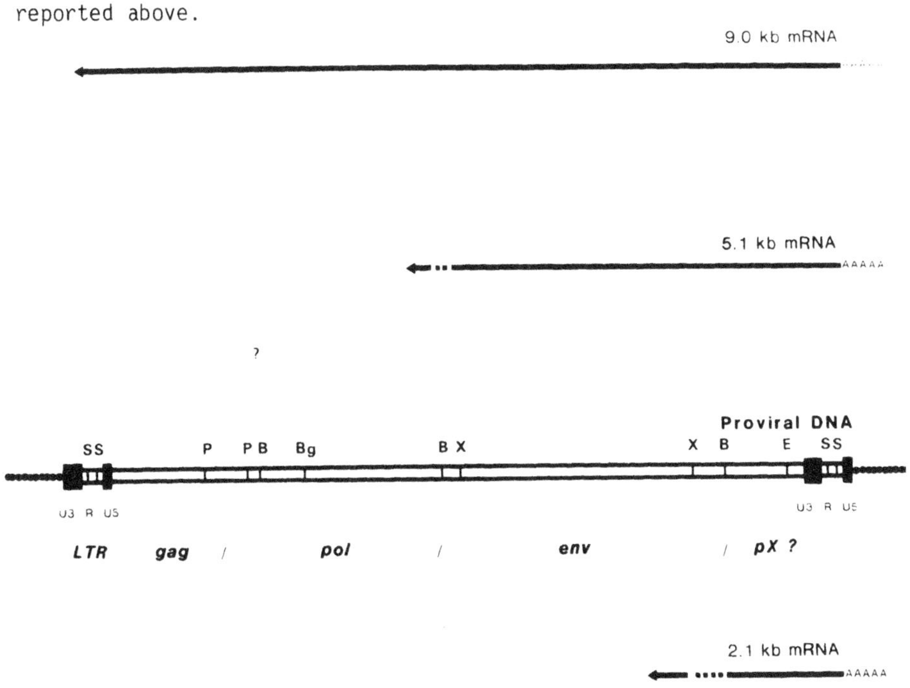

Figure 8

4. DISCUSSION

In this report we describe and map the viral mRNAs synthetized by BLV infected producing cells (figure 8). Briefly 3 species were observed : a 9.0 Kb mRNA, a 5.1 Kb mRNA and a new specie i.e. a 2.1 Kb mRNA. The 9.0 Kb mRNA is transcribed from the entire BLV provirus and may be compared to that of other retrovirus (23) and thus responsible for gag-pol gene translation. According to previous studies (24, 25) 3 major polyproteins would be synthetized from it, namely P45 pr70 and pr145. The P45 and pr70 were shown to harbor antigenicities of the gag proteins, p24, p15 and p12 ; the pr145 is a gag-pol polyprotein, origin of the polymerase.

The 5.1 Kb mRNA is the transcript of the env part of the BLV provirus extending from few nucleotides on the left hand side of the central BamHI site to the 3' end of the provirus. This region of the genome codes for a gpr72-70 containing antigenicities of the enveloppe gp51 (24, 25).

The 2.1 Kb mRNA was found to be specific of BLV infected cells. Alike the two other mRNAs, the latter was observed only in cells expressing the viral proteins and noteworthy not in non cultured tumor cells. Neither is it specific of the tumoral state as cultured tumor cells from a sporadic case of lymphosarcoma do not express such a 2.1 Kb mRNA. The hybridization patterns observed in this study indicate that this mRNA is the transcript of a region of the genome extending from the right BamHI site of the env gene to the 3' LTR. Because of a weak hybridization of the pol-env probe (n° 3) with a 2.1 kb mRNA, and if one considers this specie identical to the upperly described 2.1 kb mRNA it could be postulated that this molecule originates from a splicing event between the 5' end of the env mRNA and the pX region. The use of the technique of "sandwich hybridization" would help to confirm such a conclusion. Nevertheless this molecule is a bovine leukemia virus specific mRNA. This is in accordance with the existence of open reading frames (pX) as determined by nucleotide sequencing of both BLV and HTLV proviruses (17, 26).

Although the protein(s) coded by the pX sequences remains as yet not identified, its role in leukemogenesis can be envisioned because both BLV and HTLV are competent viruses able to code for all their structural proteins. In a way the pX could be the homology of the src gene of the Rous sarcoma virus but without any cellular proto-oncogene counterpart. In this case to play a role the pX would have to be modified (for example by mutation) and its role would reside in the initiation of the lymphoproliferative process. Arguments for such a modification of the pX are (i) only a few of the BLV infected animals develop persistent lymphocytosis and lymphosarcomas (ii) as evidenced in our epidemiological surveys in herds in which a BLV-induced lymphosarcoma occurs the leukemia risk of the other animals drastically increases (this situation mimics the emergence of an "acute BLV" in tumor cells which then is horizontally transmissible within the herd). Finally (iii) the role of the pX as "initiator" of cell multiplication by a "hit and run" mechanism is supported by the complete absence of BLV expression in tumor cells.

ACKNOWLEGDMENTS

We are indebted to Dr J. Miller and Dr Van Der Maaten for supplying the FLK-BLV cell line. We thank Dr J. Quesnel for access to a large variety of tumour bearing cattle. We greatly acknowledge the technical assistance of Mrs. C. Bourget and for the careful preparation of the manuscript Mss L. Couillaud.

REFERENCES

1. MILLER JM MILLER LD OLSON C GILLETTE KG : Virus-like particles in phytohemagglutinin-stimulated lymphocyte cultures with reference to bovine lymphosarcoma. J. Nat. Cancer Inst. (43) 1297-1305. 1969.
2. KAWAKAMI TG MOORE AL THEILEN GH MUNN RJ : Comparisons of virus like particles from leukotic cattle to feline leukosis virus. Bibl. haemat. (36) 471-475. 1970.
3. KETTMANN R PORTETELLE D MAMMERICKX M CLEUTER Y DEKEGEL D GALOUX M GHYSDAEL J BURNY A, CHANTRENNE H : Bovine leukemia virus an exogenous RNA oncogenic virus Proc. Nat. Acad. Sci. U.S.A. (73) 1014-1018. 1976.
4. KENYON SJ PIPER CE Properties of density gradient-fractionated peripheral blood leukocytes from cattle infected with bovine leukemia virus. Infect. Immun. (16) 898-903. 1977.
5.-PAUL PS, POMEROY KA, CASTRO AE JOHNSON DW MUSCOPLAT CC SORENSEN DK : Detection of bovine leukemia virus in B lymphocytes by the syncytia induction assay. J. Nat. Cancer Inst. (59) 1269-1272. 1977.
6. KETTMANN R BURNY A CLEUTER Y GHYSDAEL J. MAMMERICKX M : Distribution of bovine leukemia virus proviral DNA sequences in tissues of animals with enzootic bovine leukosis. Leuk. Res. (2) 23-32. 1978.
7. STOCK ND FERRER JF : Replicating C type virus in phytohemagglutinin-treated buffy-coat cultures of bovine origin. J. Nat. Cancer Inst. (48) 985-996 1972.

8.--BURNY A. BRUCK C, CHANTRENNE H, CLEUTER Y. DEKEGEL D, GHYSDAEL J. KETTMANN R, LECLERCQ M. LEUNEN J MAMMERICKX M PORTERELLE D : Bovine leukemia virus · molecular biology and epidemiology. In G. Klein (ed.) Viral oncology. Raven Press. New York. 1980, pp 231--289.

9.--KETTMANN R, COUEZ D. BURNY A : Restriction endonuclease mapping of linear unintegrated proviral DNA of bovine leukemia virus. J. Virol. (38) 27-33 1981.

10-DESCHAMPS J, KETTMANN R. BURNY A : Experiments with cloned complete tumor-derived bovine leukemia virus information prove that the virus is totally exogenous to its target animals species. J. Virol. (40) 605-609. 1981.

11. MAMOUN RZ ASTIER T GUILLEMAIN B DUPLAN JF : Bovine lymphosarcoma expression of BLV related proteins in cultured cells. J. gen. Virol. (64) 1895-1905. 1983.

12. NELL BG. HAYWARD NS. ROBINSON HL FANG J ASTRIN SM : Avian leukosis virus-induced tumors have common proviral integration sites and synthesize discrete new RNAs : oncogenesis by promoter insertion. Cell (23) 323-334. 1981.

13.--KETTMANN R DESCHAMPS J, COUEZ D CLAUSTRIAUX JJ, PALM R, BURNY A : Chromosome integration domain for bovine leukemia provirus in tumors J. Virol. (47) 146-160. 1983.

14.-GREGOIRE D COUEZ D DESCHAMPS J HEVERTZ S, HORS-CAYLA MC, SZPIRER J SZPIRER C BURNY A, HUEZ G, KETTMANN R : Different bovine leukemia virus-induced tumors harbor the provirus in different chromosomes. J. Virol. (50) 275-279. 1984.

15.-KETTMANN R DESCHAMPS J, CLEUTER Y, COUEZ D, BURNY A, MARBAIX G : Leukemogenesis by bovine leukemia virus : proviral DNA integration and lack of RNA expression of viral long terminal repeat and 3' proximate cellular sequences. Proc. Nat. Acad. Sci. U.S.A. (79) 2465-2469. 1982.

16.--GALLO RC : The family of human T cell leukemia viruses and their role in the cause of T cell leukemia and AIDS. This conference.

17.-BURNY A : Bovine leukemia virus : how does it act ? This conference.

18.-MAMOUN RZ. ASTIER T, GUILLEMAIN B : Establishment and propagation of a bovine leukaemia virus-producing cell line derived from the leukocytes of a leukaemic cow. J. gen. Virol. (54) 357-365. 1981.

19.-VAN DER MAATEN MJ MILLER JM : Replication of bovine leukemia virus in monolayer cell cultures. Bibl. heamat. (43) 360 362. 1976.

20.-McMASTER GK. GARMICHAEL GG : Analysis of single and double-stranded nucleic acids on polyacrylamide and agarose gels by using glyoxal and acridine orange. Proc. Nat. Acad. Sci. U.S.A. (74) 4835-4838. 1977.

21. CHANDLER PM, RIMKUS D. DAVIDSON N : Gel electrophoretic fractionation of RNAs by partial denaturation with methylmercuric hydroxide. Anal Biochem. (99) 200-206. 1979.

22.-MANIATIS T. FRITSCH EF. SAMBROOK J : Molecular cloning a laboratory manual. Cold Spring Harbor Laboratory. 1982.

23 -STEPHENSON JR : Type C structural and transformation-specific proteins. Molecular Biology of RNA Tumor Viruses. In Stephenson JR (ed.). London : Academic Press 1980, pp. 245-297.

24.-GHYSDAEL J, KETTMANN R, BURNY A : Translation of bovine leukemia virus virion RNAs in heterologous protein-synthesizing systems. J. Virol. (99) 1087-1098. 1979.

25. MAMOUN RZ, ASTIER T GUILLEMAIN B. DUPLAN JF : Bovine lymphosarcoma : processing of bovine leukaemia virus coded proteins. J. gen. Virol. (64) 2791-2795. 1983

26.-SEIKI M HATTORI S HIRAYAMA Y, YOSHIDA M : Human adult T-cell leukemia virus : complete nucleotide sequence of the provirus genome integrated in leukemia cell DNA. Proc. Nat. Acad. Sci. U.S.A. (80) 3618-3622 1983.

26

PRIMATE RETROVIRUSES AND AIDS

MURRAY B. GARDNER

Department of Pathology, University of California,
Davis, California

1. INTRODUCTION

Retroviruses have been incriminated as the primary agent of human AIDS (1,2). Further strengthening this probable etiologic association has been the discovery that an AIDS-like syndrome, which occurs spontaneously in monkeys and shows many similarities to human AIDS (3,4), is also apparently caused by an exogenous retrovirus. In this paper we briefly review the evidence for a retroviral etiology of SAIDS and compare the human and monkey syndrome and their respective retroviruses.

2. EVIDENCE FOR RETROVIRAL ETIOLOGY

The evidence for a retroviral etiology of Simian AIDS (SAIDS) derives from the following epidemiologic, virologic and serologic findings: 1) A similar novel retrovirus has been found in association with spontaneous SAIDS in at least 7 species of macaques at four Primate Centers (5). The virus is exogenous and has not yet been isolated from normal unexposed monkeys. The virus has a type D morphology, Mg++ dependent reverse transcriptase and it is related to, but antigenically and genetically distinct from the Mason-Pfizer Monkey Virus (MPMV) (6,9). By competitive radioimmunoassay (RIA), the major core (p27) protein is closely related to MPMV but the envelope glycoprotein (gp7Ø) is different. 2) Tissue culture grown virus has induced an experimental disease that closely mimics the natural disease spectrum (7,8). 3) Only this type D retrovirus and no other agent has been detected in the infective plasma sucrose gradient fractions (1.15.1.18 g/cc) and this infectivity was abolished by ether treatment (7). Other latent simian viruses (cytomegalovirus, adenovirus, parvovirus, herpes virus, HTLV-I) do not appear causative of SAIDS although they may become secondarily activated. 4) Normal disease transmission was first shown to require close physical contact (10) in keeping with spread of putative virus by body secretions such as saliva and blood. SAIDS type D virus was later found in large amounts in saliva and urine of an inapparent healthy carrier previously linked to disease outbreaks. Inoculation of healthy monkeys with this saliva virus has induced the disease. 5) Exposed monkeys have detectable humoral antibody to this type D virus and resistant monkeys may show a rise in titer. 6) The type D virus is detectable in the blood (7,8), circulating lymphocytes (6) and tumors (9) of monkeys with SAIDS. The virus appears to be cytopathic for lymphoid cells but a selective tropism for any specific subset has not as yet been demonstrated. 7) The initial MPMV isolate was also immunosuppressive when first inoculated into infant monkeys and induced a SAIDS-like disease (11,12).

Collectively, these results make a strong case for a MPMV-related family of retroviruses as the cause of monkey AIDS. Interestingly, all of the recent type D virus isolates (>30 in number) from monkeys with SAIDS at the different centers have been the MPMV variants and there have been no isolates of the parental MPMV from healthy or sick animals. Strain variation is detected in virus isolates from the different centers based on competitive RIA for envelope (gp70) and minor core (p10) proteins. Inability to isolate the original MPMV, thought to be so prevalent based on serologic survey (13), suggests that it is not now widespread and that mutations occurring in its genome over the past decade may have enhanced its immunosuppressive potency. Conclusive proof that the MPMV-related variants are the cause of SAIDS will, of course, require induction of the disease with biologically and molecularly cloned virus and prevention of disease with appropriate antisera or vaccination.

3. COMPARISON OF SAIDS WITH AIDS

The major similarities and differences between SAIDS and AIDS are summarized as follows: 1) Both diseases are infectious, exhibit similar epidemiologic, immunologic and pathologic features (14,15) and are apparently caused by exogenous retroviruses. Exposed individuals usually show humoral antibody to the virus. Virus strain variation may account for differences in disease spectrum in both man and monkey. 2) The opportunistic infections and tumors in both syndromes are alike with the exception that *Pneumocystis carinii* and disseminated KS are much less common in SAIDS.
3) Both diseases show a severe impairment of cellular and humoral immune function; in SAIDS this takes the form of a severe depletion of both T and B cells without the early reversal of the helper-suppressor cell ratio or polyclonal hypergammopathy as often seen in prodromal AIDS (3,16). On this account SAIDS most closely resembles terminal AIDS in its manifestations. However, now that monkeys relatively resistant to SAIDS are being identified, some of these hyperimmune stigmata may become evident. Although both monkey and human AIDS viruses damage rather than immortalize lymphoid cells, the SAIDS virus does not have the restricted T helper cell tropism characteristic of the HTLV family. Instead the SAIDS virus grows in a wide variety of cell types from different species (6-9).

4. COMPARISON OF RETROVIRUSES ASSOCIATED WITH SAIDS AND AIDS

Recent evidence argues strongly that human T lymphotropic retroviruses (HTLV) are the primary cause of AIDS (for summary, see 17). Specifically indicated are LAV and HTLV-III that have cytopathic effects on target T helper cells. These cytopathic variants are probably closely related and they differ immunologically from the two well characterized subgroups of HTLV, HTLV-I and HTLV-II which occasionally immortalize or transform T cells and are associated with human T cell lymphomas. There is no evidence from competitive RIA that the SAIDS virus isolates contain any endogenous or exogenous primate type C viruses, including HTLV-I (6,7). Nor is there, as yet, any evidence that these nonhuman primate type C viruses are associated with immunosuppression. The SAIDS retrovirus morphologically is indistinguishable from HTLV-III and LAV in that the extracellular particles have a similar type D structure. Identical appearing particles have also been found in a lymph node biopsy of a man with prodromal AIDS (18). However, the monkey and human viruses are antigenically unrelated because human sera reactive with the major core protein (p25) of LAV fail to react in Eliza test with the major core protein (p27) of the SAIDS virus (Chermann J.C., personal communication). Therefore, it appears that the SAIDS type D family of viruses may be the macaque counterpart of the human HTLV-III/LAV retroviruses, but the AIDS agents are unique to each species. The retroviruses causing AIDS in monkeys and humans may have had a common origin based upon their morphology, Mg++ dependent reverse transcriptase activity, and cytopathic effect on lymphoid cells. However, compared to the HTLV family, the SAIDS virus has a much broader cell tropism and is not restricted to T4 helper cells. Other primate retroviruses with type D particle morphology include the endogenous viruses of the langur and squirrel monkey, and these agents are not immunosuppressive (for summary, see 19). The langur virus, however, is related to MPMV (20,21) which suggests that Southeast Asia, the home of langurs and macaques, may have been the site of origin for MPMV and the MPMV-derived SAIDS type D retroviruses (9). Clearly then, this new simian model of AIDS offers an elegant opportunity to explore in parallel with human studies a "new biology" based on the pathophysiology of retrovirus induced immune suppression and associated disease and for determining how to prevent this problem in primates.

ACKNOWLEDGMENTS

The author wishes to thank other members of the SAIDS team at the University of California, Davis: Preston A. Marx, Kent G. Osborn, Nicholas W. Lerche, Donald H. Maul, Roy V. Henrickson, Marty Bryant, Gisela Heideker, Betsy Bencken, and Robert Munn.

REFERENCES

1. Barre-Sinoussi F, Chermann JC, Rey F, Nugeyre MT, Chamaret S, Gruest J, Dauguet C, Azler-Blin C, Vezinet-Brun F, Rouzioux C, Rozenbaum W, Montagnier L: Isolation of a T-lymphotropic retrovirus from a patient at risk for acquired immune dificiency syndrome. Science (220):868-870, 1983.
2. Gallo RC, Salahuddin SZ, Popovic M, Shearer GM, Kaplan M, Haynes BF, Palker TJ, Redfield R, Oleske J, Safai B, White G, Foster P, Markham PD: Frequent detection and isolation of cytopathic retroviruses (HTLV-III) from patients with AIDS and at risk for AIDS. Science (224):500-503, 1984.
3. Letvin NL, Eaton KA, Aldrich WR, Sehgal PK, Blake BJ, Schlossman SF, King NW, Hunt RD: Acquired immunodeficiency syndrome in a colony of macaque monkeys. Proc Natl Acad Sci (80):2718-2722, 1983.
4. Henrickson R, Maul DH, Osborn KG, Sever JL, Madden DL, Ellingsworth LR, Anderson JH, Lowenstine LJ, Gardner MB: Epidemic of acquired immunodeficiency in rhesus monkeys. Lancet (i):388-390, 1983.
5. Gardner M, Marx P, Maul D, Osborn K, Lowenstine L, Lerche N, Henrickson R, Munn B, Bencken B, Bryant M, Sever J: Simian acquired immune deficiency syndrome: An overview. In: Gottlieb MA, Groopman JE (eds) Acquired immune deficiency syndrome, UCLA Symposia on Molecular and Cellular Biology, New Series. Alan R Liss, Inc, New York, 1984, in press.
6. Daniel MD, King NW, Letvin NL, Hunt RD, Sehgal PK, Desrosiers RC: A new type D retrovirus isolated from macaques with an immunodeficiency syndrome. Science (223):602-605, 1984.
7. Marx PA, Maul DH, Osborn KG, Lerche NW, Moody P, Lowenstine LJ, Henrickson RV, Arthur LO, Gravell M, London WT, Sever JL, Levy JA, Munn RJ, Gardner MB: Simian AIDS: Isolation of a type D retrovirus and disease transmission. Science (223):1083-1086, 1984.
8. Gravell M, London WT, Hamilton RS, Sever JL, Kapikian AZ, Murti G, Arthur LO, Gilden RV, Osborn KG, Marx PA, Henrickson RV, Gardner MB: Transmission of simian AIDS with type D retrovirus isolate. Lancet (i):334-335, 1984.
9. Stromberg K, Benveniste R: Efficient isolation of endogenous rhesus retrovirus from trophoblast. Virology (128):518-523, 1983.
10. Lerche NW, Henrickson RV, Maul DH, Gardner MB: Epidemiological aspects of an outbreak of acquired immunodeficiency in rhesus macaques. Lab Anim Sci (34):146-150, 1984.
11. Fine DL, Arthur LO: Expression of natural antibodies against endogenous and horizontally transmitted macaque retroviruses in captive primates. Virology (112):49-61, 1981.
12. Fine DL, Landon JC, Pienta RJ, Kubicek MT, Valerio MJ, Loeb WG, Chopra HC: Responses of infant rhesus monkeys to inoculation with Mason-Pfizer monkey virus materials. J Natl Cancer Inst (54):651-658, 1975.

13. Fine D, Schochetman G: Type D primate retroviruses: A review. Cancer Res (38):3123-3139, 1978.
14. King NW, Hunt RD, Letvin NL: Histopathologic changes in macaques with an acquired immunodeficiency syndrome (AIDS). Amer J Path (113):382-388, 1983.
15. Osborn KG, Prahalada S, Lowenstine LJ, Gardner MB, Maul DH, Henrickson RV: The pathology of an epizootic acquired immunodeficiency in rhesus macaques. Am J Path (114):94-103, 1984.
16. Maul DH, Miller CH, Marx PA, Bleviss ML, Madden DL, Henrickson RV, Gardner MB: Simian acquired immunodeficiency syndrome: Influence of IL-2 on mitogen-induced lymphocyte blastogenesis. Submitted, 1984.
17. Editorial: The cause of AIDS? Lancet (i):1053-1054, 1984.
18. Warner TFCS, Gabel C, Hafez GR, Uno H, Borcherding WR: Type D retrovirus in prodromal AIDS? Lancet (i):860, 1984.
19. Fine DL, Schochetman G: Type D primate retroviruses: review. Cancer Res (28):3123-3139, 1978.
20. Benveniste RE, Todaro GJ: Evolution of primate oncornaviruses: An endogenous virus from langurs (*Presbytis* spp.) with related virogene sequences in other Old World monkeys. Proc Natl Acad Sci (74):4557-4561, 1977.
21. Bryant ML, Sherr CJ, Sen A, Todaro GJ: Molecular diversity among five different endogenous primate retroviruses. J Virol (28):300-313, 1978.

27

MOLECULAR COMPARISONS OF THE D-TYPE RETROVIRUSES

E. HUNTER, C. S. BARKER, J. BRADAC, S. CHATTERJEE, R. DESROSIERS AND J. W. WILLS

University of Alabama, Laboratory for Special Cancer Research, Birmingham, Alabama

1. INTRODUCTION

The D-type retroviruses represent the most recently discovered genus within the sub-family oncovirinae of the family Retroviridae. The assignment of viruses into this group has been primarily on the basis of similarities in virus structure and morphogenesis. Mason-Pfizer monkey virus (M-PMV), the prototype D-type retrovirus, was isolated from a breast carcinoma of a female rhesus monkey by Jensen et al. (12) in 1970. The virus has properties in common with both the mammalian B-type viruses (e.g. mouse mammary tumor virus, MMTV) and C-type viruses (e.g. baboon endogenous virus, BaEV) but is distinct from both (2, 3). Like MMTV, M-PMV preassembles a virus core structure or A-type particle within the cell, and thus virus particles bud from the plasma membrane with a complete nucleoid (Fig 1, panels a and b).

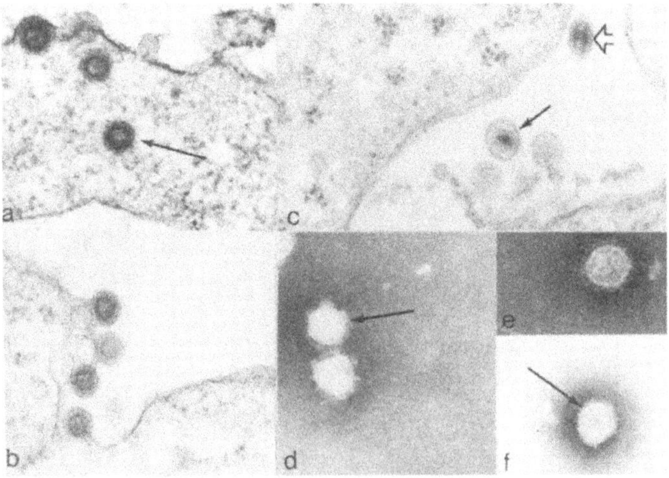

FIGURE 1. a) Intracytoplasmic A-type particles (arrow). a) and b) Budding with complete nucleoid. c) Mature virion (arrow) and virion with cylindrical core (open arrow). d), e) and f) negatively-stained virions showing knobbed-spikes (arrow).

However, the morphology of the mature D-type virion more closely resembles that of C-type viruses, in that in general the condensed, cylindrical nucleoid is centrally located (Fig.1, panel c) in contrast to the eccentric location of the B-type nucleoid. Furthermore, the virion lacks the dense fringe of glycoprotein seen on MMTV, possessing instead a halo of knobs or knobbed spikes (Fig. 1, panels d,e and f). A second feature in common with MMTV is the presence of a reverse transcriptase with a preference for magnesium over manganese (4). The latter divalent cation is preferred by most mammalian C-type retrovirus enzymes (5).

Despite the fact that M-PMV was isolated from the breast tumor of a rhesus monkey and shows many molecular similarities to MMTV, M-PMV has not been shown experimentally to be an oncogenic virus. Attempts to induce tumors by innoculation of M-PMV into rhesus monkeys (6), and other primates (quoted in 7) have been unsuccessful. M-PMV has been reported to transform rhesus foreskin cells in culture (8, 9), but this property of the virus has not been reproducible with the stocks of the virus currently available (S. C. and E. H., unpublished; L. Arthur, personal communication). Although rhesus monkeys neonatally inoculated with M-PMV or M-PMV-infected cells did not develop tumors, many developed severe lymphadenopathy, weight loss, and thymic atrophy (6). A large proportion of the inoculated animals succumbed to secondary viral or bacterial pneumonia (6). These results are particularly pertinent in light of the recent association of D-type retroviruses with Simian Aquired Immune Deficiency Syndrome (SAIDS) as will be discussed in more detail below.

In the 14 years following the identification of M-PMV, several other D-type viruses have been isolated and these are listed in Table 1. The isolates from both normal rhesus tissue (10) and cultured human cells (11, 12) are indistinguishable from M-PMV and the latter, often referred to as the "HeLa viruses", probably represented contamination of the cell lines by this primate virus (7). A distinct D-type retrovirus, morphologically resembling M-PMV, was isolated in 1977 from the lung tissue of a New World primate, the squirrel monkey. Although antigenically distinct and with no demonstrable sequence homology to M-PMV, this virus (squirrel monkey retrovirus or SMRV) was included in the D-type retrovirus group (13). The following year, a third D-type retrovirus, designated Po-1-Lu, was isolated after cocultivation of lung tissue from the Old World monkey, Presbytis obscurus, the spectacled langur (14). Po-1-Lu possesses a major capsid protein that is antigenically indistinguishable from M-PMV (14), and the genome of this isolate shows significant nucleic acid homology (20-30%) to M-PMV (15).

Table 1. D-TYPE RETROVIRUS ISOLATES

Origin	Virus	Host Tissue
OLD WORLD MONKEYS		
M. mulatta	M-PMV	Spontaneous mammary tumor of a female rhesus monkey
	X-381	Lactating mammary gland of a female monkey
	FTP-1	Placenta of a female rhesus monkey
	SAIDS-D/NE, SAIDS-D/CA	Blood of a rhesus monkey with SAIDS
	SAIDS-D/W	Fibroma of a rhesus monkey with SAIDS
P. obscurus	Po-1-Lu	Lung tissue of a spectacled langur.
NEW WORLD MONKEYS		
S. sciureus	SMRV	Lung cells of a squirrel monkey.
MAN		
H. sapiens	HeLa isolates	HeLa cell cultures

Three additional virus isolates that are related to the M-PMV and langur viruses have recently been included in the D-type retrovirus genus (16-18). These viruses, designated here SAIDS-D/NE (16), SAIDS-D/CA (17) and SAIDS-D/W (18), have been isolated from Macaque monkeys suffering from an immunodeficiency syndrome that pathologically resembles the human Aquired Immune Deficiency Syndrome, AIDS. Like M-PMV, Po-1-Lu, and SMRV, they share the biological and biochemical properties characteristic of the D-type retroviruses (Table 2). While many of these characteristics have already been discussed with regard to M-PMV, the ability of all members of the group to induce cell-cell fusion (syncytium formation) is worthy of further discussion since studies with M-PMV, SMRV, and the langur virus have shown that syncytium formation requires an intact viral genome and early protein synthesis but does not require proviral DNA synthesis (19, 20). D-type syncytium assays do not provide a measure of infectious, replication-competent virus. We have suggested previously that fusion might result from infection with a defective form of the virus (2).

Table 2. CHARACTERISTICS OF D-TYPE RETROVIRUSES

1. Bud From Cell Membrane With Complete Nucleoid
2. Assemble Intracytoplasmic A-type Particles
3. Extracellular Particles Have Central Nucleoid But Lack Prominent Surface Projections
4. Density 1.16 in Sucrose/1.21 in CsCl
5. Mg^{2+} -Dependent Reverse Transcriptase
6. Induce Cell To Cell Fusion Of Normal Cells.

The association of D-type retroviruses with SAIDS and recent observations suggesting that the retrovirus causing pulmonary adenomatosis in sheep fits into this group (22) opens up the possibility that a family of D-type viruses exists with a broad spectrum of pathogenic potential. It is imperative, therefore, to understand the molecular organization of these viruses and how they differ from one another. We present here an overview of our recent molecular studies on the D-type retroviruses in the context of previous work in this area.

2. D-TYPE RETROVIRUS PROTEIN BIOSYNTHESIS

Previous studies by others (23, 24) had suggested that M-PMV virions contained six structural polypeptides in addition to the viral reverse transcriptase; two of these, gp70 and gp20, are glycosylated and presumably represented the <u>env</u> gene products. The remaining four nonglycosylated polypeptides, p27, p14, p12 and p10, are similar in size to the <u>gag</u> gene products of other mammalian retroviruses. We have recently reexamined the composition of M-PMV virions using [^{3}H]leucine to radiolabel the virion polypeptides. As can be seen from Fig.2a, three additional polypeptides, p24, p16-18, and p6, have been resolved in polyacrylamide gels of M-PMV virions. Tryptic-peptide analyses of p24 and the leading and trailing edges of the p16-18 complex showed that all were variants of a single polypeptide. Since p24 and p16-18 are phosphoproteins, the differences in mobility may represent different levels of phosphorylation (25). The origin of p6 remains to be determined (see below).

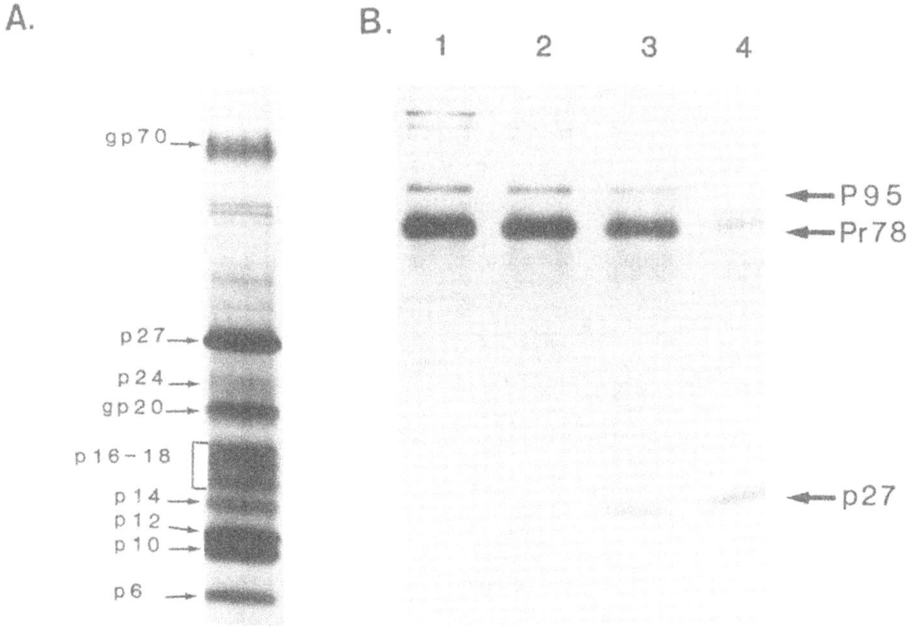

FIGURE 2. a) [^{3}H]leucine labeled virion polypeptides electrophoresed on a 12% SDS-polyacrylamide gel. b) M-PMV-infected cells were pulse-labeled (lane 1) or pulse-labeled then chased for 30 min (lane 2), 1 hr (lane 3) or 2 hr (lane 4). Detergent lysates of the cells were immunoprecipitated with antiserum to M-PMV p27.

At least 7 of the 9 virion proteins could potentially be gag gene encoded products and in order to determine which were encoded by this gene, we have identified the gag gene precursor polypeptide and assigned individual polypeptides to this molecule by tryptic peptide mapping. Immunoprecipitation of lysates from pulse-labeled, M-PMV infected cells with monospecific antiserum to the major structural protein of the virus, p27, allowed the identification of 2 major gag-related polyproteins that we have designated $Pr78^{gag}$ and $P95^{gag}$ (Fig. 2b). The intensity of both bands decreases after a chase period, with the concommitant appearance of p27. Tryptic peptide analyses of Pr78, P95 and each of the virion polypeptides showed that Pr78 contained all of the peptides of p27, pp24, pp16 - pp18, p14, p12 and p10 but not those of p6. It is likely therefore that Pr78 represents the major gag gene translation product and the precursor protein to 5 individual gag gene-encoded proteins. As we discuss below, the encoding of 5 proteins on the gag gene is unusual for mammalian viruses, being shared only by MMTV and not by any of the mammalian C-type retroviruses. From evidence presented elsewhere (25), we have concluded that P95 is analogous to the Pr110 polyprotein observed in MMTV infected cells and may represent an independent precursor for the viral protease. Although not resolved well in the particular gel shown in Fig. 2b. a third polyprotein, Pr180, was also identified in the anti-p27 immunprecipitates and the isolation of a mutant with a deletion in the pol gene (26) confirmed that Pr180 was the gag-pol precursor.

In order to determine the organization of the gag-encoded polypeptides on Pr78 we have employed the technique of pactamycin mapping (27). The results of these experiments are summarized in Fig. 3 and are compared to similar analyses for MMTV, SMRV, and BaEV.

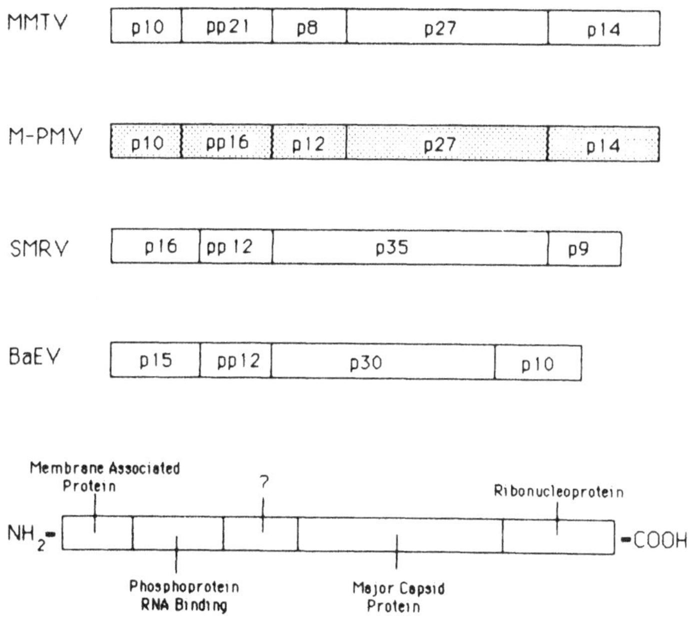

FIGURE 3. Comparison of B, C and D-type retrovirus gag-gene precursors.

Although the molecular weights of the individual structural polypeptides of various retroviruses are different, the functional domains are invariably located in the same relative positions on the precursor protein and are arranged in the order - NH_2 - Membrane Associated Protein - Phosphoprotein(RNA binding) - Major Capsid Protein - Ribonucleoprotein - COOH. In addition, we have proposed from studies on the avian retrovirus, RSV, that a fifth functional region (with an as yet undetermined function) is located to the amino-terminal side of the major capsid protein (28). In

M-PMV, p10 is a myristylated, hydrophobic and presumably membrane binding protein (E.Hunter, unpublished); the pp16 complex is a phosphoprotein; p27 is the major capsid protein and p14 is a basic,nucleic acid-binding (29) ribonucleoprotein. The fifth protein, p12, presumably plays the 'to be determined' role mentioned above.

A comparison of the organization of the M-PMV gag-precursor to that of MMTV reveals a striking similarity both in the number of polypeptides and their molecular weights (Fig.3). In MMTV p8 appears to be analogous to p12 of M-PMV (C.Dickson, personal comm.). Although we have not compared the polypeptides of M-PMV and the langur virus, it seems likely from the work of Colcher et al. (30) and Bryant et al. (24) that the two viruses will have a similar polypeptide composition. The precursor organization of SMRV on the other hand is quite different from M-PMV, it contains only 4 polypeptides (p16, pp12, p35, and p9) that have molecular weights more closely aligned with those of BaEV (31). It is possible, however, that the large major capsid protein, p35, could represent a fusion of a p12 and a p27-like polypeptide; a comparison of these polypeptides at the amino acid sequence level will be particularly informative. From the data presented above it would appear that M-PMV is more closely related to MMTV in its gag-region organization than it is to the other primate D-type retrovirus SMRV. Whether this will be reflected at the amino acid and nucleotide level and whether it points to common biological properties remains to be determined.

An analysis of M-PMV glycoprotein biosynthesis has shown that gp70 and gp20 are initially synthesized as a glycosylated polyprotein of 86,000 MW ($Pr86^{env}$) (32). The nonglycosylated form of this polyprotein, synthesized in the presence of the glycosylation inhibitor tunicamycin, is 55kd in size suggesting that the env product is highly glycosylated. Pactamycin mapping experiments place the proteins in the order: NH_2 - gp70 - gp20 - COOH, consistent with that of other retrovirus env polyproteins (27). The products of the env gene are similar in size to those of SMRV and BaEV, the major difference being the presence of carbohydrate on the smaller polypeptide, gp20.

The results of comparisons of the D-type viral proteins at the molecular level are for the most part supported by studies on their antigenic relationships. These have generally been based on competitive radio-immunoassays (RIAs). Using homologous RIAs in which the ability to compete for ^{125}I-M-PMV p27/anti-p27 binding was assessed, several investigators have been unable to distinguish between the major capsid proteins of M-PMV and Po-1-Lu (14, 33). In contrast, SMRV was found to be only partially related in these assays and MMTV or BaEV not at all (14, 33, 34). In more broadly reactive RIAs, common interspecies determinants have been identified for the latter viruses (33). Although indistinguishable in p27 assays, the langur virus shows only partial homology in homologous p10 assays and none in those employing gp70. Common interspecies determinants are shared between the gp70 of M-PMV and the other D-type isolates and with BaEV (14). This latter observaton is consistent with comparisons made at the nucleotide level described below.

3. COMPARATIVE STUDIES OF D-TYPE RETROVIRUS NUCLEIC ACIDS

The apparent relatedness of different D-type isolates at the nucleotide level depends on the comparative technique used and the level of stringency employed. For example, we have compared the RNA genomes of M-PMV, Po-1-Lu, and SMRV in two-dimensional oligonucleotide fingerprint analyses, as shown in Fig. 4.

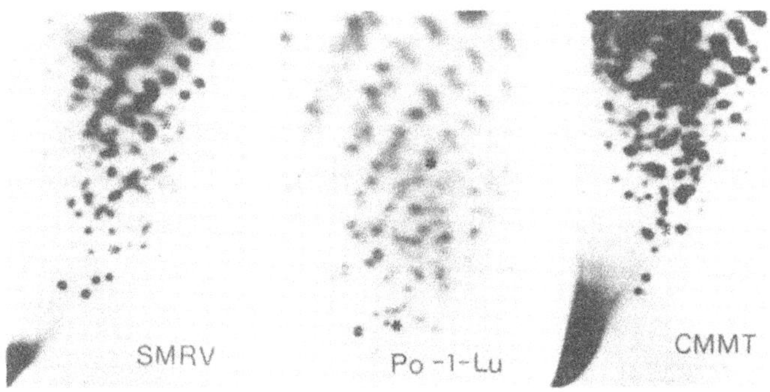

FIGURE 4. ^{32}P-labeled T_1-oligonucleotide fingerprints of SMRV, langur virus (Po-1-Lu) and M-PMV (from CMMT cells).

By this analysis, one might conclude that the viruses show no homology whatsoever, even though it is clear from the studies described above that M-PMV and the langur virus are close relatives. Hybridization in solution of complementary viral RNA or DNA probes to DNA from infected cells followed by digestion with the single strand specific nuclease (S1) indicated that M-PMV was 20-30% homologous to the langur isolate but less than 5% homologous to SMRV, even though the two viruses share antigenic determinants (36). Furthermore, these approaches provide no information on which regions of the genome contain the nucleotide sequence homologies.

In an attempt to obtain a better understanding of the genomic organization of M-PMV and its relationship to other retroviruses at the molecular level, we have molecularly cloned the M-PMV genome (37, 38). Preliminary experiments indicated that the M-PMV proviral DNA genome was cleaved three times by the restriction endonuclease HindIII, a single time by SstI, and not at all by EcoRI. In our initial approach we cloned HindIII digested M-PMV proviral DNA fragments into the bacterial plasmid, pAT153. Studies using these clones allowed a detailed restriction map to be constructed for the M-PMV genome, showed the linear proviral DNA to be 8.1kb in length and defined the length of the M-PMV LTR at 350bp (37). Using these subgenomic clones as highly specific hybridization probes we have succeeded in cloning the circular form of the unintegrated provirus via its single SstI site into the lambda cloning vector, λgtWES λB. In addition, we have cloned 5 integrated M-PMV proviruses, each representing a unique integration site, after complete EcoRI digestion of high molecular DNA from infected cells. Four of the five clones have yielded infectious virus after transfection into uninfected human or rhesus cells (38).

The molecular genetic studies described above have provided both new information on the M-PMV genome and tools to reassess the relatedness of M-PMV to other D-type and B-type retroviruses. A comparison of the restriction endonuclease cleavage maps of M-PMV, SMRV (39) and MMTV (40) (Fig. 5) in general supports the findings from liquid hybridization studies in which SMRV was found to show only limited homology and MMTV not at all (36). MMTV has a completely different pattern of cleavage for the four (hexanucleotide-recognizing) enzymes shown, while SMRV shows limited identity, apparently sharing 3 cleavage sites (marked with *).

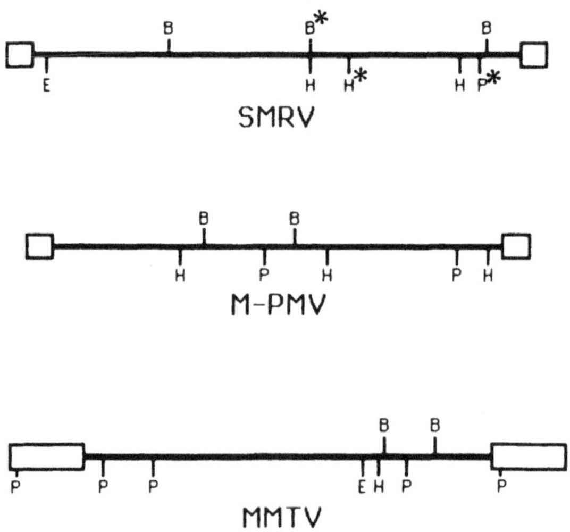

FIGURE 5. Comparative restriction maps of B and D-type retroviruses. B - BamHI, E - EcoRI, H - HindIII, P - PstI.

Two of these (BamHI and HindIII) are probably located in the sequence coding for the carboxyterminus of the pol gene product, a highly conserved region in these viruses (see below), and the third (PstI) is probably located in the sequence coding for the carboxyterminal portion of the env gene product.

In order to determine whether SMRV and M-PMV are more closely related than had previously been suggested from liquid hybridization studies, we have used the Southern blot technique which is less sensitive to mismatched base pairing but which allows the detection of sequence homologies that might not have been observed previously. The molecularly cloned genome of SMRV (39) was cleaved with a variety of restriction enzymes, transferred to nitrocellulose paper and hybridized under conditions of low stringency to a ^{32}P-labeled total M-PMV genome probe. The results of these experiments are depicted schematically in Fig. 6 and show that hybridization was observed across the entire genome of SMRV; the region of strongest hybridization corresponding to the pol gene region of this virus. Hybridization of restriction fragments of cloned BaEV proviral DNA (41), under identical conditions, results in a limited hybridization that is restricted to the env gene region of this virus (Fig. 6). This result confirms the specificity of the hybridization of M-PMV sequences to SMRV and suggests that M-PMV also shares the 600 bp region of homology previously demonstrated between BaEV and SMRV (42).

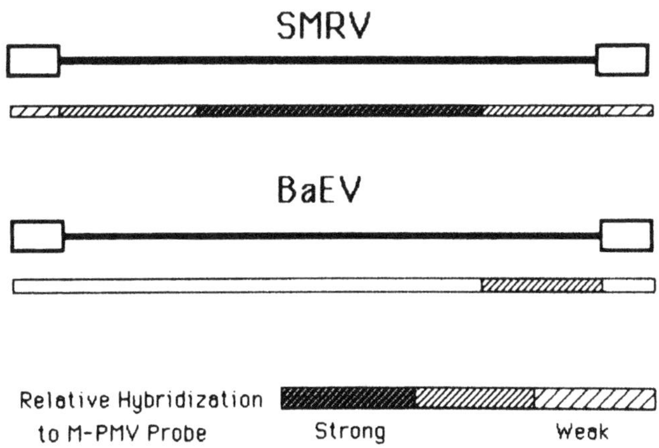

FIGURE 6. Hybridization of cloned M-PMV genomic DNA to cloned primate retroviruses under low-stringency conditions.

These studies strengthen the concept that M-PMV and SMRV have evolved from a single progenitor virus and support their inclusion in a single group. It will be interesting to determine, given the protein data discussed previously, whether the genome of MMTV can hybridize to M-PMV sequences under the low stringency conditions described here.

4. D-TYPE RETROVIRUSES ASSOCIATED WITH SIMIAN ACQUIRED IMMUNE DEFICIENCY SYNDROME

Recently a disease analogous to the human acquired immune deficiency syndrome (AIDS) has been recognized in macaque monkeys in several primate centers within the United States (16-18). At the New England Primate Center cocultivation of blood from a SAIDS-afflicted rock-macaque (*M. cyclopis*) with transformed human lymphoid cells allowed the isolation of a virus (SAIDS-D/NE) with morphogenic properties similar to those of the D-type viruses (16). A very similar virus (SAIDS-D/CA) was isolated at the California Primate Center after cocultivation of infected blood from a rhesus monkey (*M. mulatta*) with normal rhesus kidney cells (17), and a third isolate (SAIDS-D/W) has recently been reported (18). In this latter case, the immune deficiency syndrome was often accompanied by the development of a retroperitoneal fibroma, and virus was obtained after cocultivation of the fibroma tissue with canine cells (18). The major biological and biochemical properties of the isolates, summarized in Table 3, clearly place these viruses within the D-type retrovirus group.

Table 3. PROPERTIES OF THE SAIDS-D VIRUS ISOLATES

1. Assemble Intracytoplasmic A-type Particles.
2. Reverse Transcriptase Prefers Magnesium Over Manganese.
3. Fuse Human Lymphoid Cells and Normal Rhesus Cells.
4. Major Core Protein, p27, Antigenically Indistinguishable from M-PMV.
5. Nucleic Acid Homology With M-PMV and Langur Virus.

Competition radioimmunoassays have shown the major structural protein, p27, of all three SAIDS-D isolates to be indistinguishable from the p27 of M-PMV and the langur virus (L. Arthur, unpublished). However, in a type-specific RIA for the amino-terminal *gag* polypeptide, p10 of M-PMV, the SAIDS-D/W isolate can be distinguished from M-PMV and the other 2 isolates (L. Arthur - unpublished). The major antigenic difference between the SAIDS-D isolates and M-PMV is in the glycoprotein, gp70, since none of the isolates compete in an homologous M-PMV gp70 RIA. In heterologous gp70 RIAs the SAIDS-D/W isolate can again be distinguished from the New England and California isolates, the latter two being indistinguishable in all assays carried out to date (L. Arthur - unpublished).

At the nucleic acid level the new D-type viruses are clearly related to M-PMV and the langur virus. Liquid hybridization experiments in which SAIDS-D/W complementary DNA was hybridized to M-PMV and langur virus infected cell DNA prior to S_1 digestion, indicated that approximately 40% of the viral sequences were homologous (18). Using a subgenomic M-PMV probe that contained the gag and LTR regions of M-PMV it has been possible to clone the unintegrated proviral DNA of the SAIDS-D/NE virus and to obtain a restriction map of the viral genome (R. D., unpublished). A comparison of the restriction enzyme map of the SAIDS-D/NE virus with that we have established for M-PMV shows a remarkable degree of identity (Fig. 7). Of the 24 hexanucleotide recognition sites shown, 11 are shared between the SAIDS-D isolate and M-PMV. Interestingly, the majority of non-conserved sites appear to reside in those regions of the genome that would be expected to code for the gag and pol gene products of the virus, even though, in preliminary cross-hybridization experiments we have observed a uniform level of hybridization across the entire genome. This is consistent with studies by Benveniste *et al.* on DNA hybrids between M-PMV and the SAIDS-D/W DNA in which a uniform divergence across the entire viral genome was shown (18).

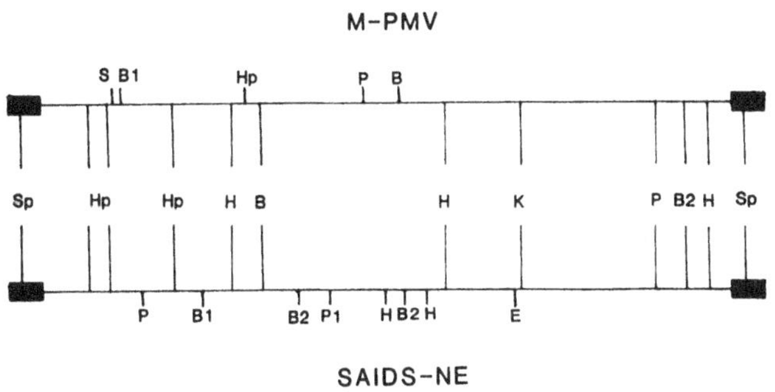

FIGURE 7. Comparative restriction maps of M-PMV and the SAIDS-D/NE isolate. B - BamHI, B1 - BglI, B2 - BglII, E - EcoRI, H - HindIII, Hp - HpaI, K - KpnI, P - PstI, P1 - PvuI, S - SstI, Sp - SphI.

Since previous studies had shown that members of the Cercopithecinae subfamily of Old World monkeys (which includes the macaques) possessed in their chromosomal DNA multiple copies of sequences related to M-PMV (36, 44), we were interested in reexamining this observation with our cloned probes. In Fig. 8, Southern blots of EcoRI digested chromosomal DNA from rhesus (lanes 5 and 6), baboon (lane 4) and African green monkey cells (lane 3) were hybridized under conditions of low stringency to pMP6 then washed under low (A), moderate (B) and then highly stringent conditions (C). Infected rhesus cells (lanes 7 and 8) provided the positive control.

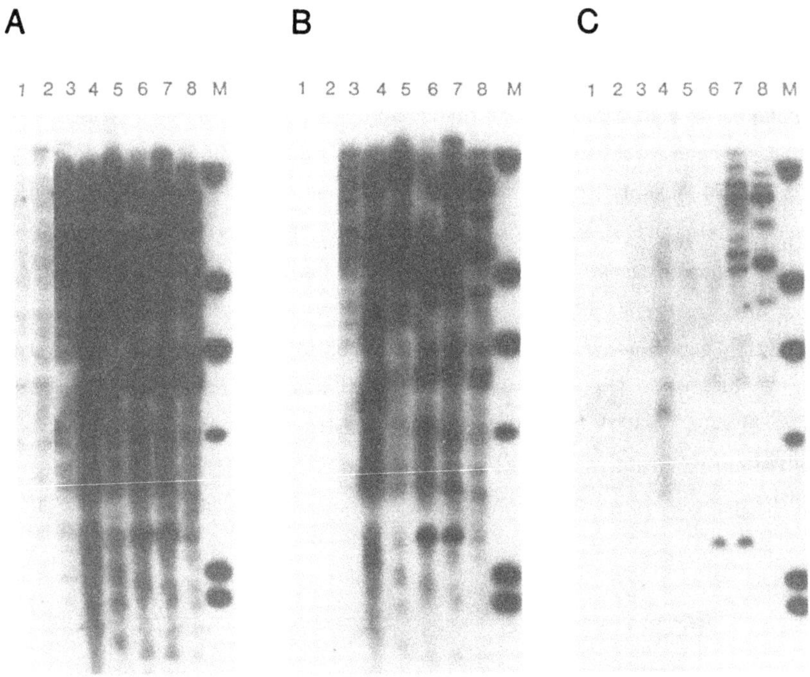

FIGURE 8. Hybridization of the gag-LTR probe of M-PMV to EcoRI digested chromosomal DNA from various species of primates.

With low and moderately stringent washes, multiple bands (30-50) of hybridizing DNA were observed in uninfected DNA from all three members of the Cercopithecinae subfamily, confirming the previous results from liquid hybridization studies (36, 44). Hybridization with human (lane 1) and chimpanzee (lane 2) chromosomal DNA was only observed at the lowest stringency. With highly stringent washes, however, only those DNAs containing exogenously introduced M-PMV sequences (lanes C7 and C8) showed positive hybridization. It is clear, therefore, that the endogenous sequences present in the chromosomal DNA of these monkeys are significantly divergent from those of M-PMV. Nevertheless, the presence of related sequences together with the propensity for retroviruses to undergo genetic recombination (45), leaves open the possibility that the pathogenic potential of Old World D-type retroviruses could evolve through frequent recombination with these endogenous cellular sequences.

Two significant questions relating to the new D-type isolates remain to be answered. The first is with regards to their role in the development of SAIDS. The SAIDS-D/CA virus has been reported to induce the disease in inoculated animals (17), whereas to date, the SAIDS-D/NE isolates have not. (No data is yet available for the SAIDS-D/W isolate). The reasons for this discrepancy remain to be determined. The second question concerns the relationship of the D-type isolates to the HTLV-III/LAV retroviruses that have recently been shown to be associated with human AIDS (46, 47). Both the simian and human viruses share important biochemical and biological properties: a reverse-transcriptase that prefers magnesium over manganese; mature particles with cylindrically shaped cores; and the ability to cause cell-to-cell fusion of human and/or primate cells. Whether these similarities are simply coincidental remains to be seen.

REFERENCES

1. Chopra HC, Mason MM: A new virus in a spontaneous mammary tumor of a rhesus monkey. Cancer Res (30): 2081-2086, 1970.
2. Jensen EM, Zelljadt I, Chopra HC, Mason MM: Isolation and propagation of a virus from a spontaneous mammary carcinoma of a rhesus monkey. Cancer Res (30): 2388-2393, 1970.
3. Kramarsky B, Sarkar NH, Moore DH: Ultrastructural Comparison of a virus from a rhesus-monkey mammary carcinoma with four oncogenic RNA viruses. Proc Natl Acad Sci, USA (68): 1603-1607, 1971.
4. Abrell JW, Smith RG, Robert MS, Gallo RC: DNA polymerase from RNA tumor viruses and human cells: Inhibition by polyuridylic acid. Science (177): 1111-1113, 1972.
5. Dion AS, Vaidya AB, Fout GS: Cation preferences for Poly(rC)-Oligo(dG)-directed DNA synthesis by RNA tumor viruses and human milk particulates. Cancer Res (34): 3509-3515, 1974.
6. Fine DL, Landon JC, Pienta RJ, Kubicek MT, Valerio MJ, Loeb WF, Chopra HC: Responses of infant rhesus monkeys to inoculation with Mason-Pfizer monkey virus materials. J Natl Cancer Inst (54): 651-658, 1975.
7. Fine D, Schochetman G: Type D primate retroviruses: A review. Cancer Res (38): 3123-3139, 1978.
8. Fine DL, Pienta RJ, Malan LB, Kubicek MT, Bennett DG, Landon JC, Valerio MG, West DM, Fabrizio DA, Chopra HC: Biologic characteristics of transformed rhesus foreskin cells infected with Mason-Pfizer monkey virus. J Natl Cancer Inst (52): 1135-1142, 1974.

9. Ahmed MJ, Yeh J, Holden HE, Korol W, Schidlovsky G, Mayyasi SA: Characterization of Mason-Pfizer monkey virus induced cell transformation in vitro. Arch Virol (55): 93-105, 1977.
10. Ahmed M, Korol W, Yeh J, Schidlovsky G, Mayyasi SA: Detection of Mason-Pfizer monkey virus infection with human KC cells carrying Rous virus genome. J Natl Cancer Inst (53): 383-387, 1974.
11. Zhdanov VM, Soloviev VO, Bektemirov JA, Ilyin K, Bykovsky AF, Mazureuko NP, Irlin IS, Yershov FI: Isolation of oncornaviruses from continuous human cell cultures. Intervirology (1): 19-26, 1973.
12. Ilyn KV, Bykovsky AF, Zhdanov VM: An oncornavirus isolated from human cancer cell line. Cancer (37): 89-96, 1973.
13. Heberling RL, Barker ST, Kalter SS, Smith GC, Helmke RJ: Isolation of an oncornavirus from a squirrel monkey (Saimiri sciureus) lung culture. Science (195): 289-292, 1977.
14. Todaro GJ, Benveniste RE, Sherr CJ, Schlom J, Schidlovsky G, Stephenson, JR: Isolation and characterization of a new type D retrovirus from the asian primate, Presbytis obscurus (Spectacled langur). Virology (84): 189-194, 1978.
15. Benveniste RE, Todaro GJ: Evolution of primate oncornaviruses: An endogenous virus from langurs (Presbytis spp.) with related virogene sequences in other Old World monkeys. Proc Natl Acad Sci, USA (74): 4557-4561, 1977.
16. Daniel MD, King NW, Letvin NL, Hunt RD, Sehgal PK, Desrosiers RC: A new type D retrovirus isolated from macaques with an immunodeficiency syndrome. Science (223): 602-605, 1984.
17. Marx PA, Maul DH, Osborn KG, Lerche NW, Moody P, Lowenstine LJ, Henrickson RV, Arthur LO, Gilden RV, Gravell M, London WT, Sever JL, Levy JA, Munn RJ, Gardner MB: Simian AIDS: Isolation of a type D retrovirus and transmission of the disease. Science (223): 1083-1086, 1984.
18. Stromberg K, Benveniste RE, Arthur LO, Rabin H, Giddens Jr. WE, Ochs HD, Morton WR, Tsai C-C: Characterization of exogenous type D retrovirus from a fibroma of a macaque with simian AIDS and fibromatosis. Science (224): 289-292, 1984.
19. Chatterjee S, Hunter E: The characterization of Mason-Pfizer monkey virus-induced cell fusion. Virology (95): 421-433, 1979.
20. Chatterjee S, Hunter E: Fusion of normal primate cells: A common biological property of the D-type retroviruses. Virology (107): 100-108, 1980.
21. Chatterjee S, Bradac J, Hunter E: Effect of tunicamycin on cell fusion induced by Mason-Pfizer monkey virus. J Virol (38): 770-776, 1981.
22. Sharp JM, Herring AJ: Sheep pulmonary adenomatosis: Demonstration of a proten which cross-reacts with the major core proteins of Mason-Pfizer monkey virus and mouse mammary tumor virus. J Gen Virol (64): 2323-2327, 1983.
23. Schochetman G, Kortright K, Schlom J: Mason-Pfizer monkey virus: Analysis and localization of virion proteins and glycoproteins. J Virol (16): 1208-1219, 1975.
24. Bryant ML, Sherr CJ, Sen A, Todaro GJ: Molecular diversity among five different endogenous primate retroviruses. J Virol (28): 300-313, 1978.
25. Bradac J, Hunter E: Polypeptides of Mason-Pfizer monkey virus: I. Synthesis and processing of the gag gene products. Submitted for publication, 1984.
26. Chatterjee S, Bradac J, Hunter E: A rapid screening procedure for the isolation of nonconditional replication mutants of Mason-Pfizer monkey virus: Identification of a mutant defective in pol. Submitted for publication, 1984.
27. Bradac J, Hunter E: Polypeptides of Mason-Pfizer monkey virus: III. Translational order of proteins on the gag and env gene products. Submitted for publication, 1984.
28. Hunter E, Bennett JC, Bhown A, Pepinsky RB, Vogt VM: Amino terminal amino acid sequence of p10, the fifth major gag polypeptide of avian sarcoma and leukemia viruses. J Virol (45): 885-888, 1983.

29. Long CW, Henderson LE, Oroszlan S: Isolation and characterization of low molecular weight DNA binding proteins from retroviruses. Virology (104): 491-496, 1980.
30. Colcher D, Teramoto YA, Schlom J: Immunological and structural relationships between langur virus and other type D retroviruses. Virology (88): 384-388, 1978.
31. Devare SG, Stephenson JR: Primate retroviruses: Intracistronic mapping of type D viral gag gene by use of nonconditional replication mutants. J Virol (29): 1035-1043, 1979.
32. Bradac J, Chatterjee S, Hunter E: Polypeptides of Mason-Pfizer monkey virus: II. Synthesis and processing of env gene products of Mason-Pfizer monkey virus. In preparation, 1984.
33. Colcher D, Teramoto, YA, Schlom J: Interspecies radioimmunoassay for the major structural protein of primate type D retrovirus. Proc Natl Acad Sci, USA (74): 5739-5743, 1977.
34. Schochetman G, Fine DL, Arthur LO, Gilden RV, Heberling RL: Characterization of a retrovirus isolated from squirrel monkeys. J Virol (24): 384-393, 1977.
35. Schlom J: Type B and Type D Retroviruses. In: Molecular Biology of RNA Tumor Viruses. Academic Press, New York, 1980, pp 447-484.
36. Benveniste RE, Todaro GJ: Evolution of primate oncornaviruses: An endogenous virus from langurs (Presbytis spp.) with related virogene sequences in other Old World monkeys. Proc Natl Acad Sci, USA (74): 4557-4561, 1977.
37. Barker CS, Wills JW, Bradac JA, Hunter E: Molecular cloning of the M-PMV genome: Molecular characterization and cloning of subgenomic fragments. Submitted for publication, 1984.
38. Barker CS, Pickel J, Tainsky M, Hunter E: Molecular cloning of the M-PMV genome: Cloning of integrated and unintegrated proviral DNAs and analysis of infectivity. In preparation, 1984.
39. Chiu L-M, Anderson PR, Aaronson SA, Tronick SR: Molecular cloning of the unintegrated squirrel monkey retrovirus genome: Organization and distribution of related sequences in primate DNAs. J Virol (47): 434-441, 1983.
40. Shank PR, Cohen JC, Varmus HE, Yamamoto, KR, Ringold GM: Mapping of linear and circular forms of mouse mammary tumor virus DNA with restriction endonucleases: Evidence for a large specific deletion occurring at high frequency during circularization. Proc Natl Acad Sci, USA (75): 2112-2116, 1978.
41. Casey J, Barker CS, Hunter E: Unpublished results.
42. Chiu I-M, Callahan R, Tronick SR, Schlom J, Aaronson SA: Major pol gene progenitors in the evolution of oncoviruses. Science (223): 364-370, 1984.
43. Desrosiers R, Barker CS, Hunter E: Molecular comparison of M-PMV and the SAIDS-D/NE isolate. In preparation, 1984.
44. Drohan W, Colcher D, Schochetman G, Schlom J: Distribution of Mason-Pfizer virus-specific sequences in the DNA of primates. J Virol (23): 36-43, 1977.
45. Hunter E: The Mechanism for genetic recombination in the avian retroviruses. Curr Top Microbiol Immunol (79): 295-309, 1978.
46. Barre'-Sinoussi F, Chermann JC, Rey F, Nugeyre MT, Chamaret S, Gruest J, Dauget C, Axler-Blin C, Vezinet-Brun F, Rouzioux C, Rozenbaum W, Mantagnier L. Isolation of a T-lymphotropic retrovirus from a patient at risk for acquired immune deficiency syndrome (AIDS). Science (220): 868-871, 1983.
47. Gallo RC, Salahuddin SZ, Popovic M, Shearer GM, Daplan M, Haynes BF, Palker TJ, Redfield R, Oleske J, Safai B, White G, Foster P, Markhem PD: Frequent detection and isolation of cytopathic retroviruses (HTLV-III) from patients with AIDS and at risk for AIDS. Science (224): 500-503, 1984.

28

WOODCHUCK HEPATITIS VIRUS AND HEPATITIS B VIRUS AS RELATED TO KNOWN RNA AND DNA TUMOR VIRUSES AND HEPATOCELLULAR CARCINOMA

CHARLES E. ROGLER, MORRIS SHERMAN AND DAVID A. SHAFRITZ

Liver Research Center and Departments of Medicine and Cell Biology, Albert Einstein College of Medicine, Bronx, New York

I. Introduction

The hepadna virus family which currently consists of four members, including Hepatitis B Virus, (HBV), woodchuck hepatitis virus (WHV), ground squirrel hepatitis virus (GSHV), and duck hepatitis B virus (DHBV), comprises a group of unique small DNA viruses with many common structural and biological features (1,2,3). Some of the major similarities include (1) a common virion structure consisting of a relaxed circular DNA of about 3.2 Kbp, (2) similar genome organization in which it appears that all the usable open reading frames which could potentially code for polypeptides >10Kd have the same polarity and order, (3) a similar replication mechanism involving reverse transcription of a full length RNA intermediate, (4) immunological cross reactivity of the surface and core antigens (5) the ability to maintain persistent infections in the liver and (6) tissue tropism primarily for the liver. Studies over the last decade have implicated two environmental agents in the pathogenesis of hepatocellular carcinoma (HCC) in man, hepatitis B virus (4) and aflatoxin B_1 (5). Initial evidence for a causal association between hepatitis B virus (HBV) infection and HCC was based on an increased frequency of HBsAg in the serum of patients with HCC (4). This relationship has been confirmed by prospective studies reporting a several hundred fold greater risk for HCC among HBV carriers as compared to noncarriers within the same population (6).

The woodchuck hepatitis virus model is the only animal virus shown to mimic the human disease with regard to the progression from persistent infection to hepatocellular carcinoma. In some areas of eastern Pennsylvania and New Jersey, wild woodchuck populations have a carrier rate of 14-40%. When maintained in captivity for 4-5 years, woodchucks with chronic active hepatitis (CAH) develop HCC at an extraordinarily high rate (up to 90%). The histologic features of chronic active hepatitis in woodchucks are very similar to those of human HBV carriers, except that woodchucks often exhibit acute inflammation as well as cirrhosis, possibly because of the relatively short interval between initial infection and development of HCC.

Early studies investigating the possible mechanism by which hepatitis virus may cause HCC led to the discovery that most HCC tissues contained integrated viral DNA in both the human and woodchuck systems (7,15). Since viral integration has been shown to play a role in oncogenesis in several systems (16,17,18), there has been intense interest in the possible role of integrated hepatitis viral DNA in HCC. Since such molecules may have a role in progression from persistent infection to HCC, we will discuss studies directed at characterizing the molecular forms of HBV and WHV DNA in chronically infected hepatocytes and hepatomas. We will also discuss histological aspects of the progression and propose possible mechanisms for transformation of hepatocytes.

II. Molecular forms of viral DNA in hepatocytes during persistent viral infection

Replicative intermediates and CCC DNA

Summers and Mason (19) have recently showed that DHBV replicates via an RNA intermediate. This process involves reverse transcription of full length DHBV pregenome RNA in immature core particles located in the cytoplasm of infected duck livers. Since all the hepadna viruses have a similar genome structure, it is likely that they all replicate via a reverse transcriptase mechanism perhaps similar to that observed in retroviruses. The viral DNA replicative intermediates required for this mechanism have also been identified for HBV (20), GSHV (21) and WHV (unpublished data). However, the transcriptional template for the generation of the RNA pregenome has not been identified. Despite the fact that virtually all hepatocytes stain for DHBV core antigen and are apparently producing virus, attempts to identify an integrated DHBV provirus in liver tissue have not been successful. A recombinant DNA library in bacteriophage lambda containing approximately 10 genomes of duck genomic DNA did not reveal a single integrated DHBV provirus when probed with a ^{32}P DHBV DNA clone (Rogler and Summers, unpublished data). However, integrated WHV and HBV have been detected in persistently infected woodchuck and human tissue, as will be discussed below.

Covalently closed circular (CCC) viral DNAs have been identified in chimpanzee HBV chronic carriers (22), WHV carriers (23) GSHV carriers (21) and DHBV carriers (24). This CCC DNA is found exclusively in the nucleus and is the most likely candidate to serve as the transcriptional template for pregenome RNA. The mechanism by which CCC viral DNAs might replicate in the nucleus is presently not understood but may be similar to the replication mechanism for nuclear CCC DNAs of papovaviruses.

Novel forms and integrated WHV DNA

Initial studies of WHV and HBV DNA in hepatomas revealed the important finding that multiple integrations of WHV and HBV DNA were often found in clonally derived hepatoma tissues (7-15). The simplest explanation for these results is that viral integration occurs in persistently infected hepatocytes before the cells become transformed and that after transformation the integrations are clonally propogated in the tumor. This, in turn, implies that oncogenesis in the liver may be a multistage process in which viral integration may be one of several steps leading to an eventual malignancy, but may not by itself be sufficient to transform the cell. This type of mechanism has recently been proposed for Epstein Barr Virus, which can immortalize normal rat kidney cells without fully transforming them (25).

In an effort to obtain direct evidence for the integration of WHV in persistently infected tissue, Rogler and Summers cloned nuclear DNA from a chronically infected woodchuck liver which showed no signs of

HCC (26). A recombinant DNA library in Charon 30 consisting of two genome equivalents of woodchuck DNA was screened and one clone containing WHV sequences integrated into cellular sequences was isolated. The viral sequences in this clone were characterized by Southern blot analysis and electron microscope heteroduplex analysis. The map of viral sequences in this clone are shown in Figure 1. The viral sequences are colinear with the WHV genome, except for deletion of approximately 550 Bp between positions 1000 and 1550 on the viral map. No inverted or direct duplications of viral sequences were observed. This integration, therefore, represents a defective genome probably incapable of supporting virus replication. However, the open reading frames coding for the viral X, pre-S, S and C genes are present, indicating that this integration could support the production of viral antigens. The right hand viral-cell junction occurs approximately at position 1550 on the genome map. This is close to the 5' end of the virion plus strand, implicating a possible functional role for the virion DNA "cohesive-end" or the single strand DNA region in integration. No rearrangements in cellular sequences at the site of viral DNA integration were detected.

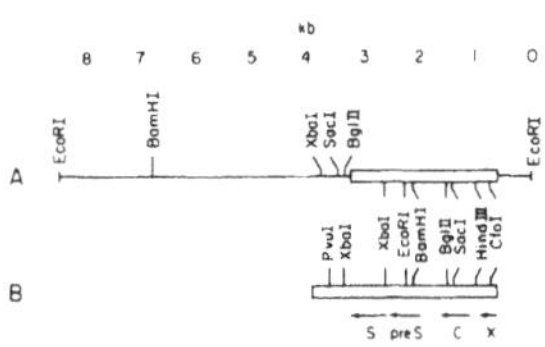

Figure 1. A. Restriction endonuclease map of clone HW 197-2: (——) woodchuck cellular sequences, (▭) WHV sequences.
B. Map of complete WHV genome and location of WHV genes.

Three additional clones containing unexpected forms of WHV were isolated during the screening of the genomic library of WHV persistently infected hepatocytes. These clones have been termed "novel forms" of WHV (23). Each "novel form" contained more than two genome equivalents of viral sequences with estensive rearrangements but no detectable cellular sequences (23). From the frequency by which "novel forms" were isolated from the library, it was estimated that they were present in approximately one copy per cell. Of a total of 11 sites at which rearrangements were mapped in the "novel form" clones, 10 occurred between viral segments of opposite polarity and one occurred between segments of the same polarity. The rearrangements are similar to those identified in integrated viral sequences cloned from woodchuck hepatocellular carcinomas (27, see below). A map of viral DNA sequences in one of the cloned "novel forms" in relation to the viral genome is illustrated in Figure 2, showing extensive rearrangement of viral DNA sequences. A similar cloning experiment with nuclear DNA from ground squirrel liver chronically infected with GSHV has yielded two additional "novel form" clones. These clones also contain rearranged viral sequences with no detectable cellular sequences (28).

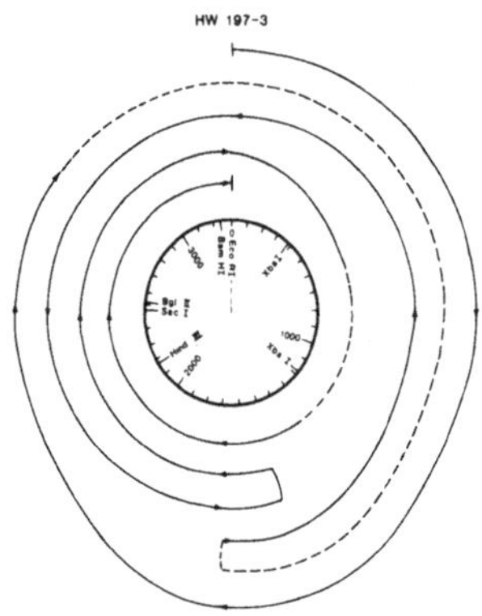

Figure 2. Structure of novel forms of WHV DNA in relationship to the intact circular viral map. The solid lines represent sections of the clone that are colinear with the viral map, and the arrows indicate progression from the left- to right-hand ends of the clone. Sections of the maps that appear as dashed lines connect sections of the genome that are adjacent in the clones. (⊢—) left end of clone; (—⊣) right end of clone. Note that several inverted duplications of viral sequences are present in a single novel form. (Reprinted, with permission, from Rogler and Summers, ref. 30).

The origin of "novel forms" and their function in persistent viral infection is currently unknown. One hypothesis is that they are derived from CCC DNA molecules in the nucleus, perhaps by rearrangement of viral sequences generated by aberrant replication or recombination mechanisms. In this case, they might represent end products of a process that gradually attenuates viral production by generating defective forms of viral DNA. Another possibility is that "novel forms" are derived from long stretches of integrated viral DNA.

HBV DNA in the liver of chronic carriers (persistent HBV infection)

Virologic aspects

In our experience, short-term carriers, i.e. patients who have been positive for HBsAg for longer than six months but less than two years, do not generally have detectable integrated HBV DNA by Southern blot analysis, irrespective of the presence of liver disease. These patients are usually HBeAg positive, DNA polymerase positive, and have circulating Dane particles. Large amounts of free viral DNA are invariably present in the liver at this stage and it is conceivable in these patients that viral DNA integration has occurred, but at low frequency and into random sites in the host genome. Such integrations would not be detected by "Southern blot" analysis, although Brechot et al, have reported integration of HBV DNA early during the infectious process (29).

In patients who are HBV carriers for several years, integrated HBV DNA has been found in a significant number of cases (15,30,31,32). In some of these patients, HBV DNA integration appears as a diffuse smear in high molecular weight DNA on Southern blot analysis, whereas in others discrete bands can be seen (Figure 3). The presence of discrete bands suggests clonal growth of a population of cells containing one or a few viral integrations. The livers of many long-term carriers have "ground glass" hepatocytes, indicating the presence of HbsAg in the cytoplasm (33). Serologically, these patients may be anti-HBe positive and may have only integrated HBV DNA and no free virion DNA in their hepatocytes. In these individuals, HBsAg may be produced from an integrated HBV DNA template.

Cellular aspects

In order to assess pathophysiologic events during persistent hepatitis B virus infection, studies were performed comparing

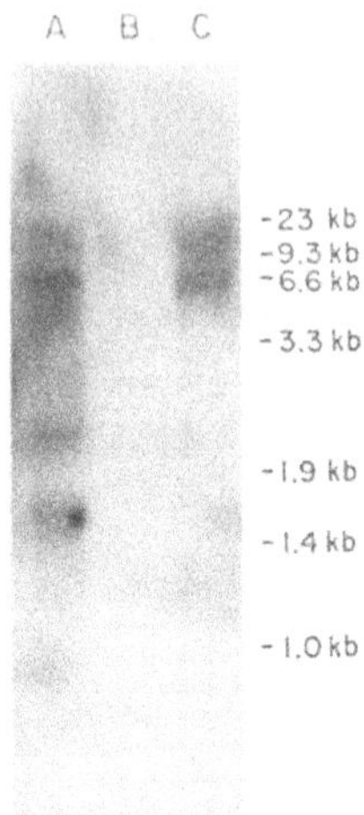

Figure 3. Detection of HBV-DNA sequences in total cellular DNA extracted from liver tissue of long-term carriers without active virus replication (Lanes A and C) and a control (Lane B).

histologic changes with the presence of HBsAg and HBcAg by immunofluorescence. The presence of various molecular forms of HBV DNA was also assessed. Our results (33), together with those of others (32,34,35), indicate that persistent HBV infection falls generally into two categories: permissive infection and non-permissive infection. The features of permissive (replicating) infection include (1) active inflammatory liver disease (chronic persistent or chronic active hepatitis), (2) HBsAg and HBcAg in individual cells distributed randomly throughout the hepatic parenchyma, and (3) free virion and lower MW replicating forms of HBV DNA. The features of non-permissive (non-replicating) infection include (1) no active inflammatory liver disease (the liver may show no histologic evidence of HBV infection or inactive cirrhosis resulting from viral infection many years earlier), (2) continued HBsAg, but not HBcAg, production, and (3) integrated HBV DNA molecules. In some cases, HBsAg production is present in nodular accumulations or clusters of cells which have the appearance of a focal clonal growth (Figure 4). The presence of such focal clonal growths perhaps represents an explanation for results we and others have made, namely that HBV integrations appear to have been clonally propagated in chronically infected human tissue.

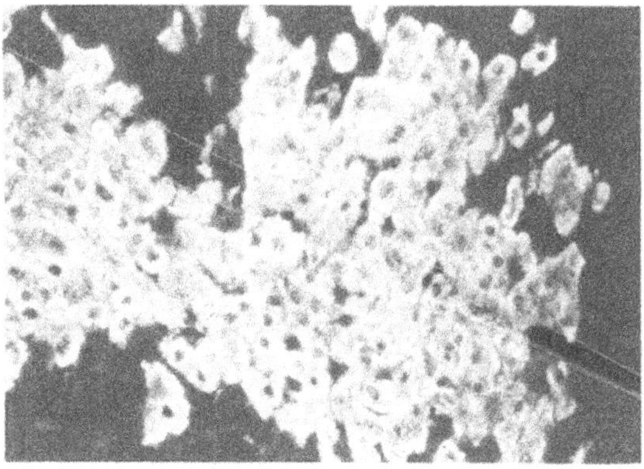

Figure 4. Detection of immunofluorescence of HBsAg in the liver of a carrier with no active virus replication. Accumulation of HbsAg is evident in the cytoplasm of many hepatocytes in focal accumulations or clusters of cells. HbcAg was not detected in replicate sections of this liver.

HBV and WHV DNA in hepatocellular carcinomas

General Considerations

Covalently closed circular, open circular and relicating forms of HBV are usually absent in tumors from HB_sAg carriers. The free HBV DNA observed in a few cases is probably due to presence of non-tumorous liver cells in the tissue specimen. Therefore, human tumors appear to be non-permissive for viral replication. Both woodchuck and human tumors have been shown to contain integrated viral DNA. Initial experiments using the Southern blot technique revealed that the tumors were clonally derived and that individual tumors could contain one or multiple integrations. Also, the amount of viral DNA in individual integrations varied greatly (7,8,10-15).

The importance of viral integration in oncogenesis has been extensively reviewed for both DNA and RNA viruses (16,17,18). Two examples of the effects of viral integration on tumorigenesis which may be particularly relevant to hepatitis and HCC are the promotor insertion mechanism, first described for ALV-induced lymphoid leukosis (36,37), and the immortalization of monkey epithelial cells by

Epstein-Barr virus (25). It is possible that integration of hepatitis virus could result in the activation of a cellular oncogene by the insertion of a viral promotor near that oncogene in accordance with the first model. On the other hand, it is possible that viral integration is just one step in a multistep process leading to the production of malignant cells.

Cloning Integration of WHV and HBV

In order to test various mechanisms of viral oncogenesis, it was necessary to clone individual integrations from primary hepatomas. In this way one could determine the position of viral promotors in relation to cell sequences in integrations and also determine whether the virus had inserted into a common cellular sequence in different tumors (promotor-insertion model). The first clones of integrated hepatitis viral DNA were obtained from two woodchuck hepatomas each of which contained only a single viral integration (27). The structure of the WHV sequences in the clones was determined by restriction endonuclease mapping and electron microscopic heteroduplex studies (27). Integrated WHV sequences were found to be highly rearranged (27), in a manner similar to the rearrangements observed in integrated SV40 DNA cloned from transformed cell lines (38,39). WHV integrations did not occur at fixed sites in either the cellular or the viral genome and deletions, duplications and inverted duplications of viral sequences were observed. Neither integrated WHV genome contained an intact unit length viral DNA segment and alterations (primarily deletions) have also been observed in cellular sequences flanking the site of WHV integration (Ogston et al., unpublished observations). A known viral promotor was located directly adjacent to cellular sequences in an orientation in which cellular sequences could be transcribed from this promotor (27).

There are several other features of these two WHV integrations (as well as a third) which require additional comment. Of the six viral-cellular junction fragments studied so far in the three clones, three are in the "cohesive end" or overlap region of the WHV genome ($\pm$

100 bp). The other three are in the region which is single-stranded in the virion particle. Koshy et. a. (40) have characterized three viral integrations cloned from a human cell line containing integrated HBV DNA. In each case they have found that the viral-cellular junction lies in the single-stranded region of the unintegrated viral genome. These authors propose a mechanism for viral DNA integration in which the single-stranded region of HBV interacts with cellular DNA during cellular replication to produce a recombination event and incorporation of viral DNA into the host genome. Ogston et. al. (27) stressed the fact that each of their WHV integrations contained sequences of the X gene region (the small open reading frame of virion DNA for which a specific polypeptide has not yet been identified). This segment of viral DNA also coincides with the "cohesive-end" of the genome, contains a TATA sequence (41) and shows gene promoter activity in vitro (42,43). Therefore, WHV integrations appear to have properties consistent with those observed for both RNA and DNA tumor viruses. Dejean et al. (44) have found similar results in a clone from a human HCC.

A schematic diagram comparing the features of a WHV integration from HCC with the integration described earlier from a non-tumorous carrier woodchuck is shown in Figure 5. In both instances a unit length WHV genome is not present. However, in the carrier integration there is merely a deletion of some viral sequences, whereas in the HCCs there are inversions, deletions and duplications of viral sequences. In addition, only the HCC integrations are associated with modifications (deletion or rearrangement) of flanking cellular sequences at the site of WHV integration (data presented below). These results provide strong evidence that integration of WHV occurs in cellular sequences during chronic WHV infection. Since rearrangements of both viral and cellular sequences were observed in clones from HCC, whereas they were not observed in the single clone from a chronic infection, these rearrangements may represent a characteristic unique to HCC. Attempts are now in progress to precisely identify, clone and characterize similar integrated HBV DNA sequences from nontumorous human and/or chimpanzee liver tissue.

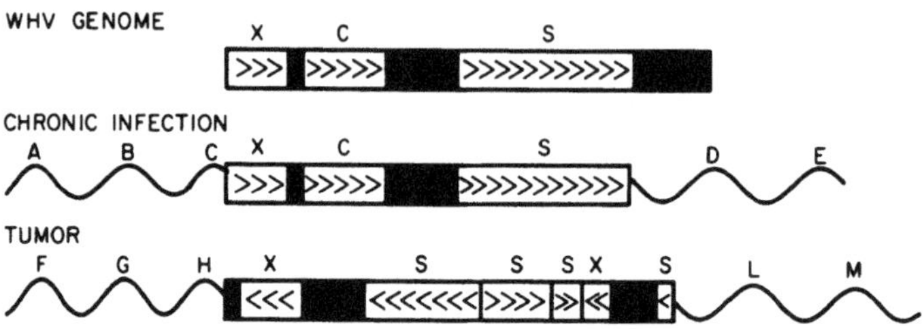

Figure 5. Schematic diagram comparing restriction maps of WHV genomic DNA (top), integrated WHV DNA from a chronic carrier woodchuck without hepatocellular carcinoma (middle) and integrated WHV-DNA from the tumor of a woodchuck carrier with hepatocellular carcinoma (bottom). The position of the viral X, C, and S gene segments is noted and the orientation of the various portions of the viral genome is denoted by >>>or<<<. Regions of the WHV genome not coding for X, C, or S are denoted by the black "filled in" areas.

Analysis of cellular sequences at the site of HBV and WHV integration

Two single copy cellular flanking sequences from two separate WHV integrations have been used to screen woodchuck tumors for integration of WHV at a common cellular site using the Southern blot technique. So far, a common cellular integration site has not been observed in approximately thirty tumors which have been screened (Ogston, Jonak and Summers, unpublished observation). Other workers who have cloned HBV integrations from hepatomas have reported similar results (personal communication). These results do not support the promotor insertion model.

In an effort to study the cellular sequences flanking HBV integrations, we have cloned two integrations from a human hepatocellular carcinoma. Experiments mapping the viral sequences in these clones revealed arrangements including deletions and partial duplications of viral sequences similar to those observed in woodchuck tumors (22). These sequences have not been characterized further;

however, both right and left hand host flanking sequences containing only single copy cellular DNA have been identified in one of these clones and have been subcloned into pBR322. These sequences of 0.78 Kb and 1.2 Kb, respectively, have been used as probes to map the cellular region flanking the HBV DNA integration in the original tumor DNA sample from which the clones were derived. The cellular flanking sequences in the tumor were compared with those of normal DNA by restriction endonuclease digestion and Southern blotting. This analysis revealed (Figure 6) that although the restriction endonuclease maps to the right of the HBV integration matched with a region of normal cellular DNA (a cellular domain), the restriction maps to the left of the HBV integration could not be matched to the predicted position in the normal cellular sequence. This meant that the cellular sequences to the left and right of the HBV integration site could not have been contiguous in the normal cellular locus before HBV integration occurred (Figure 6). These results showed that the DNA sequences up to 12kb surrounding the HBV integration have been modified, either by a large deletion or by translocation of sequences from another position in the cellular genome to this site together with integrated HBV DNA. By using both the left and right hand flanking sequence probes, we hope to determine the chromosomal location of the integration using "in situ" hybridization. Chromosomal rearrangements at the site of known celular oncogenes have been shown to occur in Burkitt's lymphoma and other neoplasms (46). It will, therefore, be interesting to determine whether this HBV associated rearrangement of cellular sequences involves a chromosomal translocation near a cellular oncogene.

Discussion and Speculation

Studies of the forms of hepatitis viral DNA present in the nuclei of persistently infected hepatocytes have provided clues as to the molecular events which may precede HCC. Studies briefly described above show that WHV DNA integrates into cellular sequences during chronic infection. Since integrated viral DNA is present in chronically infected cells, tumors which arise from these cells would

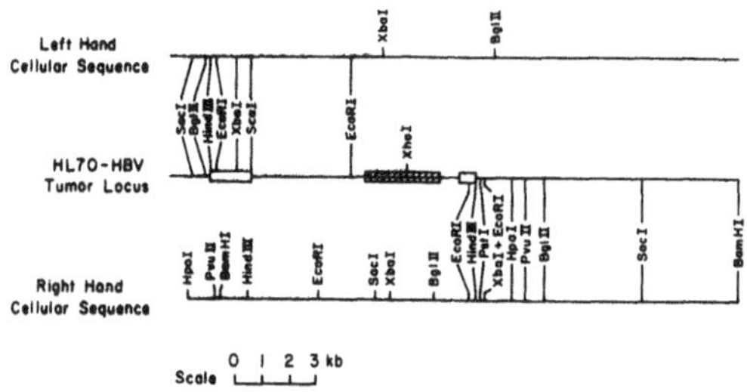

Figure 6. Schematic diagram illustrating restriction map of an integrated HBV DNA sequence with adjacent cellular flanking sequences from human tumor HL70 in comparison to normal cellular sequences mapped by use of unique right and left hand flanking sequence probes isolated from the same HBV DNA integration. See text for explanation. [open box] location of flanking probes [hatched box] integrated HBV DNA.

be expected to contain integrated viral DNA. Therefore, it may not be the initial integration that is related to oncogenesis, but rather events which occur subsequent to or as a result of viral DNA integration. One working hypothesis would be that cellular and viral sequences are rearranged after the initial integration event occurs and these rearrangements perhaps along with other factors lead to HCC.

From histological and cellular studies, it appears that there may be two types of persistent HBV infection. At one extreme, cells continue to replicate virus and show continued liver disease activity (permissive or actively replicating infection). At the other extreme, cells do not replicate the virus and show little or no liver disease activity (non-permissive or non-replicating infection). In permissive infection, the bulk of HBV DNA in hepatocytes is in free virions or replicating forms and integration into the host genome is not observable by Southern blot analysis. However, as Tiollais and coworkers have suggested (6) and Rogler and Summers have shown for woodchucks (40), integration probably occurs randomly into the host genome throughout the infectious period. Once active viral replication begins to subside, it may become possible to observe these random integrations as a smear of hybridization in the high MW region on Southern blot analysis. In some non-permissive infections, a single HBV DNA integration has been observed on Southern blots, suggesting that the cell population from which the DNA was derived is of monoclonal origin. A mixed type of persistent infection may also occur in which features of replicating and non-replicating infection are found in different cells or regions of the same liver.

Under circumstances in which hepatitis B virus remains in the liver only in the integrated form and is not replicated, it may be more difficult for host immune responses to rid the liver of infected hepatocytes than those in which viral replication continues. Under this "negative" selection pressure, there may be preferential accumulation of hepatocytes containing integrated HBV DNA especially, as compared to replicating viral DNA if the presence of the integration confers a selective advantage to the cell. Under a variety of circumstances and/or conditions which stimulate hepatocyte cell divisions over many years (host responses, humoral or hormonal factors, contact with environmental or chemical hepatotoxins or carcinogens, tumor promotors, inducers of liver regeneration, infecections with other viruses, etc.), a series of rearrangements of HBV DNA and/or cellular sequences in the host genome may occur leading to production of hepatocytes with an abnormal phenotype (cellular transformation). When such cells subsequently divide, clonal populations may be formed all containing the same integration pattern. This may appear histologically as a nodular accumulation of HbsAg producing hepatocytes ("ground-glass" cells) or a regenerative liver nodule. Continued gene rearrangement and division of such cells, under a variety of additional host factors or selection pressures, may ultimately lead to the development of an autonomously growing hepatic neoplasm (see Figure 7).

This conceptual, model, which is entirely speculative, requires integration of the HBV genome as one event in a series of steps in the transformation process but requires neither the expression of specific viral genes nor even the presence of HBV DNA in the eventual neoplasm. If such a mechanism is involved in cellular transformation, then the

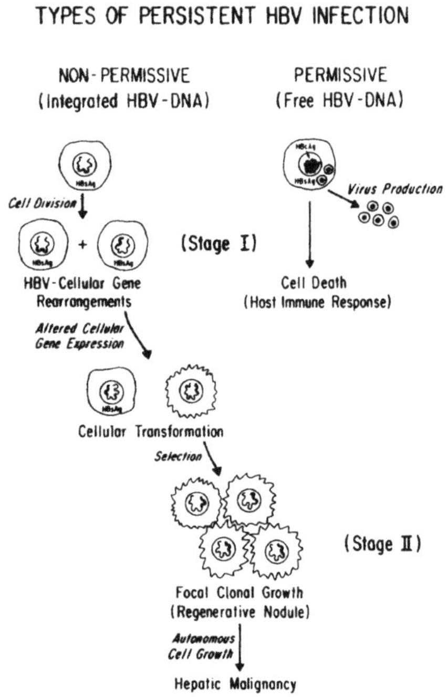

Figure 7. Conceptual model illustrating possible events following HBV infection and integration of HBV DNA into the liver cell genome which might ultimately lead to the development of hepatocellular carcinoma.

finding of integrated HBV DNA in a unique banding pattern in certain viral carriers, especially in those individuals who are no longer actively replicating virus, may have important implications in terms of risk for future development of hepatocellular carcinoma. Therefore, studies characterizing the sequence of events in modifying or rearranging HBV genes, integration of HBV DNA into the cellular genome and expression of intregrated HBV DNA sequences may ultimately be important in understanding factors involved in oncogenic transformation of human cells following virus infection.

REFERENCES

1. Robinson W, Marion P, Feitelson M, Siddiqui A: The hepadna virus group: Hepatitis B and related viruses. In: Szmuness W (ed) Viral Hepatitis 1981 Int Symp Franklin Press, Philadelphia, 1981, p57.
2. Tiollais P, Charnay P, Vyas GN. Biology of hepatitis B virus. Science (213): 406, 1981.
3. Summers J. Three recently described animal virus models for human hepatitis B virus. Hepatlogy (1): 179-183, 1981.
4. Szmuness W. Hepatocellular carcinoma and the hepatitis B virus: Evidence for a casual association. Prog Med Virol (24): 40-69, 1978.
5. Wogan GN. Aflatoxins and their relationship to hepatocellular carcinoma. In: Okuda K and Peters RL (eds) Hepatocellular Carcinoma. Wiley, New York, 1978.
6. Beasley RP, Hwang LY, Lin CC et al. Hepatocellular carcinoma and hepatitis B virus. A perspective study of 22,707 men in Taiwan. Lancet (ii): 1129-1133.
7. Snyder RL, Summers J. Woodchuck hepatitus virus and hepatocellular carcinoma. In: Essex M, Todaro G, zur Hausen M (eds) Viruses in naturally occurring cancers. Cold Spring Harbor Symposium on Cell Proliferation, 1980, (7): 447-458.
8. Summers J, Smolec JM, Werner, BG et al. Hepatitis B virus and woodchuck hepatitis virus are members of a novel class of DNA viruses. Cold Spring Harbor Conf Cell Proliferation, 1980, (7): 459-470.
9. Popper H, Shih JW-K, Gerin JL, et al. Woodchuck hepatitis and hepatocellular carcinoma: Correlation of histologic with virologic observations. Hepatology (1): 91-98, 1981.
10. Marion PL, Salazar FH, Alexander JJ, et al. State of hepatitis B viral DNA in a human hepatoma cell line. J Virol (33): 795-806, 1980.
11. Chakroborty PR, Ruiz-Opazo N, Shouval D, et al. Identification of integrated hepatitis B virus DNA and expression of viral RNA in an HBsAg-producing human hepatocellular carcinoma cell line. Nature, London (286): 531-533, 1980.
12. Brechot C, Pourcell C, Louise A, et al. Presence of integrated hepatitis B virus DNA sequences in cellular DNA of human hepatocellular carcinoma. Nature, London (286): 533-535, 1980.
13. Edman JC, Gray P, Valenzuela P, et al. Integration of hepatitis B virus sequences and their expression in a human hepatoma cell. Nature, London (286): 535-538, 1980.
14. Twist EM, Clark, HF, Aden DP, et al. Integration pattern of hepatitis B virus DNA sequences in human hepatoma cell lines. J Virol (37): 239-243, 1981.
15. Shafritz, DA, Shouval D, Sherman HI, Hadziyannis SJ, Kew MC. Integration of hepatitis B virus DNA into the genome of liver cells in chronic liver disease and hepatocellular carcinoma. New Engl J Med (305): 1067-1073, 1981.
16. Land H, Paroda LF, Weinberg, RA. Cellular oncogenes and multistep carcinogenesis. Science (222): 771-778, 1983.

17. Cooper, GM. Cellular transforming genes. Science (218): 801-806, 1982.
18. Willecke K, Schafer R. Human oncogenes. Human Genetics (66): 132-142, 1984.
19. Summers J, Mason WS. Replication of the genome of a hepatitis B-like virus by reverse transcription of an RNA intermediate. Cell (29): 403-415, 1982.
20. Fowler MJF, Monjardino J, Tsiquaye KN, Zuckerman AJ, Thomas HC. The mechanism of replication of hepatitis B virus: evidence for assymetric replication of the two DNA strands. J Med Virol (13): 83-91, 1984.
21. Weiser W, Ganem D, Seeger C, Varmus HE. Closed circular viral DNA and asymmetrical heterogenous forms in livers from animals infected with ground squirrel hepatitis virus. J Virol (48): 1-9, 1983.
22. Ruiz-Opazo N, Chakraborty PR, Shafritz DA. Evidence for supervoiled hepatitis B virus DNA in chimpanzee liver and serum Dane particles: Possible implications in persistent HBV infection. Cell (29): 129-138, 1982.
23. Rogler CE, Summers J. Novel forms of woodchuck hepatitis virus DNA isolated from chronically infected woodchuck liver nuclei. J Virol (44): 852-863, 1982.
24. Mason WS, Aldrich C, Summers J, Taylor JM. Asymmetrical replication of duck hepatitis B virus DNA in liver cells (free minus strand DNA). Proc Natl Acad Sci USA (49): 3997-4001, 1982.
25. Griffin BE, Karran L. Immortalization of monkey epithelial cells by specific fragments of Epstein-Barr virus DNA. Nature (309): 79-82, 1984.
26. Rogler CE, Summers J. Cloning and structural analysis of integrated woodchuck hepatitis virus sequences from a chronically infected liver. J Virol (50): 832-837, 1984.
27. Ogston CW, Jonak GJ, Rogler CE, Astrin SM, Summers J. Cloning and structural analysis of integrated woodchuck hepatitis virus sequences from hepatocellular carcinomas of woodchucks. Cell (29): 385-394, 1982.
28. Marion PL, Robinson WS, Rogler CE, Tapper D, Summers J. High molecular weight GSHV specific DNA in chronically infected ground squirrel liver. J Cell Biochem (suppl) (6): 203, 1982.
29. Brechot C, Hadchouel M, Scotto J, et al. State of hepatitis B virus in hepatocytes of patients with HBsAg positive and HBsAg negative liver diseases. Proc Natl Acad Sci USA (78): 3906-3910, 1981.
30. Koshy R, Maupos R, Miller R, Hofschneider PH. Detection of hepatitis B virus-specific DNA in the genomes of liver cirrhosis tissues. J Gen Virol (57): 95-102, 1981.
31. Brechot C, Scotto J, Charnay P, et al. Detection of hepatitis B virus DNA in liver and serum: a direct appriasal of the chronic carrier state. Lancet (2): 765-770, 1981.
32. Kam W, Rall LB, Smuckler EA, Schmid R, Rutter WJ. Hepatitis B viral DNA in liver and serum of asymptomatic carriers. Proc Natl Acad Sci USA (79): 7522-7526, 1982.
33. Hadziyannis SJ, Lieberman HM, Karvountzis GG, Shafritz DA. Analysis of liver disease, nuclear HBcAg, viral replication and HBV DNA in liver and serum of HbeAg versus anti-HBe positive carriers of hepatitis B virus. Hepatology (3): 656-662, 1983.

34. Hoofnagle JH. Chronic type B hepatitis (Editorial) Gastroenterology (84): 422-423, 1983.
35. Sherlock S, Thomas HC. Hepatitis B virus infection: The impact of molecular biology (Editorial) Hepatology (3): 455-456, 1983.
36. Neel BG, Hayward WS, Robinson HL, Fang J, Astrin SM. Avian leukosis virus-induced tumors have common proviral integration sites and synthesize discrete new RNAs, oncogenesis by promotor insertion. Cell (23): 323-334, 1981.
37. Neel BG, Gasic GP, Rogler CE, Shalka AM, Ju G, Hishinuma, Papas T, Astrin SM, Hayward WS. Molecular analysis of the c-myc locus in normal tissue and avian leukosis virus induced lymphomas. J Virol (44): 158-166, 1982.
38. Botchan M, Top WC, Sambrook J. The arrangement of simian virus 40 sequences in the DNA of transformed cells. Cell (9): 269, 1976.
39. Ketner G, Kelly TJ. Integrated simian virus 40 sequences in transformed cell DNA analysis using restriction endonucleases. Proc Natl Acad Sci (73): 1102, 1976.
40. Koshy R, Koch S, von Loringhoven A, Kahmann R, Murray K and Hofschneinder PH. Integration of hepatitis B virus DNA: Evidence for integration in the single-stranded gap. Cell (34): 215-223, 1983.
41. Valenzuela P, Quiroga M, Zaldivar J, et al. The nucleotide sequence of the hepatitis B viral genome and the identification of the major viral genes. In: Fields B, Jacnisch R, Fox CF (eds) Animal virus genetics. Academic Press, New York, 1980, pp 57-70.
42. Chakraborty PR, Ruiz-Opazo N, Shafritz DA. Transcription of human hepatitis B virus core antigen gene sequences in an _in vitro_ HeLa cellular extract. Virology (111): 647-652, 1981.
43. Ruiz-Opazo N. Gene Organization and Genetic Expression of Hepatitis B Virus. Ph.D. Thesis dissertation, Sue Golding Graduate Division of Medical Sciences, Albert Einstein College of Medicine of Yeshiva University, 1982.
44. Dejean A, Brechot C, Tiollais P, Wain-Hobson S. Characterization of integrated hepatitis B viral DNA cloned from a human hepatoma and the hepatoma derived cell line PLC/PRF/5. Proc Natl Acad Sci USA (80): 2505-2509, 1983.
45. Nusse R, Varmus HE. Many tumors induced by mouse mammary tumor virus contain a provirus integrated in the same region of the host chromosome. Cell (31): 99-109, 1982.
46. Yunis JJ. The chromosomal basis of human neoplasia. Science (221): 227-236, 1983.

29

ESTABLISHMENT OF VIRUS-NEGATIVE CELL LINES DERIVED FROM RADIATION- OR CHEMICALLY-INDUCED T-CELL LYMPHOMAS IN NFS/N MICE, AND GENERATION OF ONCOGENIC VIRUS FROM THESE CELL LINES FOLLOWING INFECTION OF A NON-ONCOGENIC ECOTROPIC VIRUS

K. YANAGIHARA, T. SEYAMA AND K. YOKORO
(RES. INST. NUCL. MED. & BIOL., HIROSHIMA UNIV., HIROSHIMA 734, JAPAN)

ABSTRACT

T-cell lymphomas were induced in NFS/N mice either by x-irradiation or N-nitrosoethylurea(NEU), and cell lines, from these lymphoma cases were established. Neither the expression of infectious endogenous viruses nor MuLV-related activities were detectable by various standard assays in both primary lymphomas and cell lines. Further, there was no amplification of env gene of endogenous viruses(xenotropic and MCF), or no amplification of rearrangement of myc and ras gene family as demonstrated by Southern blot assay.

Oncogenic MCF virus was generated from non-producer lymphoma cell lines of NFS/N origin infected with a non-oncogenic ecotropic virus(E4). This may represent the possible mechanism of occasional emergence and the isolation of oncogenic viruses in non-viral T-cell lymphomagenesis in certain mouse strains.

INTRODUCTION

T-cell lymphomas can readily be induced in many mouse strains by exposing young mice to ionizing radiation, chemical carcinogens or certain hormones. However, the detailed induction mechanism is still left obscure. The demonstration of "indirect mechanism of lymphoma" by Kaplan and his associates(1), the successful transmission of radiation-, chemically-, or hormonally-induced lymphomas by cell-free extracts derived from lymphoma tissues, or the isolation of lymphomagenic C-type viruses from lymphomatous tissues, all support to the belief that a virus is the direct etiological agent and that lymphomagenic agents act merely as the trigger for the activation of a latent lymphomagenic virus already present in the host. However, the etiological role of endogenous MuLV in radiation- or chemically-induced lymphomagenesis is not yet fully understood. More recently reports have appeared showing activation of the ras gene family in carcinogen- or radiation-induced T-cell lymphomas(2,3). Further, new cellular oncogene, Tlym-1 has been isolated by transfection of mouse T-cell lymphoma(4). However, the activation mechanism of cellular oncogene is unknown. The present study was undertaken to gain an insight into mechanism of lymphomagenesis using NFS/N strain mice whose genome of endogenous MuLV is incomplete and is hardly expressed(5).

MATERIALS AND METHODS

Animals: Inbred NFS/N mice of both sexes were used throughout in the present study. These mice were originally obtained from Mr. M. Saito, Central Institute for Experimental Animals, Kawasaki, Japan, in 1982, and has since been propagated in our laboratories by brother-sister mating.

Induction of T-cell lymphomas: T-cell lymphomas were induced in young NFS/N mice either by a fractionated total-body x-irradiation(170R x 4, at a 7 day interval) or continuous oral administration of NEU with a concentration of 200ppm dissolved in the drinking water. The lymphoma incidence in both groups was about 90% with an average latent period of 3-5 months.

Cell cultures: Suspensions of lymphoma cells from individual cases were prepared in the culture medium, washed and seeded in 60mm plastic dishes at a concentration of $1\text{-}2 \times 10^7$ cells per dish. After cell lines were established in floating state, a serial passage, twice a week, was carried out by transfering of 5×10^5 cells. These cell lines were maintained in RPMI1640 medium supplemented with heat-inactivated 10% fetal bovine serum, antibiotics and 5×10^{-5}M 2-mercaptoethanol.

Virus assays: Culture fluids were collected during the exponential growth phase, clarified by centrifugation at 3,000xg for 30 min and passed membrane filter of 0.45μm pore size, aliquoted and stored at -80°C. Infectivity assays and co-cultivation assays were performed as described previously(6). Immunofluorescence assays for the viral antigen, and electron microscopic observations for the detection of virus particles were carried out as previously described(6). RNA dependent DNA polymerase assay was performed using the procedure described by Ono et al. (7) with minor modifications.

DNA analysis: DNA was extracted from cells according to the method of Cooper et al.(8). DNA(20μg) was digested with 40U restriction enzyme for 18hr at 37°C according to reaction conditions recommended by supplier. The fragments were separated on Tris-borate-agarose gels(0.7%), transfered to nitrocellulose, and hybridized with virus env-specific DNAs, or oncogene DNAs which had been isolated from the plasmid clones and labeled with ^{32}P-phosphate by nick translation. The hybridization was performed at 42°C for 16hr in 50ml of 0.8M Nacl, 100mM PIPES(pH6.8), 100μg/ml denatured salmon testis DNA, 5 x Denhardt's solution, 100mg/ml dextran sulfate, 50% formamide, and then the nitrocellulose filter was washed three times with 0.2 x SSC at 50°C for 30min.

RESULTS AND DISCUSSION

Establishment of lymphoma cell lines and characterization of their properties

Seven permanent cell lines from primary lymphoma cases, three from x-ray-induced and four from NEU-induced lymphomas, were established. Each cell line was cloned, and designated as RTL and CTL, respectively. The doubling time of these cell lines was about 15-20 hours. All cell lines were lymphomagenic in syngeneic mice, killing recipients in 2 to 3 weeks after cell inoculation, similar to those reported by others(9). Examination of surface markers(Thy 1.2, Lyt-1, sIgM(μ), and sIgG),and of terminal deoxynucleotidyl transferase(TdT) activity indicated that they are consisted of neoplastic cells of moderately differentiated T-cell lineage. Cytogenetic study revealed the presence of trisomy of # 15 chromosome in some cells of every line.

Examination for the expression of various MuLVs in lymphoma cell lines

The expression of endogenous MuLVs in lymphoma cell lines was examined by transmission electron microscopy, cytoplasmic viral antigen, RNA dependent DNA polymerase(RDDP) activity and virus infectivity assays(Table 1). The generation of C-type virus particles from RTL and CTL cell lines was never detected. All cell lines were negative for RDDP activity as well as the expression of intracytoplasmic viral antigen, except one cell line, CTL 4 showed a low RDDP activity. Induction experiments, with IUdR and BUdR also failed to induce replicating MuLV from any of these cell lines. Likewise, the expression of endogenous viruses was never detected in the thymus, spleen and bone marrow of any preleukemic or leukemic NFS/N mice treated either with x-rays or NEU. A similar finding has been reported by Fischinger(10) in cell lines established from radiation-induced lymphomas in NIH/Swiss mice. These results suggest that expression of the endogenous virus is tightly suppressed in NFS mice, and there is no relationship between expression of infectious viruses and lymphomagenic process and the maintenance of neoplastic state in both x-ray- and NEU-treated mice of this strain.

Table 1. Detection of various murine leukemia virus(MuLV) expressions in lymphoma cell lines derived from radiation(RTL)-and chemically(CTL)-induced lymphomas

Cell line (source of MuLV)	Expression of cytoplasmic viral antigens	Presence of C type particles	RDDP activity	Titer						Induction
				Direct infection			Cocultivation infection			IudR
				XC plaque	Mink S^+L^-	MCF	XC plaque	Mink S^+L^-	MCF	
RTL 1	–	0	–	–	–	–	–	–	–	–
RTL 2	–	0	–	–	–	–	–	–	–	–
RTL 3	–	0	–	–	–	–	–	–	–	–
CTL 1		0	–	–	–	–	–	–	–	–
CTL 2	N.T.	0	–	–	–	–	–	–	–	–
CTL 3	–	0	–	–	–	–	–	–	–	–
CTL 4	–	0	–	–	–	–	–	–	–	–

Analyses of various MuLV env specific genes and of cellular oncogenes present in the DNA of lymphoma cells

We have analyzed the association of endogenous virus in lymphomagenesis at gene level. In the first trial, DNAs were extracted and purified from abovementioned NFS lymphoma cell lines and from cells of other sources as controls. As shown in Fig.1, these DNAs were digested with BglII plus EcoRl and hybridized to ^{32}P-labeled pXenv DNA probe(11). There was no amplification or rearrangement of xenotropic env gene in x-ray or NEU-induced lymphoma cell DNAs as compared with those of normal thymocytes, making a clear band of 2.0Kb. DNAs derived from rat thymoma and human T cell leukemia never hybridized with this probe(Fig.1). Although data is not shown, DNA of NFS lymphoma cells and normal thymocytes hybridized equally with MCF env DNA probe(0.7Kb between a BamH1 and EcoR1 site in env of the p247-1b plasmid DNA) (12), making a faint band of 0.4Kb. In addition, these DNAs never hybridized with env DNA of ecotropic virus(13) as was expected.

Fig.1. Hybridization of endogenous MuLV-related sequences to the xenotropic env-specific DNA probe

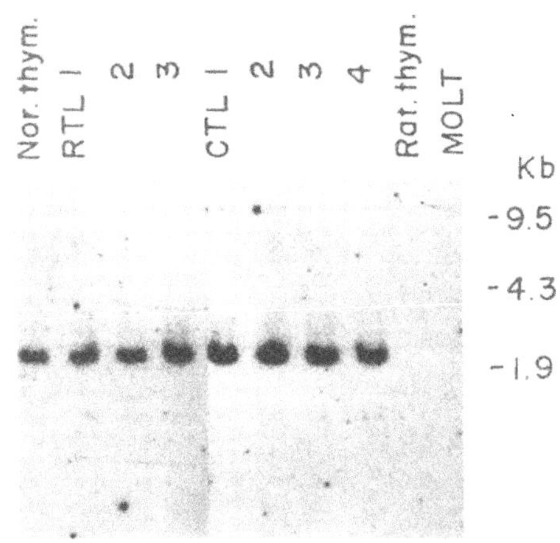

In the second trial, the expression of various cellular oncogenes, such as C-H-ras, C-N-ras, C-K-ras and C-myc genes, in DNA of lymphoma cells was examined also with Southern blot assay. As shown in Fig.2, cellular DNAs were digested with BamH1. The probe used was an EcoR1 fragment from BS-9(14). There was no evidence for either amplification or rearrangement of C-H-ras gene in lymphoma cells as compared to normal thymocytes, showing clear band at about 3.3-3.9Kb. When a fragment of N-ras clone (clone pAT8.8)(15), obtained by digesting the clone with EcoR1 and BamH1, is used as probe, it hybridized with EcoR1-digested

DNA of T24 cell line, making a strong band of 10Kb, whereas similarly treated DNAs of NFS lymphomas and normal thymocytes hybridized with the probe, making clear bands at 3.7,6.7 and 12Kb. In addition to these analyses, the expression and amplification of K-ras and myc genes were also tested using respective probe [HiHi-3(16) and V-myc(17)]. In these analyses too, none of NFS lymphoma DNA showed any abnormal pattern.

Fig. 2. Analysis of the C-ras sequences present in DNA of radiation-, and carcinogen-induced NFS/N T-cell lymphomas

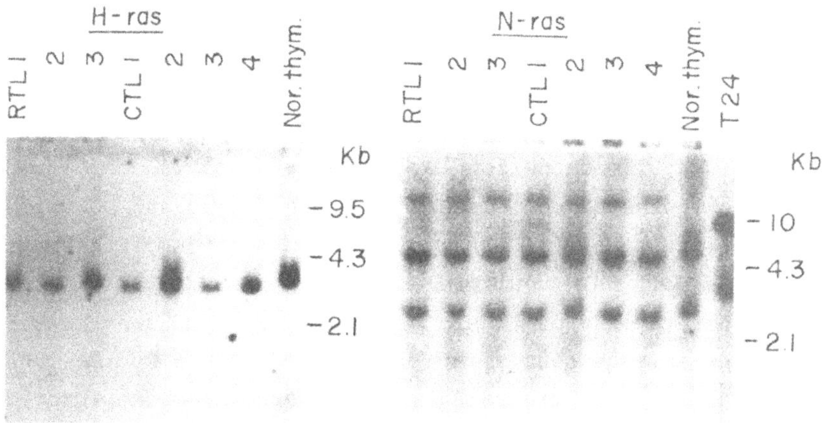

Results so far obtained indicated that no recognizable changes could be found at DNA level. However, most recently, activated C-K-ras and N-ras has been identified in radiation-, and chemically-induced T-cell lymphomas, respectively(2,3). Presently, we are trying to assess the transcriptional dose of gene information to messenger RNA by the Northern blot assay.

Generation of lymphomagenic type-C virus from non-producer lymphoma cell lines following infection of a non-oncogenic ecotropic virus

Experimental design and a part of results are shown in Fig.3. Non-virus producing cell lines derived either from x-ray- or NEU-induced lymphomas were infected in vitro, with a non-oncogenic ecotropic virus(E4).

Fig. 3. Generation of lymphomagenic type-C viruses from NFS/N non-producer lymphoma cell lines infected with an ecotropic virus (E4)

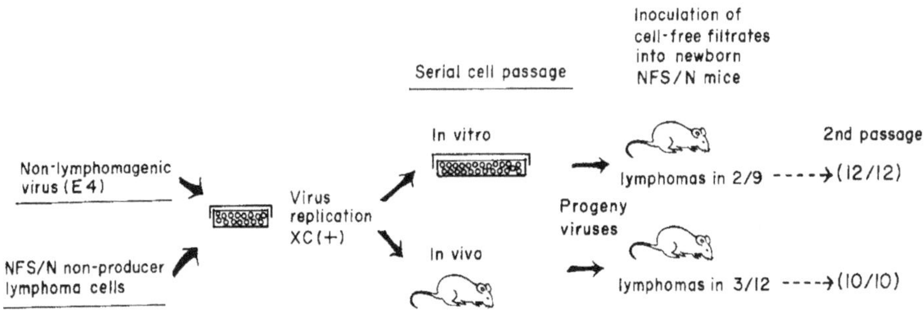

Infection was established, and the generation of the progeny virus was easily detectable by XC plaque assay on cell-free filtrates of infected cell lines. But xenotropic and MCF viruses were not detectable at this point. Inoculation of these filtrates as well as of culture media into newborn NFS mice resulted in the development of thymic or non-thymic lymphomas in varying incidence in each case with a latency of 3 to 6 months. Furthermore, cell-free filtrates(20%w/v) prepared from the induced lymphoma tissue showed much stronger lymphomagenic potency, and, MCF virus and various phenotypically mixed viruses could be detected in some of these lymphoma cells. As shown in the lowest row of the Table 2, infection of a cell line, derived from radiation-induced fibrosarcoma in a NFS mouse, with E4 virus was also resulted in the release of progeny virus. However, the cell-free filtrates of progeny virus-producing sarcoma cells never showed lymphomagenicity. These findings indicate that originally infected non-oncogenic E4 virus might has been incorporated certain oncogenic informations present in cell genome of non-virus producing lymphoma cells; most probably through recombination between viral genes of E4 and modified endogenous viral gene of physically- or chemically-induced lymphoma cells. This kind of event may take place rather frequently in vivo, following irradiation or chemical treatment, namely, these agents

Table 2. Generation of lymphomagenic viruses by infection of chemically-, or radiation-induced NFS/N non-producer lymphoma cell lines with a non-oncogenic ecotropic virus(E4)

Cells	MuLV	Passage level	Titer of infectious virus XC plaque	Mink S^+L^-	MCF	Lymphoma Incidence (%)	Type of lymphoma Thymic	Non-thymic	Latency (days)
CTL1	E4	3	3.32	–	–	0/6 (0)			
		5	3.88	–	–	1/9 (11)	0	1	86
		7	3.27	–	–	4/12 (33)	1	3	161
CTL2	E4	2	2.82	–	–	4/9 (44)	3	1	123
		5	4.01	–	–	3/9 (33)	2	1	91
		6	3.14	–	–	5/17 (29)	1	4	138
RTL1	E4	5	3.77	–	–	4/11 (36)	0	4	128
		10	2.82	–	–	7/22(32)	0	7	163
		15	3.16	–	–	1/6 (17)	0	1	113
RTL3	E4	5	3.04	–	–	5/8 (63)	0	5	184
		10	3.65	–	–	3/14 (21)	0	3	134
		15	2.98	–	–	4/8 (50)	0	4	117
RTL3			–	–	–	0/21			
	E4		4.03	–	–	0/23			
144II*	E4	2	3.12	–	–	0/9			
		5	3.00	–	–	0/11			

*: A cell line derived from radiation-induced fibrosarcoma developed in a NFS/N mouse.

may cause cell transformation by mutating certain genes, including proviral DNA of endogenous viruses, and at the same time, the activation of infectious ecotropic virus. Under these circumstances, an increase of the chance for generation of a lymphomagenic recombinant virus can be easily conceived, and those phenomena may also mislead a concept that a lymphomagenic virus play the principal role in induction of lymphomas by radiation or chemical agents. Nevertheless, we are still inclined to consider that the emergence of a lymphomagenic virus, represented by MCF virus, is incidental to the lymphomagenic treatment, and a lymphoma develops by other means which is still to be explored.

Acknowledgement

We are most grateful to Prof. T. Takano, Keio Univ., Tokyo, for his generous cooperation in the present studies. We thank Dr. D.R. Lowy and Dr. M.A. Martin for DNA clone of virus env specific gene; Dr. R.W. Ellis, Dr. A.Hall, Dr. E.H. Chang and Dr. Y. Taya for DNA clones of oncogenes; Dr. H. Nakamura for a rabbit anti-TdT serum, and Dr. Y. Takamori for RDDP assay. This work was supported by Grant-in-Aid for Cancer Research from the Ministry of Education, Science and Culture, Japan, and Foundation for Promotion of Cancer Research, Japan.

References

1. Kaplan HS: On the natural history of the murine leukemias. Cancer Res (27): 1325-1340, 1967.
2. Guerrero I, Calzada P, Mayer A, Pellicer A: A molecular approach to leukemogenesis: Mouse lymphomas contain an activate C-ras oncogene. Proc Natl Acad Sci USA (81): 202-205, 1984.
3. Vousden KH, Marshall CJ: Three different activated ras genes in mouse tumours; evidence for oncogene activation during pro gression of a mouse lymphoma. The EMBO Journal (3): 913-917, 1984.
4. Lane MA, Sainten A, Doherty KM, Cooper GM: Isolation and characterization of a stage-specific transforming gene, Tlym-1, from T-cell lymphomas. Proc Natl Acad Sci USA (81): 2227-2231, 1984.
5. Chattopadhyay SK,Lowy DR, Teich NM, Livine AS, Rowe WP: Evidence that the AKR murine leukemia-virus genome is complete in DNA of the high-virus AKR mouse and incomplete in the DNA of the "virus-negative" NIH mouse. Proc Natl Acad Sci USA (71): 167-171, 1974.
6. Yanagihara K, Hamada K, Seyama T, Imamura N, Yokoro K: In vitro studies of the mechanism of leukemogenesis. II. Characterization of endogenous murine leukemia viruses isolated fro AKR thymic epithelial reticulum cell lines. J Virology (41): 360-366, 1982.
7. Ono K, Ohashi A, Yamamoto A, Matsukage A, Nishioka N, Takahashi T, Nakayama C, Saneyoshi M: Discrimination of reverse transcriptase from cellular DNA polymerase by kinetic analysis. Cell Molecul Biol (25): 323-328, 1980.
8. Cooper GM, Okenquist S, Silverman L: Transforming activity of chemically transformed and normal cells. Nature(284): 418-421, 1980.
9. Lieberman M, Decleve A, Castagnoli PR, Boniver J, Finn OJ, Kaplan HS: Establishment, characterization and virus expression of cell lines derived from radiation- and virus-induced lymphomas of C57BL/Ka mice. Int J Cancer (24): 168-177, 1979
10. Fischinger RJ, Thiel HJ, Ihle JN, Lee JC, Elder JH: Detection of a recombinant murine leukemia virus-related glycoprotein on virus-negative thymoma cells. Proc Natl Acad Sci USA (78): 1920-1924, 1981.
11. Buckler CE, Hoggan MD, Chan HW, Sears JF, Khan AS, Moore JL, Hartley JW, Rowe WP, Martin MA: Cloning and characterization of an envelope-specific probe from xenotropic murine leukemia proviral DNA. J Virology (41): 228-236, 1982.
12. Chattopadyay SK, Cloyd MW, Linemeyer DL, Lander MR, Rands E, Lowy DR: Cellular origin and role of mink cell focus-forming viruses in murine thymic lymphomas. Nature (295): 25-31,1982
13. Chattopadhyay SK, Lander MR, Rands E, Lowy DR: Structure of endogenous murine leukemia virus DNA in mouse genomes. Proc Natl Acad Sci USA (77): 5774-5778, 1980.
14. Ellis RW, DeFeo D, Maryak JM, Young HA, Shin TY, Chang EH, Lowy DR, Scolnick EM: Dual evolutionary origin for the rat genetic sequences of harvey murine sarcoma virus. J Virology (36): 408-420, 1980.

15. Hall A, Marshall CJ, Spurr NK, Weiss RA: Identification of transforming gene in two human sarcoma cell lines as a new member of the ras gene family located on chromosome 1. Nature (303): 396-400, 1983.
16. Ellis RW, DeFeo D, Shin TY, Gonda MA, Young HA, Tsuchida N, Lowy DR, Scolnick EM: The p21 src genes of Harvey and Kirsten sarcoma viruses originate from divergent members of a family of normal vertebrate genes. Nature (292): 506-511, 1981.
17. Alitalo K, Bishop JM, Smith DH, Chen EY, Colby WW, Levinson AD: Nucleotide sequence of the v-myc oncogene of avian retrovirus MC29. Proc Natl Acad Sci USA (80): 100-104, 1983.

30

PERSPECTIVES AND PROSPECTS OF MOLECULAR BIOLOGY IN THE CONTROL OF HUMAN MALIGNANCIES

PETER J. FISCHINGER

National Cancer Institute, Bethesda, Maryland

1. INTRODUCTION

Recent dramatic advances in the areas of molecular biology, and the isolation of human retroviruses associated with cancer, set the stage for a number of new opportunities in the diagnosis, treatment and prevention of cancer. The involvement of unique cellular genes which are directly related to cancer causation, i.e. oncogenes, has opened new approaches in the examination of how the transformed state is maintained. As has been made amply clear in this volume, oncogenes function either by over-producing their normal protein product or by producing a mutated protein. Based on large volumes of past epidemiological data, cancer was always considered a multistep process; present studies with transforming genes also implicate the participation of multiple genes in the final tumor state. One of the greatest benefits of oncogenes has been the unification of diverse concepts derived from studies in biological and chemical carcinogenesis into a single cohesive hypothesis at the level of molecular genetics.

The prospects of control of human cancer can be considered as a two-step process. The first aspect is the translation of known concepts and measures into practice. Based on this simple premise, the National Cancer Institute has set goals for the year 2000 to reduce the rate of cancer deaths by one half of what it is today. This could be realized by preventive measures which take cognizance of life styles in which certain cancers already occur at very low rates. The second element is the transfer of the state-of-the-art treatment for all cancer patients immediately from the inception of the diagnosis. These projections did not include the possible application which could derive from the concepts discussed in this volume. The prospects of molecular diagnosis of susceptibility or carrier state of neoplastic disease, the possible attack on the product of the oncogene itself, and the feasibility of primary prevention of cancer caused by human retroviruses, are very much bolstered by the recent enormous increase in new data. It may be reasonable to expect that further reduction of cancer mortality would accrue from the application of these findings. Although it is clear that these findings are at present at the research level, a number of ongoing indications in the above areas may allow for reasonable speculations.

2. DIAGNOSIS OF MOLECULAR STATES PREDISPOSING TO CANCER

Three major thrusts contribute to the possibility of detecting genetic states which would presage a high probability of tumor development. These are the identification and the activation of oncogenes in human tumors, the diagnosis by restriction fragment length polymorphisomes (RFLP), and the documentation of a general involvement of chromosomal alterations in neoplasms (1, 2, 3).

A remarkable breakthrough has been the recent unambiguous diagnosis of the unsymptomatic autosomal dominant carriers of Huntington's disease. This was accomplished by going to a human DNA library and searching for RFLP differences with anonymous, nonrepetitive DNA probes comparing patients to normals. Although the responsible gene for this disease is still unknown, a small segment of chromosome 4 shows two unique restriction endonuclease cut patterns which are predictive of the disease. Thus carriers can be clearly identified so that further offspring with a lethal dominant gene can be prevented (4). A somewhat more complex state has also been recently reported for phenylketonuria. Not only does the affected individual display unique RFLP patterns, but also the parental carrier states can be described at the molecular level (5).

It is well known that a number of human tumors of childhood have a clear cut genetic basis. Specific chromosomal lesion patterns have been described which identify the child at risk for developing these malignancies. Chromosomal aberrations have now been described in almost all human tumors, and data depictive of extensive reproducible patterns, involving deletions, translocations, inversions, trisomies, and gene amplifications, have been recently summarized (3). Although leukemias and lymphomas have been particularly well documented, about 40 kinds of human solid tumors have been described to have a familial pattern (6).

Three well-studied human tumors which appear as both inherited and sporadic all involve chromosomal deletions associated with recessive genes (Table 1). The best studied case is the retinoblastoma which has a deletion of the q14 band of chromosome 13, the site of the now identified Rb gene. The homozygous condition has two identical alleles which can arise in one of four ways such as a loss of normal chromosome with or without a reduplication, a mitotic recombination, or lastly a translocation. In the sporadic cases, the deletion may not be visible and is considered to arise on a molecular level by several possible mechanisms. Recent data implicate the participation of cellular oncogenes in the process. A high degree of transcription of the N-*myc* oncogene occurs with or without N-*myc* amplification, the latter state associated with progressive tumor growth (7,8). The outcome of the above is that the child at risk could be identified even before the tumor appears. The probability of detection is very high in familial cases, but could also be quite high in the sporadic case if testing were to occur.

The second condition is the Wilm's tumor, where a similar deletion of the p13 band of chromosome 11 results in homozygosity, probably by a translocation mechanism. The mechanism itself was determined by using DNA probes directed to the tip of the short arm of number 11 chromosome, and by comparing the resulting RFLP's. In nontumor tissues, the deletion is generally visible in familial forms but is invisible or heterozygous in sporadic cases. Presumably a submicroscopic deletion occurred nonetheless, because the translocation in one tumor between chromosomes 11 and 12 resulted in the loss of the c-*Ha*-*ras1* protooncogene (9). In all forms of the disease, the genetic identification of the patient is better than 50% with existing technology.

The neuroblastoma is analogous to the above because it also involves a recessive gene on chromosome 1 which is deleted and/or inactivated. As in the retinoblastoma system, the N-*myc* oncogene is transcribed and amplified, and in one instance, ras activation was shown to occur (11). The identification of the patient from tumor tissue at least is uniformly positive. A major feature of the above three systems is that on a microscopically visible level, a deletion is predictive of high tumor risk in children who have as yet not been affected. Secondly, the finesse of analysis can extend to the molecular level by a derivation of DNA probes representing areas of chromosomes where deletions are taking place, thus allowing for a much finer dissection.

Based on the above relatively rare familial cancers, an extrapolation may be feasible in several high incidence human solid tumors. In the familial Gardner's syndrome there is a large number of polyps in the colon, of which one or more sooner or later undergo malignant change. The presence of a specific genetic lesion has not been determined. The examination of colorectal tumors for the presence of activated oncogenes have shown a rate of K-ras activation as high as in any other malignancy (1). In human lung carcinoma, a genetic basis can only be speculated upon. One of the confounding features of this cancer is that although risk increases with long-term, heavy tobacco use, only 10-20% of the heaviest smokers will actually develop this tumor. Because of high incidence and lethality from this tumor in an ever younger population, it may be reasonable to assume that a segment of the population may be at a selectively higher risk, which may have a genetic basis. In the small cell lung cancer (SCLC) the band p14 on chromosome 3 has been depicted as the breakpoint in the resulting 3(p14, p23) deletion (12). This change occurs in essentially all SCLC tumors examined. As in many other solid tumors the K-ras oncogene is activated in transfection assays. Additionally, the myc gene has been found to be amplified as well (1). It is important to note that in both of the above tumors, normal body cells do not have activated oncogenes, implying that this event is closely associated with the malignancy itself. Although specific RFLP's have not been examined, these tumors may be amenable to an intensive effort. The number of RFLP probes has been rising rapidly so that more extensive examinations are feasible. As in the childhood tumors, a specific genetic change may be assessible at the molecular level to determine whether higher risk for tumor exists with certain patterns even if the nature of the gene complex is still unknown.

3. ATTACK ON THE ONCOGENE PRODUCT

The mutations responsible for the activation of the <u>ras</u> family of oncogenes imply an altered protein product. Based on the superb precision of monoclonal antibodies, the altered epitopic site could be theoretically recognized as distinct from the epitope on the proto-oncogene product. Such a monoclonal antibody could be originally directed against a sequence-specified, artificial peptide with the appropriate amino acid change. The specific antibody could then be labeled with a radionuclide chelate and be used for diagnosis or treatment. Alternatively, conjugation of toxins to the antibody may be used to kill tumor cells carrying the activated oncogene product. In fact, a number of prototype studies are going on in which tumor specific surface antigens are recognized by specific, armed monoclonal antibodies to visualize and/or kill metastases.

The attack on the product of the activated oncogene is, however, conceptually different from the above. Tumor specific antigens are known to be derepressed neo-antigenic cellular proteins or glycolipids. Past studies indicate a significant degree of heterogeneity in the amount of antigen present on individual tumor cells, present even in a single section of tumor stained with antibody and peroxidase. Modulation and turning off of tumor specific antigens is the norm in the presence of an immunologically hostile environment. Tumor cells will therefore escape the intended treatment. However, because the product of the oncogene is at the core of the reaction, the tumor cell cannot turn off oncogene products with impunity. If the cell would stop the production of the oncogene product, it would exhibit a normal phenotype. In fact, under circumstances in which a highly active oncogene in a tumor cell is de-amplified, and its transcription repressed by drug treatment, the normal differentiated functions reappear (13). Accordingly, the retention of the oncogene antigen by the tumor cell allows for its being killed, whereas the turning off should result in a reversion to normalcy.

A key element may be the question of access of antibody to the oncogene antigen. Although some oncogene protein products are at the cell surface, others are cytoplasmic or nuclear. One of the possible approaches could be to use the concepts of receptor mediated endocytosis to get the armed antibody or its fragments into the cell (14). Active experiments of this type are being pursued at present.

4. FEASIBILITY OF DEVELOPING VACCINES TO HUMAN RETROVIRUSES

The epidemiology of human exposure to human T-cell lymphotropic retrovirus (HTLV) family indicates geographic areas of virus prevalence and a close association with an increase in certain lymphoid neoplasms. Recently the acute problem of the autoimmune deficiency syndrome (AIDS) has also been associated with the variant, HTLV III agent, which induces a cytopathic rather than a proliferative response (15). The exposure to HTLV III is limited clearly defined risk populations which could be amenable to protective measures.

Up to now no effective vaccine exists against a retrovirus despite the fact that in some species, such as the cat, feline leukemia virus (FeLV) induces the majority of all tumors in the cat and causes an AIDS as well. In all retroviruses, the viral subunit coded by the envelope (<u>env</u>) gene, which is the external glycoprotein, is known to contain neutralization specific epitopes. The contiguous transmembrane protein (p15E) in some viruses may directly mediate immune suppression. However, recent data indicate that a complex of the above proteins allows for a proper presentation of the epitopes to the immune system, whereas either antigen alone did not elicit adequate protective antibody. Trials in the veterinary science area are ongoing both in the US and Great Britain, and appear highly promising. A corollary to the above is that in some circumstances, treatment with high titer passive neutralizing antibody could prevent establishment of virus carrier state, or have a cytoreductive effect on tumor itself (16).

Because of the unique nature of retroviral replication, vaccines containing nucleic acid would not be advisable. Two major factors which militate this position are the presence of long terminal repeats which are required for the integration of even defective genomes and which could have an adverse effect if integration occurs next to a cellular oncogene as in the typical "promoter insertion" model. Secondly, the event is relatively more common than originally suspected, and new human acute retroviruses could result from an oncogene capture. A special case involving modern biotechnology may be the infectious recombinant virus. Typically, vaccinia virus is genetically modifed so that a new viral glycoprotein env gene can be introduced within its thymidine kinase gene. The foreign env gene is then expressed under the control of the vaccinia promoters. Antibodies have been made to a number of viral proteins in this way, and experimental protection could be achieved (17).

Other new technologies, such as the expression of recombinant DNA derived viral glycoprotein genes in bacterial yeast and mammalian vector systems, show promise. A special feature of retroviruses is that, although the neutralizing epitope is on the protein backbone, proper additions of carbohydrate groups are needed to present the protein with proper folding topology (18). Accordingly, eukaryotic expression vectors may be needed to get a correct antigen. Similar to the above, artificial peptides can be constructed. The regions of the protein which are hydrophilic and which elicit immune responses can be predicted. The past experience has been that, although antipeptide antibodies can be reactive with the virus, neutralization or protection is very difficult to achieve. However, new approaches of cyclizing peptides and better carriers, are on the horizon. Regardless of which technique will prove most advantagous, the key element is that vaccination against retroviruses may be feasible today. The presence of high-risk test groups in AIDS could allow for controlled trials of a vaccine. The resulting learning process will have significant ramifications on the expanded vaccine approaches, which could be geared to protect against lymphomas and leukemias in select areas of high virus exposure.

In summary, a reduction of neoplastic diseases may be feasible using modern molecular biology. Early diagnosis of the genetically predisposed person could be beneficial, especially in terms of avoidance of specific environmental insults. Monoclonal antibodies directed to activated oncogene products could make an impact on treatment. For the first time primary prevention of retrovirus-associated human neoplastic disease can be seriously considered in select cluster vaccine programs.

REFERENCES

1. Slamon DJ, deKerniow JB, Verma IM, Cline MJ: Expression of cellular oncogenes in human malignancies. Science (224): 256-262, 1984.
2. Botstein D, Davis RW, Skolnick MH, White RL: Construction of a genetic linkage map in man using restriction fragment length polymorphisms. Am J Hum Genet (32): 314-331, 1980.
3. Yunis JJ: The chromosomal basis of human neoplasia. Science (221): 227-236, 1983.
4. Gusella JF, Wexler NS, Conneally PN, Naylor SL, Anderson MA, Tanzi RE, Wathins PC, Ottina K, Wallace MR, Sakaguchi AY, Young AB, Shoulson I, Bonilla E, Martin JB: A polymorphic DNA marker genetically linked to Huntington's disease. Nature (306): 234-238, 1983.
5. Woo SLC, Lidsky AS, Guttler F, Chandra T, Robson KJH: Cloned human phenylalanine hydroxylase gene allows prenatal diagnosis and carrier detection of classical phenylketonuria. Nature (306): 151-155, 1983.
6. Mulvihill JJ: The genetic repertory of human neoplasia. In: Mulvihill JJ, Miller RW, Fraumeni JF (Eds) Genetics of Human Cancer. Raven Press, New York, pp 137-143, 1977.
7. Schwab M, Alitalo K, Klempnauer KH, Varmus HE, Bishop JM, Gilbert F, Brodeur G, Goldstein M. and Trent J: Amplified DNA with limited homology to myc cellular oncogene is shared by human neuroblastoma cell lines and a neuroblastoma tumor. Nature (305): 245-248, 1983.
8. Lee W-H, Murphree AL, Benedict WF: Expression and amplification of the N-myc gene in primary retinoblastoma. Nature (309): 458-460, 1984.
9. Orkin SH, Goldman DS, Sallan SE: Development of homozygosity for chromosome 11p markers in Wilm's tumour. Nature (309): 172-174, 1984.
10. Reeve AE, Housiau PJ, Gardner RJM, Chewings WE, Grindley RM, Millow LJ: Loss of a Harvey ras allele in sporadic Wilm's tumour. Nature (309): 174-176, 1984.
11. Shumazu K, Goldfarb M, Perucho M, Wigler M: Isolation and preliminary characterization of the transforming gene of a human neuroblastoma cell line. Proc Natl Acad Sci USA (80): 2112-2116, 1983.
12. Whang-Peng, J., Kao-Shan, C.S., Lee E.C., Bunn, P.A., Carney, D.N., Gazdar, A.F., and Minna, J.D.: Specific chromosome defect associated with human small lung cancer: Deletion 3p(14-23). Science (215): 181-182,1982.
13. Westin EH, Wong-Staal F, Gelmann EP, Dalla Favera R, Papas T, Lautenberger JA, Eva A, Reddy EP, Tronick SR, Aaronson SA, Gallo RC: Expression of cellular homologs of retroviral onc genes in human hematopoietic cells. Proc Natl Acad Sci USA (75): 2490-2494. 1982.
14. Goldstein JL, Brown MS: The LDL receptor locus and the genetics of familial hypercholesteroremia. Ann Genet (13): 259-289, 1979.
15. Sarngadharan, MG, Popovic, M, Bruch L, Schupbach J, and Gallo RC: Antibodies reactive with human T-lymphotrophic retrovirus (HTLV III) in the serum of patients with AIDS. Science (224): 506-508, 1984.
16. Jarrett O: Pathogenesis of feline leukemia virus related diseases. In: Goldman JM and Jarrett O (Eds.) Mechanisms of Viral Leukemogenesis. Churchill Livingstone, London, pp 135-154, 1984.
17. Smith GL, Mackett M, and Moss B: Infectious vaccinia recombinants that express hepatitis B surface antigen. Nature (302): 72-74, 1983.
18. Burny A: Leukaemogenesis by bovine leukeamia virus. In: Goldman J.M. and Jarrett, O. (Eds.) Mechanisms of Viral Leukemogenesis. Churchill Livingstone, London, pp 229-260, 1984.

Table 1. Predictive identification of susceptibility by chromosomal or

Disease	Genetic Component	Chromosome Location	Nature of Lesion
Retinoblastoma[i]	Recessive gene	13 (q14)	Hemizygous Homozygous Deletion mitotic recombination
Wilms tumor[i]	Recessive gene	11 (p13) (t11;12) (p13;q13)	Homozygous, Deletion of p13, Translocation
Neuroblastoma	Recessive gene	1 (p1, p36)	Deletion
Gardner's Syndrome (polyposis coli)	Epidemiological evidence	6 or 12	Unknown
Lung Carcinomas	Suspected only	3, p14, p21, p23 (SCLC) also 11, 12	Deletion
Huntington's Disease	Autosomal dominant gene	4	Gene is unknown Two forms of RFLP[iii]

[i]Occur both as inherited and sporadic forms
[ii]Frequency in 10-20% of tumors examined
[iii]Restriction fragment length polymorphism
[iv]Small cell lung cancer

molecular markers to select neoplastic and non-neoplastic diseases.

Non Affected Tissues	Identification Method	Oncogenes in Affected Tissue	Identification of Patient
Deletion 13 q14, sporadic type is heterozygous	Various	N-*myc* transcribed or amplified	Positive in 50-100%
Deletions other forms are Heterozygous	Probe, tip of short arm of 11	c-Has-ras1 lost in translocation	Positive in ≥50%
Heterozygous	Various	N-*myc* transcribed, amplified, *ras* activated	Positive from all tumors tested
Heterozygous Normal onc	Oncogene probes	K-*ras* activated	Presence of polyps
Normal onc	Chromosomal oncogene probes	*myc* amplified K-*ras* activated	Chromosomal changes in ~100% of SCLC's
Lesion is in all tissues	Probe G8 anonymous nonrepetitive DNA	Not applicable	Positive in ≥99%

31

IMPLICATIONS FOR THE CONTROL OF HUMAN CANCER

J.W. BERG

Department of Epidemiology, AMC Cancer Research Center, Denver, Colorado; and Departments of Pathology, Biometrics and Preventive Medicine, University of Colorado School of Medicine, Denver, Colorado

It should be apparent to the readers of this volume that a sense of urgency characterized this field. Much of this, of course, is attributable to the immediate clinical problems of AIDS and the viral-induced T-cell leukemia. There should be no need here to reiterate in detail what other contributors have presented regarding these diseases, namely that diagnosis and detection of carriers are possible, that vaccines for prevention are forseeable but that current knowledge about the viruses does not yet project to major changes and advances in treatment.

Overall, another kind of urgency comes from the wide new areas that have been opened for investigation. As several contributors described, human cancer is central now not only because of its own importance but as a guide to understanding the mechanisms and stages of normal growth and development. In my view, this vision of new areas of investigation and new ways of thinking about human cancer is the most important aspect of the current research described herein. By contrast, the "advances" in human cancer control in the past 30 years have been minor variations of old themes involving little change in our underlying concepts of causes, approaches to treatment or, in my own field, of methods and goals of diagnosis. The gains were often empirical without an underlying theoretical basis. One means of recognizing an important new conceptual framework, such as we see emerging here, is that it seems to provide new explanations as well as suggesting new investigations. The current work is especially striking and unusual because it is concerned equally with basic molecular biology, animal models, and clinical cancer. What have been separate worlds for decades now are seen to merge. One consequence of this is that those of us concerned with human cancer must strive to understand not only what the scientists are telling us about their observations of human disease but we must also reinterpret our day-to-day working concepts and presumptions. We should expect and encourage basic changes in the way we think about cancer causes (epidemiology), cancer development, cancer diagnosis (pathology) and the goals of cancer treatment.

One cannot expect to predict all of the ways new insights will affect an old science, but certain immediate implications seem obvious. These arise from the re-interpretation of old facts in this new terminology and framework of thinking. For example, the once vague ideas as to how malaria might be involved in the pathogenesis of Burkitt's lymphoma now are replaced by a specific role, part of a logical and verifiable series of steps. The result is one of a small family of carcinogenic chromosomal translocations, and so a cancer. In several senses, cancer epidemiology now has a new paradigm. First, we have new tools to look at new "clusters" of cancer. Besides looking for histories of exposure to a common chemical agent (almost the only successful technique in the past) the patients can be studied for other common health problems with more assurance that the findings could be relevant. Further, the cancers themselves and the tissues of origin can be studied for common genetic abnormalities and/or abnormal expression of a common proto-oncogene. Beyond this there is more reason than ever for epidemiologists to be concerned with the whole sequence of events connecting a particular exposure or a particular genetic inheritance to overt cancer. The more explicit our ideas are of what the stages of carcinogenesis are, the more chance we have to discover their causes and by implication the methods of preventing or reversing key steps and thereby aborting the cancer process.

There are other and more widely applicable reasons, of course, for learning which cancers are characterized by particular translocations. The most practical reason is that it now looks as if uniformity of chromosomal change may imply not only uniformity of microscopic appearance and uniformity of clinical behavior but uniformity of response to treatment. In particular, it suggests an explanation for the recent successes in the treatment of many childhood cancers and also the reason equivalent gains are not being seen for carcinomas in adults. The former would have a Burkitt's-like uniformity of proto-oncogene expression, the latter characteristically express several proto-oncogenes in abnormal manner or in abnormal amounts.

We can translate the differences of morphology and biochemical expression that we find within a single cancer as well as among a set of similarly-named cancers from different patients into a wide range of combinations of expression of oncogenes representing, in turn, a large number of accumulated genetic changes that, along a large number of different pathways, have generated many different clones of malignant cells. Whether it is a necessary part or not of their capability for malignant behavior, most will continue to give rise to variants with different characteristics, different appearances, different affinity for particular sites of metastasis, and different degrees of resistance to various chemotherapeutic agents.

The paradigm here would be classic chronic myelogenous leukemia (CML) where the steps in progression are particularly explicit and clear. The chronic leukemia itself is an intermediate stage. In most instances, the patient dies because the chronic neoplasm with relatively mature looking cells gives rise to a more primitive cell line producing a "blast crisis." The chronic phase is uniform as cancers go with a usual chromosomal rearrangement, a usual microscopic picture of at least partial differentiation of most circulating cancer cells, and usually a clinical course marked by minimal symptoms until blast crisis occurs. With blast crisis, however, the uniformity disappears at all levels so that the blasts can show even lymphoid traits and the responses to treatment are variable both between patients and in the same patient at different times. This is the stage as noted above at which we find most carcinomas. The key point to me, however, is that the CML on occasion can be seen to arise from an earlier stage in which there is no cancerous proliferation of cells but where the marrow stem cells, polyclonal to begin with, have been replaced by a monoclonal but otherwise normally maturing cell complex marked by the Philadelphia chromosomal translocation. Thus, there seem to be three separate steps to lethal malignancy: (1) monoclonality, (2) overproliferation of minimally deviant cells, (3) addition of further and diverse deviations resulting in a much more malignant cancer. The question now is not whether carcinomas of particular organs individually go through similar stages; most almost certainly do. The problem is whether there will be enough uniformity in these stages to be exploited for control purposes. I think that there may be despite the great variability among clinically manifest cancers. Immediate challenges are to see if the earliest precursors of common cancers, the hyperplasias, the dysplasias, adenomas, etc., show preferential abnormal expression of a proto-oncogene characteristic of a particular organ or cancer type and also to determine when monoclonality develops.

On our way to these goals we can at least point to one critical point in the evolution for many common cancers. For human bowel cancer, it occurs early as the formation of adenomas. Once an adenoma is formed, it seems to have the same risk of further malignant progression independent of genetics or geography. It is the propensity for adenoma formation that marks the nearly 100% risk of cancer in the genetically predisposed polyposis patient or that separates the low-cancer-risk individual in Japan from his high-risk brother who has migrated to the United States. For broncogenic cancers in smokers, there is an intermediate decision point. Microscopically in situ carcinoma can be found in the bronchi of all heavy smokers, yet in only about 1 in 8 does clinical cancer develop before some other disease, often smoking related, kills the individual. For prostatic cancer the crucial switch seem to appear even later to convert an invasive but indolent cancer into a clinically apparent one. In all parts of the world, aging of males is accompanied by the development in at least half the population of what looks to the pathologist like cancer. The difference between populations at high and at low risk for growth and metastases of fully malignant cells is a difference in frequency of anaplastic, aggressive cell lines presumably by conversion of the usual and ubiquitous low grade cancer.

If we view the early stages in the progression as resulting from specific and still simple growth abberations, may we not conceive of chemical growth control just as we hope vitamin A analogs can reverse such precancerous states as squamous metaplasia in bronchi. My own feeling is that this hope is better founded than the hope of chemically identifying the presence of such precancerous states in urine or blood. That is not because the cells of these lesions may not be making unusual products but because, as was found to be true for CEA, many types of injuury result in cells reversing to earlier stages of development as part of the response and repair process. Expression of proto-oncogenes should be no exception to this since their very presence in the genome and conservation across species argues for an important role both in normal growth and development and in the parallel repair processes. One therefore should not expect the production of any onco-fetal antigen to be specific for cancer, however important it would be to find one that was even nearly specific. If there is to be continued search for cancer-specific products, perhaps the most logical candidates are nucleic acids and proteins directly related to characteristic proto-oncogenes since many cancers seem to arise just because of qualitative or quantitative alterations in those genes' expression.

The new information and concepts presented here should have a particularly important impact on the concept of cancer grade. Morphologists have long graded cancer by the degree of resemblance to normal cells. The more the resemblance, the lower the grade and supposedly the less aggressive the cancer. Biochemical parallels exist in the testing of breast cancer for hormone receptors or studying bladder tumors for blood-group antigen expression. It has even been suggested that the best estimate of deviation comes from a total profile of expressed enzymes. While all of these measures of deviation have some correlation with prognosis and response to treatment they all are imperfect. One measure of their unsatisfactory predictive value is that there is far less concensus about grading cancers than about classifying them other ways. This may be the time for revision of the grading scheme to classify cancers by their degree of difference not from just the normal mature, post-mitotic cell but from <u>some</u> cell type in the normal sequence of development. This would include for skin cancers not only their difference from mature squamous cells but also from the basal reserve cells that supply cell replacements in adult life and even, if appropriate, distance from some embryonic precursor of the basal cells. In this theoretical framework basal cell cancers might be lower grade than squamous cell skin cancers logically as well as practically if they differed less from their own normal counterpart. Proto-oncogenes are important here because their abnormalities are likely to be the actual cellular lesions. Other differences may be secondary but they also may not be deviations but normal parts of the phenotype at the stage most closely corresponding to the cancer cell. In this redefinition of grade, an embryonal cancer cell could be low grade if it was only a minimal deviation from a normal cell of the early embryo.

There are more immediate implications for pathologists, however. Now our diagnostic goal is recognition by appearance. We advance our art by learning more and more subtle distinctions. Sometimes these are sought only after clinicians have noted different types of the behavior within a group of cancers we have labeled all with the same name. Sometimes we ourselves work out relations between different appearances and different clinical behaviors. Most often perhaps we start with differences of appearance and try subsequently to find clinical correlations. One way or another we keep expanding our diagnostic vocabulary. Too often, unfortunately, as currently with lymphoma nomenclature, new classfications are not always reproducible nor generally accepted. With Burkitt's tumor a unique clinical picture finally led to recognition of a unique appearance under the microscope. Now we learn that both are directly related to malexpression of a particular proto-oncogene.

Moreover, there are strong suggestions that other lymphoid and hematopoietic neoplasms show the same kind of correlation. It may well be that the aim of all tumor classification really is the identification of which genes are being expressed. This might imply that test tubes, gels and blots will replace microscopes in cancer diagnosis, but I believe that visual recognition in the old fashioned sense of looking at cells and tissues will prove to be good enough and efficient enough to survive even if patterns of stains in two-dimensional gels also become diagnostic tools and lead us to more meaningful classifications.

In summary, I see the discoveries discussed herein as being special. Suddenly our picture of cancer is so much more explict that it invites and justifies new ways of thinking about the disease. It brings laboratory and clinical concepts together and, more importantly, it brings investigators in the two areas much closer, abolishing a separation that was an embarassment to most "comprehensive" cancer centers. New goals are in sight for cancer diagnosis and cancer treatment. Epidemiology as the search for causes has both new justification for concentrating on the earliest stages of cancer development and new tools to work with.

All this may not be enough to solve the problem of human cancer and it certainly does not justify setting an early date for the achievement of that ultimate goal, but it should mean faster progress than hitherto, particularly in these early stages when so many important questions suddenly seem answerable.

INDEX

A

B

T

U

V

CPSIA information can be obtained
at www.ICGtesting.com
Printed in the USA
BVHW040803250520
580268BV00003B/34

9 781461 296201